W9-CPF-014

JAN - - 2018

DATE DUE

			PRINTED IN U.S.A.

Aging
SOURCEBOOK

First Edition

Health Reference Series

First Edition

Aging

SOURCEBOOK

Basic Consumer Health Information about the Physiology of Aging, Healthy Aging through Physical Activity, Healthy Eating, and Anti-Aging Methods, and Health Concerns due to Aging and Aging-Associated Diseases Such as Cancers, Cardiovascular Disorders, Eye Disorders, Gastrointestinal Disorders, Hormonal Imbalances, Mental Disorders, Musculoskeletal Disorders, Neurodegenerative Disorders, Respiratory Disorders, and Renal Disorders

Along with Information about Geriatric Healthcare, Assisted Living, Home Modification, Legal and Financial Assistance, a Glossary of Related Terms, and a List of Resources for Additional Help and Information

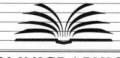

OMNIGRAPHICS

615 Griswold, Ste. 901, Detroit, MI 48226

Bibliographic Note
Because this page cannot legibly accommodate all the copyright notices, the Bibliographic Note portion of the Preface constitutes an extension of the copyright notice.

* * *

OMNIGRAPHICS
Siva Ganesh Maharaja, *Managing Editor*
***

Copyright © 2018 Omnigraphics

ISBN 978-0-7808-1583-4
E-ISBN 978-0-7808-1584-1

Library of Congress Cataloging-in-Publication Data

Names: Omnigraphics, Inc., issuing body.

Title: Aging sourcebook: basic consumer health information about the physiology of aging and associated diseases and medical conditions, including cancers, degenerative disorders, and psychological issues, with guidelines for geriatric care, healthy aging, and aging in place, emphasizing physical activity, diet, sexuality, assistive technologies, caregiver responsibilities, and advanced care planning; along with a glossary of related terms and a directory of resources for more information.

Description: First edition. | Detroit, MI: Omnigraphics, [2018] | Series: Health reference series | Includes bibliographical references and index.

Identifiers: LCCN 2017034130 (print) | LCCN 2017035067 (ebook) | ISBN 9780780815841 (eBook) | ISBN 9780780815834 (hardcover: alk. paper)

Subjects: LCSH: Older people--Health and hygiene. | Aging.

Classification: LCC RA777.6 (ebook) | LCC RA777.6 .A38 2018 (print) | DDC 613/.0438--dc23

LC record available at https://lccn.loc.gov/2017034130

Electronic or mechanical reproduction, including photography, recording, or any other information storage and retrieval system for the purpose of resale is strictly prohibited without permission in writing from the publisher.

The information in this publication was compiled from the sources cited and from other sources considered reliable. While every possible effort has been made to ensure reliability, the publisher will not assume liability for damages caused by inaccuracies in the data, and makes no warranty, express or implied, on the accuracy of the information contained herein.

This book is printed on acid-free paper meeting the ANSI Z39.48 Standard. The infinity symbol that appears above indicates that the paper in this book meets that standard.

Printed in the United States

HARPER COLLEGE LIBRARY
PALATINE, ILLINOIS 60067

Table of Contents

Part III: Aging-Associated Diseases and Medical Conditions

Part IV: Geriatric Healthcare

Part V: Senior Living Options and End-of-Life Care

Part VI: Legal and Economic Issues Related to Aging

Part VII: Additional Help and Information

Preface

About This Book

According to the Office of the Surgeon General, the number of Americans who celebrated their 65th birthday has reached a record-breaking 46 million, with an expected projection of 74 million by 2030. This is in large part thanks the baby boomer generation, which has swelled the ranks of seniors. However, medical advances and healthier lifestyle choices have also led to individuals living longer. The vast ranks of older adults in the United States continue to contribute to society in a variety of ways, but, as they move into advanced old age, their needs will create new challenges for their families, medical and public health professionals, and the wider community.

Aging Sourcebook, First Edition provides information about physiology of aging, impact of stress on aging, and how the brain's health can make a difference. It also discusses about healthy aging through physical activities, healthy food habits, and immunizations. The book provides information on aging-associated diseases and medical conditions such as cancers, cardiovascular disorders, eye disorders, instability, mental disorders, musculoskeletal disorders, neurodegenerative disorders, respiratory disorders, and more. It also offers tips on using medicines safely and improving the quality of life. Suggestions for Medicare assistance for treatments, getting help with caregiving, financial counseling, and end-of-life care are also provided. The book concludes with a glossary of terms related to aging and a directory of organizations that provides information about aging.

How to Use This Book

This book is divided into parts and chapters. Parts focus on broad areas of interest. Chapters are devoted to single topics within a part.

Part I: Physiology of Aging defines aging and discusses the biology of aging process and factors contributing to life span. The role of genetics, metabolism, and immune system in the physiology of aging is described. This part contains statistics related to the aging population across the globe and in the United States, and the cost of healthcare for the aged.

Part II: Healthy Aging gives an overview of ways in which one can age in a healthy manner. This part emphasizes exercise, physical activity, and eating habits. Various concerns such as mental health, forgetfulness, coping with the loss of loved ones, and emotional health are discussed. Details on immunizations to prevent flu and shingles are also provided.

Part III: Aging-Associated Diseases and Medical Conditions describes various age-related problems like cancers, cardiovascular disorders, eye problems, gastrointestinal disorders, hormonal imbalances, mental disorders, musculoskeletal disorders, neurodegenerative conditions, respiratory problems, renal disorders, and substance abuse.

Part IV: Geriatric Healthcare provides general information and guidelines on healthcare for aging individuals. Essential details about pain management, medications, assistive technologies like hearing aids, complementary care, and personal safety measures are provided. The benefits of leading an active lifestyle are explained.

Part V: Senior Living Options and End-of-Life Care discusses various options on assisted living, home care, nursing home care, and retirement communities. Long-term and end-of-life care are explained in detail.

Part VI: Legal and Economic Issues Related to Aging examines legal issues with respect to advance care planning and getting your affairs in order. It also provides information on health coverage, financial assistance, and claiming earned benefits through pension.

Part VII: Additional Help and Information provides a glossary of important terms related to aging and a directory of resources that offer information about aging.

Bibliographic Note

This volume contains documents and excerpts from publications issued by the following government agencies: Agency for Healthcare Research and Quality (AHRQ); Bureau of Justice Statistics (BJS); Centers for Disease Control and Prevention (CDC); Centers for Medicare and Medicaid Services (CMS); *Eunice Kennedy Shriver* National Institute of Child Health and Human Development (NICHD); Internal Revenue Service (IRS); National Cancer Institute (NCI); National Center for Complementary and Alternative Medicine (NCCAM); National Eye Institute (NEI); National Heart, Lung, and Blood Institute (NHLBI); National Institute of Arthritis and Musculoskeletal and Skin Diseases (NIAMS); National Institute of Diabetes and Digestive and Kidney Diseases (NIDDK); National Institute of Mental Health (NIMH); National Institute on Aging (NIA); National Institute on Deafness and Other Communication Disorders (NIDCD); National Institute on Drug Abuse (NIDA); National Institutes of Health (NIH); *NIH News in Health*; Office of Disease Prevention and Health Promotion (ODPHP); Office on Women's Health (OWH); U.S. Administration on Aging (AOA); USA.gov; U.S. Department of Veterans Affairs (VA); U.S. Environmental Protection Agency (EPA); and U.S. Food and Drug Administration (FDA).

It may also contain original material produced by Omnigraphics and reviewed by medical consultants.

About the Health Reference Series

The *Health Reference Series* is designed to provide basic medical information for patients, families, caregivers, and the general public. Each volume takes a particular topic and provides comprehensive coverage. This is especially important for people who may be dealing with a newly diagnosed disease or a chronic disorder in themselves or in a family member. People looking for preventive guidance, information about disease warning signs, medical statistics, and risk factors for health problems will also find answers to their questions in the *Health Reference Series*. The *Series*, however, is not intended to serve as a tool for diagnosing illness, in prescribing treatments, or as a substitute for the physician/patient relationship. All people concerned about medical symptoms or the possibility of disease are encouraged to seek professional care from an appropriate healthcare provider.

A Note about Spelling and Style

Health Reference Series editors use *Stedman's Medical Dictionary* as an authority for questions related to the spelling of medical terms and the *Chicago Manual of Style* for questions related to grammatical structures, punctuation, and other editorial concerns. Consistent adherence is not always possible, however, because the individual volumes within the *Series* include many documents from a wide variety of different producers, and the editor's primary goal is to present material from each source as accurately as is possible. This sometimes means that information in different chapters or sections may follow other guidelines and alternate spelling authorities. For example, occasionally a copyright holder may require that eponymous terms be shown in possessive forms (Crohn's disease vs. Crohn disease) or that British spelling norms be retained (leukaemia vs. leukemia).

Medical Review

Omnigraphics contracts with a team of qualified, senior medical professionals who serve as medical consultants for the *Health Reference Series*. As necessary, medical consultants review reprinted and originally written material for currency and accuracy. Citations including the phrase, "Reviewed (month, year)" indicate material reviewed by this team. Medical consultation services are provided to the *Health Reference Series* editors by:

Dr. Vijayalakshmi, MBBS, DGO, MD
Dr. Senthil Selvan, MBBS, DCH, MD
Dr. K. Sivanandham, MBBS, DCH, MS (Research), PhD

Our Advisory Board

We would like to thank the following board members for providing initial guidance on the development of this series:

- Dr. Lynda Baker, Associate Professor of Library and Information Science, Wayne State University, Detroit, MI

- Nancy Bulgarelli, William Beaumont Hospital Library, Royal Oak, MI

- Karen Imarisio, Bloomfield Township Public Library, Bloomfield Township, MI

- Karen Morgan, Mardigian Library, University of Michigan-Dearborn, Dearborn, MI

- Rosemary Orlando, St. Clair Shores Public Library, St. Clair Shores, MI

Health Reference Series *Update Policy*

The inaugural book in the *Health Reference Series* was the first edition of *Cancer Sourcebook* published in 1989. Since then, the *Series* has been enthusiastically received by librarians and in the medical community. In order to maintain the standard of providing high-quality health information for the layperson the editorial staff at Omnigraphics felt it was necessary to implement a policy of updating volumes when warranted.

Medical researchers have been making tremendous strides, and it is the purpose of the *Health Reference Series* to stay current with the most recent advances. Each decision to update a volume is made on an individual basis. Some of the considerations include how much new information is available and the feedback we receive from people who use the books. If there is a topic you would like to see added to the update list, or an area of medical concern you feel has not been adequately addressed, please write to:

Managing Editor
Health Reference Series
Omnigraphics
615 Griswold, Ste. 901
Detroit, MI 48226

Part One

Physiology of Aging

Chapter 1

Aging under the Microscope

Chapter Contents

Section 1.1

What Is Aging?

This section includes text excerpted from "Biology of Aging—Aging under the Microscope," National Institute on Aging (NIA), National Institutes of Health (NIH), January 21, 2017.

The Aging Process

We may want to live forever, but who looks forward to getting old? We hope we're vigorous right up until the very end. Still, day-to-day, many of us make unhealthy choices that could put our future at risk.

From the beginning of time, people have tried to understand aging. Almost every culture has a mythology to explain it. As we grow up, tales of eternal youth pique our curiosity. And, it is these musings that may provide just the spark needed to ignite a budding scientist. There's the little girl, excited to visit her grandmother, who asks her parents how someone so spunky and fun could be so old. Or, the 3rd grader who, after watching in awe as a caterpillar spins a cocoon and then days later emerges as a butterfly, peppers the teacher with questions about this magical transformation. These are the types of questions and kinds of experiences that could stimulate a lifelong quest to explore what happens as we age.

Technology today supports research that years ago would have seemed possible only in a science fiction novel. Over centuries, theories about aging have emerged and faded, but the true nature of the aging process is still uncertain. The fact is—aging is a part of everyone's life. But the facts of aging—what is happening on a biochemical, genetic, and physiological level—remain rich for exploration.

What Aging Means

In the broadest sense, aging reflects all the changes that occur over the course of life. You grow. You develop. You reach maturity. To the young, aging is exciting—it leads to later bedtimes and curfews, and more independence. By middle age, another candle seems to fill up the top of the birthday cake. It's hard not to notice some harmless

4

cosmetic changes like gray hair and wrinkles. Middle age also is the time when people begin to notice a fair amount of physical decline. Even the most athletically fit cannot escape these changes. Take marathon runners, for example. A study funded by National Institutes of Health (NIH) found that their record times increased with age—aging literally slowed down the runners. Although some physical decline may be a normal result of aging, the reasons for these changes are of particular interest to gerontologists.

Gerontologists look for what distinguishes normal aging from disease, as well as explore why older adults are increasingly vulnerable to disease and disability. They also try to understand why these health threats take a higher toll on older bodies. Since 1958, NIA's Baltimore Longitudinal Study of Aging (BLSA) has been observing and reporting on these kinds of questions. As with any longitudinal study, the BLSA repeatedly evaluates people over time rather than comparing a group of young people to a group of old people, as in a cross-sectional study. Using this approach, BLSA scientists have observed, for example, that people who have no evidence of ear problems, or noise-induced hearing loss, still lose some of their hearing with age—that's normal. Using brain scans to learn if cognitive changes can be related to structural changes in the brain, BLSA scientists discovered that even people who remain healthy and maintain good brain function late in life lose a significant amount of brain volume during normal aging.

However, some changes that we have long thought of as normal aging can be, in fact, the signs of a potential disease. Take, for example, sudden changes in personality. A common belief is that people become cranky, depressed, and withdrawn as they get older. But an analysis of long-term data from the BLSA showed that an adult's personality generally does not change much after age 30. People who are cheerful and assertive when they are younger will likely be the same when they are age 80. The BLSA finding suggests that significant changes in personality are not due to normal aging, but instead may be early signs of disease or dementia.

The rate and progression of cellular aging can vary greatly from person to person. But generally, over time, aging affects the cells of every major organ of the body. Changes can start early. Some impact our health and function more seriously than others. For instance, around the age of 20, lung tissue starts to lose elasticity, and the muscles of the rib cage slowly begin to shrink. As a result, the maximum amount of air you can inhale decreases. In the gut, production of digestive enzymes diminishes, affecting your ability to absorb foods properly and maintain a nutritional balance. Blood vessels in your heart accumulate

5

fatty deposits and lose flexibility to varying degrees, resulting in what used to be called "hardening of the arteries" or atherosclerosis. Over time, women's vaginal fluid production decreases, and sexual tissues atrophy. In men, aging decreases sperm production, and the prostate can become enlarged.

Scientists are increasingly successful at detailing these age-related differences because of studies like the BLSA. Yet studies that observe aging do not identify the reasons for age-related changes, and, therefore, can only go so far toward explaining aging. Questions remain at the most basic level about what triggers aging in our tissues and cells, why it occurs, and what are the biological processes underlying these changes. Scientists look deep into our cells and the cells of laboratory animals to find answers. What they learn today about aging at the cellular and molecular levels may, ultimately, lead to new and better ways to live a longer, healthier life.

Section 1.2

Genetics: Is Aging in Our Genes?

This section includes text excerpted from "Biology of Aging—Genetics: Is Aging in Our Genes?" National Institute on Aging (NIA), National Institutes of Health (NIH), January 21, 2017.

You may get your hair color from your father's side of the family and your great math skills from your mother. These traits are "in the genes," so to speak. Likewise, longevity tends to "run in families"—your genetic makeup plays an important role in how you age. You can see evidence of this genetic connection in families with siblings who live into their 90s or families that have generation after generation of centenarians. These long-lived families are the basis for many genetic studies.

Identifying the genes associated with any trait is difficult. First, just locating the gene requires a detailed understanding of the trait, including knowledge of most, if not all, of the contributing factors and pathways related to that trait. Second, scientists must have clear ways of determining whether the gene suspected to have a relationship with the trait has a direct, indirect, or even no effect on that trait.

Identifying longevity genes is even more complex than determining genes for height or hair color, for example. Scientists do not know all the factors and pathways that contribute to longevity, and measuring a gene's effect on long-lived animals, including humans, would literally take a lifetime! Instead, scientists have identified hundreds of genes that affect longevity in short-lived animal models, like worms and flies. Not all of these genes promote long life. Sometimes mutating or eliminating a gene, increases lifespan, suggesting that the normal function of the gene limits longevity. Findings in animal models point to places for scientists to look for the genes that may influence longevity in humans.

How Can We Find Aging Genes in Humans?

The human genetic blueprint, or genome, consists of approximately 25,000 genes made up of approximately 3 billion letters (base pairs) of deoxyribonucleic acid (DNA). Small deviations in the base pairs naturally occur about once in every 1,000 letters of DNA code, generating small genetic variants. Scientists are finding that some of these variants (polymorphisms) are actually associated with particular traits or chance of developing a specific disease. People with a certain trait, for example, those living past age 100, may be more likely to have one variant of a gene, while people without the same trait may be more likely to have another variant. While it is very difficult to prove that a gene influences aging in humans, a relationship, or "association," may be inferred based upon whether a genetic variant is found more frequently among successful agers, such as centenarians, compared with groups of people who have an average or short lifespan and healthspan.

Several approaches are used to identify possible genes associated with longevity in humans. In the candidate gene approach, scientists look for genes in humans that serve similar functions in the body as genes already associated with aging in animal models, so-called "homologs" or "orthologs" to animal genes. For instance, after finding longevity genes involved in the insulin/IGF-1 pathway of animal models, researchers look for the comparable genes in the insulin/IGF-1 pathway of humans. Scientists then determine whether the genes are linked to longevity in humans by looking to see if a variant of the genes is prevalent among people who live healthy, long lives but not for people who have an average healthspan and lifespan.

In a National Institute on Aging (NIA)-funded project, researchers studied 30 genes associated with the insulin/IGF-1 pathway in humans to see if any variants of those genes were more common in

7

women over 92 years old compared to women who were less than 80 years old. Variants of certain genes—like the *FOXO3a* gene—predominated among long-lived individuals, suggesting a possible role with longer lifespan. This finding provides evidence that, like in animal models, the insulin/IGF-1 pathway has a role in human aging. These genes may be important to future development of therapies to support healthy aging.

Another approach, the genome-wide association study, or GWAS, is particularly productive in finding genes involved in diseases and conditions associated with aging. In this approach, scientists scan the entire genome looking for variants that occur more often among a group with a particular health issue or trait. In one GWAS study, NIH-funded researchers identified genes possibly associated with high and low blood fat levels, cholesterol, and, therefore, risk for coronary artery disease. The data analyzed were collected from Sardinians, a small genetically alike population living off the coast of Italy in the Mediterranean, and from two other international studies. The findings revealed more than 25 genetic variants in 18 genes connected to cholesterol and lipid levels. Seven of the genes were not previously connected to cholesterol/lipid levels, suggesting that there are possibly other pathways associated with risk for coronary artery disease. Heart disease is a major health issue facing older people. Finding a way to eliminate or lower risk for heart disease could have important ramifications for reducing disability and death from this particular age-related condition.

Scientists are also currently using GWAS to find genes directly associated with aging and longevity. Because the GWAS approach does not require previous knowledge of the function of the gene or its potential relationship with longevity, it could possibly uncover genes involved in cellular processes and pathways that were not previously thought to play roles in aging. Since no single approach can precisely identify each and every gene involved in aging, scientists will use multiple methods, including a combination of the GWAS and candidate gene approaches to identify genes involved in aging.

As scientists continue to explore the genetics of aging, its complexity becomes increasingly evident. Further studies could illustrate the varying ways genes influence longevity. For example, some people who live to a very old age may have genes that better equip them to survive a disease; others may have genes that help them resist getting a disease in the first place. Some genes may accelerate the rate of aging, others may slow it down. Scientists investigating the genetics of aging do not foresee a "Eureka!" moment when one gene is discovered as the principal factor affecting health and lifespan. It is more likely that we will identify several combinations of many genes that affect aging, each to a small degree.

Section 1.3

Metabolism: Does Stress Really Shorten Your Life?

This section includes text excerpted from "Biology of Aging—Metabolism: Does Stress Really Shorten Your Life?" National Institute on Aging (NIA), National Institutes of Health (NIH), August 21, 2017.

What Stress Is

Have you ever looked at side-by-side photos of a person before and after a particularly trying time in his or her life, for instance, before and a few years after starting a highly demanding job? The person likely appears much older in the later photo. The stress of the job is thought to contribute to the prematurely aged appearance. You might feel stress from work or other aspects of your daily life, too. Stress is everywhere. Even when you feel relaxed, your body is still experiencing considerable stress—biological stress. And, it is this type of stress that is widely studied by gerontologists for its effects on aging and longevity.

Biological stress begins with the very basic processes in the body that produce and use energy. We eat food and we breathe, and our body uses those two vital elements (glucose from food and oxygen from the air) to produce energy, in a process known as metabolism. You may already think of metabolism as it pertains to eating—"My metabolism is fast, so I can eat dessert," or "My metabolism has slowed down over the years, so I'm gaining weight." Since metabolism is all about energy, it also encompasses breathing, circulating blood, eliminating waste, controlling body temperature, contracting muscles, operating the brain and nerves, and just about every other activity associated with living.

These everyday metabolic activities that sustain life also create "metabolic stress," which, over time, results in damage to our bodies. Take breathing—obviously, we could not survive without oxygen, but oxygen is a catalyst for much of the damage associated with aging because of the way it is metabolized inside our cells. Tiny parts of the cell, called mitochondria, use oxygen to convert food into energy. While mitochondria are extremely efficient in doing this, they produce potentially harmful by-products called oxygen free radicals.

Free Radicals and Aging

A variety of environmental factors, including tobacco smoke and sun exposure, can produce them, too. The oxygen free radicals react with and create instability in surrounding molecules. This process, called oxidation, occurs as a chain reaction: the oxygen free radical reacts with molecule "A" causing molecule "A" to become unstable; molecule "A" attempts to stabilize itself by reacting with neighboring molecule "B"; then molecule "B" is unstable and attempts to become stable by reacting with neighboring molecule "C"; and so on. This process repeats itself until one of the molecules becomes stable by breaking, or rearranging itself, instead of passing the instability on to another molecule.

Some free radicals are beneficial. The immune system, for instance, uses oxygen free radicals to destroy bacteria and other harmful organisms. Oxidation and its by-products also help nerve cells in the brain communicate. But, in general, the outcome of free radicals is damage (breaks or rearrangements) to other molecules, including proteins and deoxyribonucleic acid (DNA). Because mitochondria metabolize oxygen, they are particularly prone to free radical damage. As damage mounts, mitochondria may become less efficient, progressively generating less energy and more free radicals.

Scientists study whether the accumulation of oxidative (free radical) damage in our cells and tissues over time might be responsible for many of the changes we associate with aging. Free radicals are already implicated in many disorders linked with advancing age, including cancer, atherosclerosis, cataracts, and neurodegeneration.

Fortunately, free radicals in the body do not go unchecked. Cells use substances called antioxidants to counteract them. Antioxidants include nutrients, such as vitamins C and E, as well as enzyme proteins produced naturally in the cell, such as superoxide dismutase (SOD), catalase, and glutathione peroxidase.

Many scientists are taking the idea that antioxidants counter the negative effects of oxygen free radicals a step further. Studies have tested whether altering the antioxidant defenses of the cell can affect the lifespan of animal models. These experiments have had conflicting results. NIA-supported researchers found that inserting extra copies of the *SOD* gene into fruit flies extended the fruit flies' average lifespan by as much as 30 percent. Other researchers found that immersing roundworms in a synthetic form of SOD and catalase extended their lifespan by 44 percent. However, in a comprehensive set of experiments, increasing or decreasing antioxidant enzymes in laboratory mice had no effect on lifespan. Results from a limited number of human clinical trials involving antioxidants generally have not supported the premise that adding antioxidants to the diet will support longer life. Antioxidant supplementation remains a topic of continuing investigation.

Section 1.4

Immune System: Can Your Immune System Still Defend as You Age?

This section includes text excerpted from "Biology of Aging—Immune System: Can Your Immune System Still Defend You as You Age?" National Institute on Aging (NIA), National Institutes of Health (NIH), August 21, 2017.

Immune System and Its Functions

Elementary schools are breeding grounds for the common cold. Kids pass their germs around as often as they share their lunch. For children, catching a cold may not be a big deal. They might take it easy for a few days while their immune system kicks into action and fights off infection. But for their older teachers and grandparents, each cold can be more of a challenge. It may take a week, or longer to get back to feeling 100 percent. Does that mean that the immune system gets weaker as we age? That's what gerontologists are trying to figure out.

Our immune system is a complicated network of cells, tissues, and organs to keep us healthy and fight off disease and infection. The immune system is composed of two major parts: the innate immune system and the adaptive immune system. Both change as people get older. Studies to better understand these changes may lead to ways of supporting the aging immune system.

Innate immunity is our first line of defense. It is made up of barriers and certain cells that keep harmful germs from entering the body. These include our skin, the cough reflex, mucous membranes, and stomach acid. If germs are able to pass these physical barriers, they encounter a second line of innate defense, composed of specialized cells that alert the body of the impending danger. Research has shown that, with age, innate immune cells lose some of their ability to communicate with each other. This makes it difficult for the cells to react adequately to potentially harmful germs called pathogens, including viruses and bacteria.

Immune System and Inflammation

Inflammation is an important part of our innate immune system. In a young person, bouts of inflammation are vital for fighting off disease. But as people age, they tend to have mild, chronic inflammation, which is associated with an increased risk for heart disease, arthritis, frailty, type 2 diabetes, physical disability, and dementia, among other problems. Researchers have yet to determine whether inflammation leads to disease, disease leads to inflammation, or if both scenarios are true. Interestingly, centenarians and other people who have grown old in relatively good health generally have less inflammation and a more efficient recovery from infection and inflammation when compared to people who are unhealthy or have average health. Understanding the underlying causes of chronic inflammation in older individuals—and why some older people do not have this problem—may help gerontologists find ways to temper its associated diseases.

The adaptive immune system is more complex than the innate immune system and includes the thymus, spleen, tonsils, bone marrow, circulatory system, and lymphatic system. These different parts of the body work together to produce, store, and transport specific types of cells and substances to combat health threats. T cells, a type of white blood cell (called lymphocytes) that fights invading bacteria, viruses, and other foreign cells, are of particular interest to gerontologists.

T cells attack infected or damaged cells directly or produce powerful chemicals that mobilize an army of other immune system substances and cells. Before a T cell gets programmed to recognize a specific harmful germ, it is in a "naïve" state. After a T cell is assigned to fight off a particular infection, it becomes a "memory" cell. Because these cells remember how to resist a specific germ, they help you fight a second round of infection faster and more effectively. Memory T cells remain in your system for many decades.

A healthy young person's body is like a T cell producing engine, able to fight off infections and building a lifetime storehouse of memory T cells. With age, however, people produce fewer naïve T cells, which makes them less able to combat new health threats. This also makes older people less responsive to vaccines, because vaccines generally require naïve T cells to produce a protective immune response. One exception is the shingles vaccine. Since shingles is the reactivation of the chickenpox virus, this particular vaccine relies on existing memory T cells and has been particularly effective in older people. Researchers are investigating ways to develop other vaccines that are adjusted for the changes that happen in an older person's immune system.

Negative, age-related changes in our innate and adaptive immune systems are known collectively as immunosenescence. A lifetime of stress on our bodies is thought to contribute to immunosenescence. Radiation, chemical exposure, and exposure to certain diseases can also speed up the deterioration of the immune system. Studying the intricacies of the immune system helps researchers better understand immunosenescence and determine which areas of the immune system are most vulnerable to aging. Ongoing research may shed light on whether or not there is any way to reverse the decline and boost immune protection in older individuals.

Chapter 2

Aging across the Globe

In 2010, an estimated 524 million people were aged 65 or older—8 percent of the world's population. By 2050, this number is expected to nearly triple to about 1.5 billion, representing 16 percent of the word's population. Although more developed countries have the oldest population profiles, the vast majority of older people—and the most rapidly aging populations—are in less developed countries. Between 2010 and 2050, the number of older people in less developed countries is projected to increase more than 250 percent, compared with a 71 percent increase in developed countries.

This remarkable phenomenon is being driven by declines in fertility and improvements in longevity. With fewer children entering the population and people living longer, older people are making up an increasing share of the total population. In more developed countries, fertility fell below the replacement rate of two live births per woman by the 1970s, down from nearly three children per woman around 1950. Even more crucial for population aging, fertility fell with surprising speed in many less developed countries from an average of six children in 1950 to an average of two or three children in 2005. In 2006, fertility was at or below the two-child replacement level in 44 less developed countries.

Most developed nations have had decades to adjust to their changing age structures. It took more than 100 years for the share of France's

This chapter includes text excerpted from "Global Health and Aging," National Institute on Aging (NIA), National Institutes of Health (NIH), October 2011. Reviewed September 2017.

population aged 65 or older to rise from 7 percent to 14 percent. In contrast, many less developed countries are experiencing a rapid increase in the number and percentage of older people, often within a single generation (Figure 2.1). For example, the same demographic aging that unfolded over more than a century in France will occur in just two decades in Brazil. Developing countries will need to adapt quickly to this new reality. Many less developed nations will need new policies that ensure the financial security of older people, and that provide the health and social care they need, without the same extended period of economic growth experienced by aging societies in the West. In other words, some countries may grow old before they grow rich.

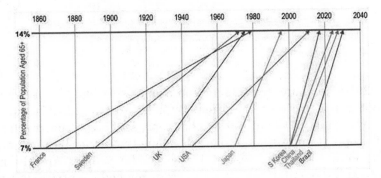

Figure 2.1. *Time Required or Expected for Percentage of Population Aged 65 and over to Rise from 7 Percent to 14 Percent*

In some countries, the sheer number of people entering older ages will challenge national infrastructures, particularly health systems.

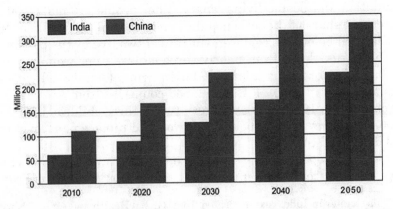

Figure 2.2. *Growth of the Population Aged 65 and Older in India and China: 2010–2050*

This numeric surge in older people is dramatically illustrated in the world's two most populous countries: China and India (Figure 2.2). China's older population—those over age 65—will likely swell to 330 million by 2050 from 110 million in 2011. India's population of 60 million in 2011 is projected to exceed 227 million in 2050, an increase of nearly 280 percent. By the middle of this century, there could be 100 million Chinese over the age of 80. This is an amazing achievement considering that there were fewer than 14 million people this age on the entire planet just a century ago.

Chapter 3

Aging in the United States

U.S. Population Is Aging

The growth in the number and proportion of older adults in the United States is unprecedented in the nation's history. By 2050, it is anticipated that Americans aged 65 or older will number nearly 89 million people, or more than double the number of older adults in the United States in 2010.

The rapid aging of the U.S. population is being driven by two realities: Americans are living longer lives than in previous decades and, given the post-World War II baby boom, there are proportionately more older adults than in previous generations. Many Americans are now living into their 70s, 80s, and beyond. The leading edge of the baby boomers reached age 65 in 2011, launching an unparalleled phenomenon in the United States. Since January 1, 2011, and each and every day for the next 20 years, roughly 10,000 Americans will celebrate their 65th birthdays. In 2030, when the last baby boomer turns 65, the demographic landscape of the nation will have changed significantly. One of every five Americans—about 72 million people—will be an older adult.

This chapter contains text excerpted from the following sources: Text beginning with the heading "U.S. Population Is Aging" is excerpted from "The State of Aging and Health in America 2013," Centers for Disease Control and Prevention (CDC), May 31, 2016; Text under the heading "Emerging Issues in the Health of Older Adults" is excerpted from "Older Adults," Office of Disease Prevention and Health Promotion (ODPHP), U.S. Department of Health and Human Services (HHS), August 23, 2017.

The aging of the nation's population has wide-ranging implications for virtually every facet of American society. At each point in the lifespan of baby boomers, the United States has felt and been changed by the impact of their numbers and needs—from booming sales in commercial baby food during the late 1940s, to the construction of thousands of new schools during the 1950s, to the housing construction boom of the 1970s and 1980s. The significant proportion of Americans represented by the baby boomers continues to exert its influence. In large measure, this influence will have its most profound effects on the nation's public health, social services, and healthcare systems. Public health plays a key role in advocating for those in need, linking individuals and communities to available services, and promoting healthy aging because of its effects on personal, societal, cultural, economic, and environmental factors. The public health sector is ideally positioned to meet the growing needs and demands of a rapidly aging nation.

U.S. Population Is Becoming More Racially and Ethnically Diverse

Along with the dramatic aging of the U.S. population during the next several decades will be significant increases in racial and ethnic diversity. Although young people in the United States currently reflect diversity more strikingly than their older counterparts, the racial and ethnic makeup of older adults is changing as well. In 2010, 80 percent of adults aged 65 years or older in the United States were non-Hispanic white. By 2030, that percentage will have declined, and older non-Hispanic white adults will make up 71.2 percent of the population, whereas Hispanics will make up 12 percent, non-Hispanic blacks nearly 10.3 percent, and Asians 5.4 percent. By 2050, the racial and ethnic diversity of older U.S. adults will have changed even more profoundly. Older non-Hispanic white adults, long deemed the "majority population," will account for only about 58 percent of the total population aged 65 or older, a decline of more than 20 percent from 2010. During the same period, the proportion of older Hispanics will almost triple—from 7 percent in 2010 to nearly 20 percent in 2050. The proportion of older Asian-Americans will more than double during 2010–2050, from 3.3 percent to 8.5 percent, and the proportion of older African-Americans will increase from 8.3 percent to 11.2 percent. At all ages, the health status of Hispanics, Asian-Americans, African-Americans, and other minority population groups, such as American Indians/Alaska Natives and Native Hawaiians/Other Pacific Islanders, has long lagged behind that of non-Hispanic whites. For a variety of reasons, older adults in these groups may experience the effects of health disparities more than younger people. Language barriers, reduced access to healthcare, low socioeconomic status, and differing cultural norms can be major challenges to promoting health in an increasingly diverse older population.

The Burden of Chronic Disease for Older Adults

Leading Causes of Death

During the twentieth century, effective public health strategies and advances in medical treatment contributed to a dramatic increase in average life expectancy in the United States. The 30-year gain in life expectancy within the span of a century had never before been achieved. Many of the diseases—including tuberculosis, diarrhea and enteritis, and syphilis—are no longer the threats they once were. Although they may still present significant health challenges in the United States, these diseases are no longer the leading killers of American adults. However, other diseases have continued to be leading causes of death every year since 1900. By 1910, heart disease became the leading cause of death every year except 1918–1920, when the influenza epidemic took its disastrous toll. Since 1938, cancer has held the second position every year. Heart disease and cancer pose their greatest risks as people age, as do other chronic diseases and conditions, such as stroke, chronic lower respiratory diseases, Alzheimer disease, and diabetes. Influenza and pneumonia also continue to contribute to deaths among older adults, despite the availability of effective vaccines.

Diminished Quality of Life and Loss of Independence

The burden of chronic diseases encompasses a much broader spectrum of negative health consequences than death alone. People living with one or more chronic diseases often experience diminished quality of life, generally reflected by a long period of decline and disability associated with their disease.

Chronic diseases can affect a person's ability to perform important and essential activities, both inside and outside the home. Initially, they may have trouble with the instrumental activities of daily living (IADLs), such as managing money, shopping, preparing meals, and taking medications as prescribed. As functional ability—physical, mental, or both—further declines, people may lose the ability to perform

21

more basic activities, called activities of daily living (ADLs), such as taking care of personal hygiene, feeding themselves, getting dressed, and toileting. The inability to perform daily activities can restrict people's engagement in life and their enjoyment of family and friends. Lack of mobility in the community or at home significantly narrows an older person's world and ability to do the things that bring enjoyment and meaning to life. Loss of the ability to care for oneself safely and appropriately means further loss of independence and can often lead to the need for care in an institutional setting. The need for caregiving for older adults by formal, professional caregivers or by family members—and the need for long-term care services and supports—will increase sharply during the next several decades, given the effects of chronic diseases on an aging population.

Major Contributor to Healthcare Costs

The nation's expenditures for healthcare, already the highest among developed countries, are expected to rise considerably as chronic diseases affect growing numbers of older adults. Today, more than two-thirds of all healthcare costs are for treating chronic illnesses. Among healthcare costs for older Americans, 95 percent are for chronic diseases. The cost of providing healthcare for one person aged 65 or older is three to five times higher than the cost for someone younger than 65.

By 2030, healthcare spending will increase by 25 percent, largely because the population will be older. This estimate does not take into account inflation and the higher costs of new technologies. Medicare spending is projected to increase from $555 billion in 2011 to $903 billion in 2020.

Ways to Promote and Preserve the Health of Older Adults and Reduce Costs

Death and decline associated with the leading chronic diseases are often preventable or can be delayed. Multiple opportunities exist to promote and preserve the health of older adults. The challenge is to more broadly apply what is already known about reducing the risk of chronic disease. Death is unavoidable, but the prevalence of chronic illnesses and the decline and disability commonly associated with them can be reduced.

Although the risk of developing chronic diseases increases as a person ages, the root causes of many of these diseases often begin early in life. Practicing healthy behaviors from an early age and getting recommended screenings can substantially reduce a person's risk of developing chronic diseases and associated disabilities. Research has shown that people who do not use tobacco, who get regular physical activity, and who eat a healthy diet significantly decrease their risk of developing heart disease, cancer, diabetes, and other chronic conditions. Unfortunately, current data on health-related behaviors among people aged 55–64 years do not indicate a positive future for the health of older Americans.

If a meaningful decline in chronic diseases among older adults is to occur, adults at younger ages, as well as the nation's children and adolescents, need to pursue health-promoting behaviors and get recommended preventive services. Communities can play a pivotal role in achieving this goal by making healthy choices easier and making changes to policies, systems, and environments that help Americans of all ages take charge of their health.

Addressing Challenges for People with Multiple Chronic Conditions

More than a quarter of all Americans and two of three older Americans have multiple chronic conditions, and treatment for this population accounts for 66 percent of the country's healthcare budget. The nation's healthcare system is largely designed to treat one disease or condition at a time, but many Americans have more than one, and often several, chronic conditions. For example, just 9.3 percent of adults with diabetes have only diabetes. Other common conditions include arthritis, asthma, chronic respiratory disease, heart disease, and high blood pressure.

People with chronic diseases may also have other health problems, such as substance use or addiction disorders, mental illness, dementia or other cognitive impairments, and developmental disabilities. The varied nature of these conditions leads to the need for multiple healthcare specialists, a variety of treatment regimens, and prescription medications that may not be compatible. People with multiple chronic conditions face an increased risk of conflicting medical advice, adverse drug effects, unnecessary and duplicative tests, and avoidable hospitalizations, all of which can further endanger their health. Figure 3.1 shows the rates of multiple chronic conditions among Medicare fee-for-service beneficiaries.

To address these risks, the U.S. Department of Health and Human Services (HHS) developed a strategic framework to improve health outcomes for people with multiple chronic conditions. Federal agencies

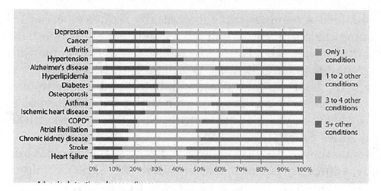

Figure 3.1. *Multiple Chronic Conditions among Medicare Fee-for-Service Beneficiaries*

and key partners will use this framework to improve and coordinate care for people with multiple chronic conditions, make the best use of effective self-care strategies, and support research to fill knowledge gaps.

New Directions in Public Health for Older Americans

As more and more Americans reach the age of 65, society is increasingly challenged to help them grow older with dignity and comfort. Meeting these challenges is critical to ensuring that baby boomers can look forward to their later years. Three key areas that public health professionals are beginning to address among older adults are binge drinking, emergency preparedness, and health literacy. These areas have long been the target of healthcare and aging services professionals.

Older Adults and Excessive Alcohol Use

Excessive alcohol use, including binge drinking, accounts for more than 21,000 deaths among adults 65 or older each year in the United States. Binge drinking is defined as women consuming four or more drinks and men consuming five or more drinks on a single occasion. In 2006, excessive drinking cost the U.S. economy $223.5 billion, or $1.90 a drink. Excessive drinking increases a person's risk of developing high blood pressure, liver disease, certain cancers, heart disease, stroke, and many other chronic health problems, as well as a person's risk of car crashes, falls, and violence. Excessive alcohol use can also interact with prescription and over-the-counter medications and affect compliance with treatment protocols for chronic conditions, thus undermining the effective management of chronic diseases.

However, older adults who binge drank reported engaging in this behavior more frequently than their younger counterparts—an average of five to six times a month. They also reported consuming an average of about six drinks when they did, thereby increasing their risk of developing many health and social problems.

Centers for Disease Control and Prevention (CDC) is assessing the public health effect of excessive drinking, including binge drinking. They are also working with states and communities to translate strategies for preventing excessive alcohol consumption recommended in *The Guide to Community Preventive Services (Community Guide)* into public health practice. These recommendations include increasing the price of alcohol, regulating the number and concentration of alcohol retailers in a community, holding alcohol retailers liable for harms resulting from illegal sales to underage or intoxicated persons, maintaining government controls of alcohol sales (avoiding privatization), using electronic screening and brief intervention for excessive alcohol use, and limiting the days and hours when alcohol is sold.

CDC is also helping to increase screening and counseling for excessive alcohol use in clinical settings, as recommended for adults by the U.S. Preventive Services Task Force (USPSTF). Taken together, these prevention measures can help reduce excessive alcohol use and the many health and social harms related to it. They can also help the United States meet the Healthy People 2020 leading health indicator of reducing binge drinking among all U.S. adults.

Using Data to Better Protect Vulnerable Older Adults in Emergencies

Some older adults may have difficulty keeping themselves safe and healthy during an emergency or natural disaster. Conditions such as impaired mobility, multiple chronic health conditions, or difficulty with memory may cause some older adults to need extra help planning for and dealing with situations such as hurricanes or floods. Emergencies and disasters can also disrupt the help that many older adults rely on for independent living, such as help from friends, family, and home-based medical care.

To help states, communities, and partner organizations plan for the needs of older adults, CDC released *Identifying Vulnerable Older Adults and Legal Preparedness Options for Increasing Their Protection During All-Hazards Emergencies: A Cross-Sector Guide for States and Communities.* This guide presents practical strategies and legal options for protecting older adults during all-hazards emergencies. A key strategy in this guide is "characterizing the population." This phrase means using community and state data about demographics, health status, medical conditions, service requirements, and other needs to paint a picture of the older adult population so their needs are properly considered in planning. Some of the key indicators in this report, such as disability, oral health, taking medicine for high blood pressure, and influenza and pneumococcal vaccinations, are particularly important when trying to understand the medical needs and health status of a community. This knowledge helps to ensure that appropriate medical equipment, pharmaceuticals, and preventive measures can be taken in a shelter environment, evacuation, or shelter-in-place event.

Improving Health Literacy among Older Adults

Why Does Health Literacy Matter?

Every day, people confront situations that involve life-changing decisions about their health. These decisions are made in places such as grocery and drug stores, workplaces, playgrounds, doctors' offices, clinics and hospitals, and around the kitchen table. Obtaining, communicating, processing, and understanding health information and services are essential steps in making appropriate health decisions. However, research indicates that today's health information is presented in ways that are not usable by most adults. *Limited health literacy* occurs when people cannot find and use the health information and services they need.

- Nearly 9 of 10 adults have trouble using the everyday health information that is routinely available in our healthcare facilities, retail outlets, media, and communities.

- Among adult age groups, those aged 65 or older have the smallest percentage of people with proficient health literacy skills and the largest percentage with "below basic" health literacy skills.

- Without clear information and an understanding of the information's importance, people are more likely to skip necessary medical tests, end up in the emergency room more often, and have a harder time managing chronic diseases such as diabetes or high blood pressure

What Is Health Literacy?

Health literacy was defined by *Healthy People 2010* as, "the degree to which individuals have the capacity to obtain, process, and understand basic health information and services needed to make appropriate health decisions." *Healthy People 2020* is tracking health literacy improvement, which is defined as how many healthcare providers make sure their instructions are easy for patients to understand.

How Can We Improve Health Literacy?

Recent federal policy initiatives have brought health literacy to a tipping point. The skills of individual patients are not the only important part of health literacy. This concept includes what health systems and professionals do to make health information and services understandable for everyone, regardless of their literacy skills. We can build our own health literacy skills and help others—such as community members, health professionals, and anyone who communicates about health—build their skills. Every organization involved in health information and services needs its own health literacy plan to improve its organizational practices.

Emerging Issues in the Health of Older Adults

- Person-centered care planning that includes caregivers.

- Quality measures of care and monitoring of health conditions.

- Fair pay and compensation standards for formal and informal caregivers.

- Minimum levels of geriatric training for health professionals.

- Enhanced data on certain subpopulations of older adults, including aging lesbian, gay, bisexual, and transgender (LGBT) populations.

Chapter 4

Aging and Its Impact on the Body

Chapter Contents

Section 4.1

Changes to Your Heart with Age

This section includes text excerpted from "Heart Health,"
National Institute on Aging (NIA), National Institutes of
Health (NIH), August 21, 2017.

Your Heart

Your heart is a strong muscle about the size of the palm of your
hand. Just like an engine makes a car go, the heart keeps your body
running. The heart has two pumps. The stronger pump uses arteries
to send blood with oxygen away from the heart, throughout the body.
The other pump uses veins to bring blood back to the heart and sends
it to the lungs to get more oxygen. An electrical system in the heart
controls the heart pumps (the heart beat or pulse).

Check Your Blood Pressure

As you get older, it is important for you to have your blood pressure
checked regularly, even if you are healthy. You may feel fine, but if not
treated, high blood pressure can lead to stroke and problems with your
heart, eyes, and kidneys. Exercise and reducing salt in your diet can
help, but often medication is needed to manage high blood pressure
and the related problems.

Changes to Your Heart with Age

Aging can cause changes in the heart and blood vessels. For example, as you get older, your heart can't beat as fast during physical
activity or stress as when you were younger. However, the number of
heart beats per minute (heart rate) at rest does not change as you age.

Many of the problems older people have with their heart and blood
vessels are really caused by disease, not by aging. For example, an
older heart can normally pump blood as strong as a younger heart;
less ability to pump blood is caused by disease. But, changes that happen with age may increase a person's risk of heart disease. The good

news is there are things you can do to delay, lower, or possibly avoid or reverse your risk.

A common problem related to aging is "hardening of the arteries," called arteriosclerosis. This problem is why blood pressure goes up with age.

Age can cause other changes to the heart. For example:

- Blood vessels can become stiffer, and some parts of the heart wall will thicken to help with blood flow.

- Your valves (one-way, door-like parts that open and close to control the blood flow inside your heart) may become thicker and stiffer, causing leaks or problems with pumping blood out of the heart.

- The size of the sections of your heart may increase.

Other factors, such as thyroid disease or chemotherapy, may weaken the heart muscle. Things you can't control, like your family history, might also increase your risk of heart disease. But even so, leading a heart-healthy lifestyle might help you avoid or delay serious illness.

Heart Disease

There are many different kinds of heart disease. The most common is atherosclerosis, the buildup of fatty deposits or plaques in the walls of arteries. As plaque builds up, there is less space for blood to flow normally and deliver oxygen throughout the body, including to the heart. Depending on where the build-up is, it can cause a heart attack, leg pain, or a stroke. Atherosclerosis is not part of normal aging and can be serious. There are choices you can make to prevent or delay heart disease, including:

- Don't smoke

- Stay at a healthy weight

- Avoid spending hours every day sitting

- Exercise

- Keep your diabetes, high blood pressure, and/or high cholesterol under control

- Manage your stress

- Don't drink a lot of alcohol

Some Medical Tests

Your doctor will check your blood pressure and do a blood test to check your cholesterol, a fat that can add to plaques in your arteries. He or she might also do a blood test for CRP (C-reactive protein) and suggest you have an ECG or EKG, an electrocardiogram. This is a test that looks at electrical activity in your heart.

Signs of Heart Disease

Early heart disease often doesn't have symptoms, or the symptoms may be barely noticeable. This is especially true in older adults. That's why regular check-ups with your doctor are important.

Contact your doctor right away if you feel any chest pain. However, as you get older, chest pain is a less common sign of heart disease, so be aware of other symptoms. Tell your doctor if you feel:

- Pain in the shoulders, arms, neck, jaw, or back
- Shortness of breath when active or at rest
- Chest pain during physical activity that gets better when you rest
- Lightheaded
- Dizzy
- Confusion
- Headaches
- Cold sweats
- Nausea/vomiting
- Easily tired or fatigued
- Swelling in the ankles, feet, legs, stomach, and/or neck
- Less able to exercise or be physically active
- Problems doing your normal activities

Problems with a rapid or irregular heartbeat are much more common in older adults than younger people and need to be treated. See a doctor if you feel a fluttering in your chest or have the feeling that your heart is skipping a beat or beating too hard, especially if you are weaker than usual, dizzy, or tired. If you have any signs of heart disease, your doctor may send you to see a cardiologist, a doctor who specializes in the heart.

Section 4.2

Brain Health: You Can Make a Difference!

This section includes text excerpted from "Brain Health:
You Can Make a Difference!" Eldercare Locator, U.S.
Administration on Aging (AOA), November 20, 2014.
Reviewed September 2017.

There are many lifestyle choices you can make to maintain a healthy body as you age. But what about the steps you can take to support a healthy brain as you grow older? This section will provide you with some information and guidance to help you make smart choices about your brain health with each passing year.

Memory and Learning

As you grow older, you may notice differences in the way your mind works. You may have difficulty finding the correct words, multitasking or paying attention. The good news is that even if you have already noticed some of these changes, you are still able to learn new things, create new memories, and improve vocabulary and language skills.

Potential Threats to Brain Health

Health Conditions

Some health conditions can negatively affect your brain. Heart disease, high blood pressure, and diabetes can alter, or damage blood vessels throughout your body, including the brain. Alzheimer disease and other types of dementia also harm the brain. While no one knows how to prevent dementia, many approaches that are good for your health in other ways, including engaging in exercise and eating a healthy diet, are being tested.

Medicines

Some medications and certain combinations of drugs can affect your thinking and the way your brain works. Older adults taking medications should be particularly careful when consuming alcohol, as drugs may interact negatively with it.

Alcohol

Drinking alcohol can slow or impair communication among your brain cells. This can cause slurred speech, a fuzzy memory, drowsiness, and dizziness; it can also lead to long-term difficulties with your balance, memory, coordination, and body temperature.

Smoking

The risks associated with smoking are heart attacks, stroke, and lung disease.

Brain Injury

Older adults are at higher risk of falling and other accidents that can cause brain injury.

Actions You Can Take to Help Protect Your Brain

Take Charge

- Get recommended health screenings regularly.
- Manage health conditions, such as diabetes, high blood pressure, and high cholesterol.
- Be sure to talk with your doctor or pharmacist about the medications you take and any possible side effects on memory, sleep, and how your brain works.
- To learn more about how to move or exercise in a healthy way, ask your healthcare provider about your personal situation.

Eat Right

Try to maintain a balanced diet of fruits and vegetables, whole grains, lean meats (including fish and poultry), and low-fat or nonfat dairy products. Monitor your intake of solid fat, sugar, and salt, and eat proper portion sizes.

Get Moving

Being physically active may help reduce the risk of conditions that can harm brain health, such as diabetes, heart disease, depression, and stroke; it may also help improve connections among your brain cells. Older adults should get at least 150 minutes of exercise each week.

Drink Moderately, If at All

Staying away from alcohol can reverse some negative changes related to brain health.

Don't Smoke

Quitting smoking at any age will be beneficial to the health of your mind and body. Nonsmokers have a lower risk of heart attacks, stroke and lung diseases, as well as increased blood circulation.

Be Safe

To reduce the risk of falling, exercise to improve balance and coordination, take a falls prevention class, and make your home safer.

Think and Connect

Keep your mind active by doing mentally stimulating activities like reading, playing games, learning new things, teaching or taking a class and being social. Older adults who remain active and engaged with others by doing activities like volunteering report being happier and healthier overall.

Taking the First Step

You can start to support your brain health with some small, first steps, and build from there.

- Begin an exercise routine, such as a daily walk, with the goal of increasing the amount of time and speed.

- Add an extra serving of fruit and vegetables each day.

- Make an appointment for a health screening or a physical exam.

- Seek out volunteer opportunities that interest you.

- Sign up for a class or program at your community college or community center.

Section 4.3

Vision

This section includes text excerpted from "Aging and
Your Eyes," National Institute on Aging (NIA), National
Institutes of Health (NIH), July 6, 2017.

Are you holding the newspaper farther away from your eyes than
you used to? Join the crowd—age can bring changes that affect your
eyesight. Some changes are more serious than others, but for many
problems, there are things you can do to protect your vision. The key
is to have regular eye exams so you can spot problems early.

How Can You Protect Your Eyesight?

Have your eyes checked regularly by an eye care professional—
either an ophthalmologist or optometrist. People over age 60 should
have dilated eye exams yearly. During this exam, the eye care professional will put drops in your eyes to widen (dilate) your pupils so
that he or she can look at the back of each eye. This is the only way
to find some common eye diseases that have no early signs or symptoms. If you wear glasses or contact lenses, your prescription should
be checked, too. See your doctor regularly to check for diseases like
diabetes and high blood pressure. These diseases can cause eye problems if not controlled or treated.

See an eye care professional right away if you:

- Suddenly cannot see or everything looks blurry
- See flashes of light
- Have eye pain
- Experience double vision
- Have redness or swelling of your eye or eyelid

Common Eye Problems

The following common eye problems can be easily treated. But,
sometimes they can be signs of more serious issues.

- **Presbyopia** is a slow loss of ability to see close objects or small print. It is normal to have this problem as you get older. People with presbyopia often have headaches or strained, tired eyes. Reading glasses usually fix the problem.

- **Floaters** are tiny specks or "cobwebs" that seem to float across your vision. You might see them in well-lit rooms or outdoors on a bright day. Floaters can be a normal part of aging. But, sometimes they are a sign of a more serious eye problem, such as retinal detachment. If you see many new floaters and/or flashes of light, see your eye care professional right away.

- **Tearing** (or having too many tears) can come from being sensitive to light, wind, or temperature changes, or having a condition called dry eye. Wearing sunglasses may help. So, might eye drops. Sometimes tearing is a sign of a more serious eye problem, like an infection or a blocked tear duct. Your eye care professional can treat these problems.

- **Eyelid problems** can result from different diseases or conditions. Common eyelid problems include red and swollen eyelids, itching, tearing, and crusting of eyelashes during sleep. These problems may be caused by a condition called blepharitis and treated with warm compresses and gentle eyelid scrubs.

Eye Diseases and Disorders

The following eye conditions can lead to vision loss and blindness. They may have few or no early symptoms. Regular eye exams are your best protection. If your eye care professional finds a problem early, often there are things you can do to keep your eyesight.

- **Cataracts** are cloudy areas in the eye's lens causing blurred or hazy vision. Some cataracts stay small and don't change your eyesight a lot. Others become large and reduce vision. Cataract surgery can restore good vision. It is a safe and common treatment. If you have a cataract, your eye care professional will watch for changes over time to see if you would benefit from surgery.

- **Corneal diseases and conditions** can cause redness, watery eyes, pain, problems with vision, or a halo effect of the vision (things appear to have an aura of light around them). Infection and injury are some of the things that can hurt the cornea. Treatment may be simple—for example, changing your eyeglass prescription or using eye drops. In severe cases, surgery may be needed.

- **Dry eye** happens when tear glands don't work well. You may feel stinging or burning, a sandy feeling as if something is in the eye, or other discomfort. Dry eye is more common as people get older, especially for women. Your eye care professional may tell you to use a home humidifier or air cleaner, special eye drops (artificial tears), or ointments to treat dry eye.

- **Glaucoma** often comes from too much fluid pressure inside the eye. If not treated, it can lead to vision loss and blindness. People with glaucoma often have no early symptoms or pain. You can protect yourself by having dilated eye exams yearly. Glaucoma can be treated with prescription eye drops, lasers, or surgery.

- **Retinal disorders** are a leading cause of blindness in the United States. Retinal disorders that affect aging eyes include:

- **Age-related macular degeneration (AMD).** AMD can harm the sharp, central vision needed to see objects clearly and to do common things like driving and reading. During a dilated eye exam, your eye care professional will look for signs of AMD. There are treatments for AMD. If you have AMD, ask if special dietary supplements could lower your chance of it getting worse.

- **Diabetic retinopathy.** This problem may occur if you have diabetes. Diabetic retinopathy develops slowly and often has no early warning signs. If you have diabetes, be sure to have a dilated eye exam at least once a year. Keeping your blood sugar, blood pressure, and cholesterol under control can prevent diabetic retinopathy or slow its progress. Laser surgery can sometimes prevent it from getting worse.

- **Retinal detachment.** This is a medical emergency. When the retina separates from the back of the eye, it's called retinal detachment. If you see new floaters or light flashes, or if it seems like a curtain has been pulled over your eye, go to your eye care professional right away. With treatment, doctors often can prevent loss of vision.

What Is Low Vision?

Low vision means you cannot fix your eyesight with glasses, contact lenses, medicine, or surgery. Low vision affects some people as they age. You may have low vision if you:

- Can't see well enough to do everyday tasks like reading, cooking, or sewing
- Have difficulty recognizing the faces of your friends or family
- Have trouble reading street signs
- Find that lights don't seem as bright

If you have any of these problems, ask your eye care professional to test you for low vision. Special tools can help people with low vision to read, write, and manage daily tasks. These tools include large-print reading materials, magnifying aids, closed-circuit televisions, audio tapes, electronic reading machines, and computers with large print and a talking function.

Other tips that may help:

- Brighten the lighting in your room.
- Write with bold, black felt-tip markers.
- Use paper with bold lines to help you write in a straight line.
- Put colored tape on the edge of your steps to help you see them and prevent you from falling.
- Install dark-colored light switches and electrical outlets that you can see easily against light-colored walls.
- Use motion lights that turn on when you enter a room. These may help you avoid accidents caused by poor lighting.
- Use telephones, clocks, and watches with large numbers; put large-print labels on the microwave and stove.

Remember to ask your eye doctor if your vision is okay for safe driving.

Tips for Healthy Eyes

- Protect your eyes from too much sunlight by wearing sunglasses that block ultraviolet (UV) radiation and a hat with a wide brim when you are outside.
- Stop smoking.
- Make smart food choices.
- Be physically active and maintain a healthy weight.

- Maintain normal blood pressure.

- Control diabetes (if you have it).

If you spend a lot of time at the computer or focused on one thing, you can forget to blink. Every 20 minutes, look away about 20 feet for 20 seconds to prevent eye strain.

Section 4.4

Hearing Loss

This section includes text excerpted from "Hearing Loss: A Common Problem for Older Adults," National Institute on Aging (NIA), National Institutes of Health (NIH), July 24, 2017.

Hearing loss is a common problem caused by noise, aging, disease, and heredity. People with hearing loss may find it hard to have a conversation with friends and family. They may also have trouble understanding a doctor's advice, responding to warnings, and hearing doorbells and alarms.

Approximately one in three people between the ages of 65 and 74 has hearing loss, and nearly half of those older than 75 has difficulty hearing. But some people may not want to admit they have trouble hearing. Older people who can't hear well may become depressed or may withdraw from others to avoid feeling frustrated or embarrassed about not understanding what is being said. Sometimes older people are mistakenly thought to be confused, unresponsive, or uncooperative because they don't hear well.

Hearing problems that are ignored or untreated can get worse. If you have a hearing problem, see your doctor. Hearing aids, special training, certain medicines, and surgery are some of the treatments that can help.

Signs of Hearing Loss

Some people have a hearing problem without realizing it. You should see your doctor if you:

- Have trouble hearing over the telephone

- Find it hard to follow conversations when two or more people are talking
- Often ask people to repeat what they are saying
- Need to turn up the TV volume so loud that others complain
- Have a problem hearing because of background noise
- Think that others seem to mumble
- Can't understand when women and children speak to you

Types of Hearing Loss

Hearing loss comes in many forms. It can range from a mild loss, in which a person misses certain high-pitched sounds, such as the voices of women and children, to a total loss of hearing.

There are two general categories of hearing loss:

- **Sensorineural hearing loss** occurs when there is damage to the inner ear or the auditory nerve. This type of hearing loss is usually permanent.

- **Conductive hearing loss** occurs when sound waves cannot reach the inner ear. The cause may be earwax buildup, fluid, or a punctured eardrum. Medical treatment or surgery can usually restore conductive hearing loss.

Sudden Hearing Loss

Sudden sensorineural hearing loss, or sudden deafness, is a rapid loss of hearing. It can happen to a person all at once or over a period of up to 3 days. It should be considered a medical emergency. If you or someone you know experiences sudden sensorineural hearing loss, visit a doctor immediately.

Age-Related Hearing Loss (Presbycusis)

One type of hearing loss, called presbycusis, or age-related hearing loss, comes on gradually as a person ages. It seems to run in families and may occur because of changes in the inner ear and auditory nerve. Having presbycusis may make it hard for a person to tolerate loud sounds or to hear what others are saying.

Age-related hearing loss most often occurs in both ears, affecting them equally. Because the loss is gradual, someone with presbycusis may not realize that he or she has lost some of his or her ability to hear.

Ringing in the Ears (Tinnitus)

Tinnitus, also common in older people, is typically described as ringing in the ears, but it also can sound like roaring, clicking, hissing, or buzzing. It can come and go. It might be heard in one or both ears, and it may be loud or soft. Tinnitus can accompany any type of hearing loss and can be a sign of other health problems, such as high blood pressure or allergies, or a side effect of medications.

Causes of Hearing Loss

Loud noise is one of the most common causes of hearing loss. Noise from lawn mowers, snow blowers, or loud music can damage the inner ear, resulting in permanent hearing loss. Loud noise also contributes to tinnitus. You can prevent most noise-related hearing loss. Protect yourself by turning down the sound on your stereo, television, or headphones; moving away from loud noise; or using earplugs or other ear protection.

Earwax or fluid buildup can block sounds that are carried from the eardrum to the inner ear. If wax blockage is a problem, try using mild treatments, such as mineral oil, baby oil, glycerin, or commercial ear drops to soften earwax. A punctured ear drum can also cause hearing loss. The eardrum can be damaged by infection, pressure, or putting objects in the ear, including cotton-tipped swabs. See your doctor if you have pain or fluid draining from the ear.

Viruses and bacteria (including the ear infection otitis media), a heart condition, stroke, brain injury, or a tumor may affect your hearing.

Hearing loss can also result from taking certain medications. "Ototoxic" medications damage the inner ear, sometimes permanently. Some ototoxic drugs include medicines used to treat serious infections, cancer, and heart disease. Some antibiotics are ototoxic. Even aspirin at some dosages can cause problems. Check with your doctor if you notice a problem while taking a medication.

Heredity can cause hearing loss, as well. But not all inherited forms of hearing loss take place at birth. Some forms can show up later in life. For example, in otosclerosis, which is thought to be a hereditary disease, an abnormal growth of bone prevents structures within the ear from working properly.

Ways to Cope with Hearing Loss

If you notice signs of hearing loss, talk to your doctor. If you have trouble hearing, you should:

- Let people know you have a hearing problem.

- Ask people to face you and to speak more slowly and clearly. Also, ask them to speak louder without shouting.

- Pay attention to what is being said and to facial expressions or gestures.

- Let the person talking know if you do not understand what he or she said.

- Ask the person speaking to reword a sentence and try again.

Tips for Talking with Someone with Hearing Loss

Here are some tips you can use when talking with someone who has a hearing problem:

- In a group, include people with hearing loss in the conversation.

- Find a quiet place to talk to help reduce background noise, especially in restaurants and at social gatherings.

- Stand in good lighting and use facial expressions or gestures to give clues.

- Face the person and speak clearly.

- Speak a little more loudly than normal, but don't shout.

- Speak at a reasonable speed.

- Do not hide your mouth, eat, or chew gum while speaking.

- Repeat yourself if necessary, using different words.

- Try to make sure only one person talks at a time.

- Be patient. Stay positive and relaxed.

- Ask how you can help.

The most important thing you can do if you think you have a hearing problem is to seek professional advice. Your family doctor may be able to diagnose and treat your hearing problem. Or, your doctor may refer you to other experts, like an otolaryngologist (ear, nose, and throat doctor), or an audiologist (health professional who can identify and measure hearing loss).

Devices to Help with Hearing Loss

Your doctor or specialist may suggest you get a hearing aid. Hearing aids are electronic, battery-run devices that make sounds louder. There are many types of hearing aids. Before buying a hearing aid, ask if your health insurance will cover the cost. Also ask if you can have a trial period so you can make sure the device is right for you. An audiologist or hearing aid specialist will show you how to use your hearing aid.

Assistive listening devices, alerting devices, and cochlear implants can help some people with hearing loss. Alert systems can work with doorbells, smoke detectors, and alarm clocks to send you visual signals or vibrations. For example, a flashing light can let you know someone is at the door or the phone is ringing. Some people rely on the vibration setting on their cell phones to alert them to calls.

Cochlear implants are electronic devices for people with severe hearing loss. They don't work for all types of hearing loss.

Section 4.5

Menopause

This section includes text excerpted from "Menopause," *Eunice Kennedy Shriver* National Institute of Child Health and Human Development (NICHD), December 3, 2012. Reviewed September 2017.

Menopause refers to the time in a woman's life when she stops having a menstrual period and is no longer fertile. The time leading up to menopause is called the menopausal transition, or perimenopause.

During perimenopause, a woman's ovaries start to produce less estrogen and progesterone. Changes in these hormones cause symptoms of menopause. Periods occur less often and eventually stop. Although this typically is a gradual process that happens over time, in some cases, a woman's periods will stop suddenly. Throughout perimenopause, ovulation—the release of eggs from the ovaries—also occurs less and less frequently.

Menopause is the point at which a woman has not had a period in 12 consecutive months. The time after menopause is called postmenopause, a phase that lasts for the rest of a woman's life.

All women experience menopause, usually between ages 45 and 55. The average age of menopause is 51, but it occurs earlier in some women. Women who smoke may go through menopause earlier than women who don't smoke.

However, perimenopause can begin several years earlier when levels of estrogen and progesterone first begin to fluctuate. Surgical or medical menopause is the term for a decrease in estrogen that is a result of surgery to remove the ovaries or uterus, or medical treatments such as chemotherapy or hormone therapy to treat breast cancer.

What Are Common Symptoms?

- Perimenopause begins with a change in a woman's menstrual cycle. During perimenopause, a woman's periods may be irregular in that they could last for a longer or shorter amount of time or be lighter or heavier. Although such changes are expected, women should consult a healthcare provider if they experience heavy bleeding, periods that occur very close together, spotting, or periods that last longer than a week.

- A common symptom of menopause is the appearance of hot flashes (sometimes called a hot flush). Hot flashes occur because of changing estrogen levels in a woman's body. A hot flash consists of a sudden feeling of heat and may include flushing of the face and neck, red blotches on the chest and arms, and sweating followed by shivering. A hot flash can last 30 seconds to 10 minutes.

- During menopause, many women experience vaginal dryness, which can make sexual intercourse uncomfortable and can lead to vaginal or urinary tract infections. In addition, the bladder muscles may weaken, which could lead to urine leakage when sneezing, coughing, laughing, or running. This condition is called urinary incontinence.

- Some women find that they're not as interested in sex, while others find that they enjoy sex more during the years around menopause. It's important to note that women can still become pregnant during perimenopause and should take appropriate contraceptive measures. Also, menopause does not change the risk of contracting a sexually transmitted disease.

- In addition, getting a good night's sleep can sometimes be difficult for menopausal women. Whether sleep is disrupted due to night sweats or other reasons, long-term lack of sleep can lead to fatigue, lack of energy, and memory problems.

- Mood changes such as irritability or anxiety can occur when a woman is going through menopause. These symptoms could be due to shifts in hormones or lifestyle factors, such as caring for elderly parents, that are likely to occur during this time in a woman's life.

- Other physical changes occur that can put menopausal women at risk for osteoporosis and heart disease. The loss of estrogen causes women to lose bone density, a condition called osteoporosis. This can cause the bones to become weak and prone to breakage.

- Heart disease may develop after menopause due to the loss of estrogen or to other problems related to normal aging. Weight gain, high blood pressure, and diabetes all put stress on the heart and can increase the risk of a heart attack or stroke.

What Causes It?

In the natural process of menopause, a woman's ovaries stop releasing eggs and making the hormones estrogen and progesterone. When this occurs, a woman stops having her period and is no longer fertile.

Menopause can also occur after surgical removal of a woman's ovaries or following chemotherapy or hormone therapy for the treatment of breast cancer.

How Is It Diagnosed?

Women typically notice the signs and symptoms of menopause without a formal diagnosis from their healthcare provider. A change in menstrual patterns and the appearance of hot flashes are usually the first signs.

Although blood tests are not required, healthcare providers can run blood or urine tests to determine levels of the hormones estradiol, follicle-stimulating hormone (FSH), and luteinizing hormone (LH). At menopause, the ovaries become less responsive to FSH and LH hormones, so the body makes more of these hormones to compensate. Estradiol and other hormones decrease around menopause as well.

A healthcare provider can use the test results to tell if a woman is in menopause.

During and after menopause, a woman should get regular physical, pelvic, breast, colorectal, and skin exams to monitor her health.

What Are the Treatments?

Menopause is a normal part of aging and every woman goes through it. It can't be prevented and normally doesn't require treatment. However, some symptoms of menopause can be lessened or perhaps even eliminated with treatment. Likewise, the risk of disorders or diseases associated with menopause, such as osteoporosis and heart disease, may benefit from treatment.

Physicians used to routinely prescribe hormone replacement therapy (HRT) with estrogen and, sometimes, progesterone to treat the general symptoms of menopause. However, this is no longer routine after several large studies showed that HRT can raise the risk of breast cancer, heart attacks, strokes, and blood clots.

If you are having trouble with menopause symptoms, talk to your healthcare provider about the benefits and risks of what is now called menopausal hormone therapy (MHT). According to the National Institute on Aging (NIA), only women at low risk for stroke, heart disease, blood clots, and breast cancer are considered candidates for MHT—and only those who have entered menopause recently. MHT can be given in the forms of pills, creams, or skin patches. Most medical professionals recommend an individualized MHT plan for each woman based on the age of menopause. It is important to know that MHT may cause side effects, such as bleeding, bloating, breast tenderness or enlargement, headaches, mood changes, and nausea.

The loss of estrogen may also be associated with changes in cholesterol levels and increased risk of heart disease. If you have high blood pressure or diabetes or are overweight, your healthcare provider may prescribe dietary changes or drugs to reduce your risk of heart disease, heart attack, and stroke.

Treatment for Osteoporosis and Bone Loss Related to Menopause

Because bone loss increases in the first two years after menopause, healthcare providers may order a bone density test, such as a dual-energy X-ray absorptiometry (DEXA) scan. If you have osteoporosis or are at risk for it, your healthcare provider may prescribe bone-strengthening drugs or supplements to help prevent future bone loss and fractures.

Medications commonly prescribed to treat osteoporosis include:

- Bisphosphonates
- Calcium + vitamin D
- Calcitonin
- Parathyroid hormone
- Raloxifene

There are also many things you can do as part of a healthy lifestyle to help prevent bone loss:

- Eat a healthy, low-fat, low-cholesterol diet that features lots of vegetables, fruits, and whole-grain foods.
- Make sure to get at least 1,200 mg of calcium and 800–1,000 international units (IUs) of vitamin D each day.
- Avoid drinking more than one alcoholic drink per day.
- Don't smoke.
- Avoid consuming caffeine.
- Achieve and maintain a healthy weight.
- Exercise most days of the week, including exercise that elevates your heart rate, and weight-bearing exercises such as weight lifting or walking.

Treatment of Hot Flashes and Night Sweats

Several prescription drugs are available to relieve hot flashes and night sweats:

- Clonidine, a blood pressure drug
- Gabapentin, a seizure drug that has been shown to reduce hot flashes
- Menopausal hormone therapy (MHT)

There are also several practical things you can do on a daily basis to relieve these symptoms:

- Sleep in a cool room in light clothing.

- Keep a fan on in your bedroom at night.

- Sip a cold drink of water or juice.

- Avoid smoking, caffeine, and alcohol.

- When you feel a hot flash coming on, take several slow, deep breaths.

Treatment of Irregular or Missed Periods

While irregular or missed periods are normal during perimenopause or the menopausal transition, women with very heavy bleeding or periods close together may want to talk to a healthcare provider about regulating their periods with one of the following:

- Low-dose birth control pills to regulate menstrual bleeding

- MHT

Treatment of Vaginal Dryness

- A water-based lubricant (not petroleum jelly)

- MHT

Treatment of Sleep Problems

- Be physically active most days of the week during the day.

- Go to bed and get up at the same time each day.

- Set aside time to wind down and relax before bed, whether by reading or taking a warm bath.

- Avoid alcohol or eating a large meal right before bedtime.

- Avoid caffeine after the morning.

- Avoid drinking fluids before bed.

Other FAQs

What Is Menopausal Hormone Therapy (MHT)?

Menopausal hormone therapy (MHT) used to be called hormone replacement therapy (HRT). MHT is an umbrella term for the several different combinations of hormones available in different forms and doses. Some women use MHT to relieve some of the symptoms of menopause, such as hot flashes, night sweats, vaginal dryness, and mood swings. Women who still have their uterus take the hormones estrogen and progesterone, while a woman whose uterus has been removed just needs estrogen.

MHT may be given in the form of a skin patch, vaginal tablet or cream, oral pill, implant, injection (shot), vaginal ring insert, gel, or spray.

If your healthcare provider determines that you are a candidate for MHT, he or she will prescribe the best form and dose to treat your particular symptoms.

What Are the Benefits and Risks of MHT?

MHT can relieve hot flashes, night sweats, vaginal dryness, and mood swings. It also can help prevent bone loss, improve cholesterol levels, and lower the chances of colorectal cancer. But, like all hormones, MHT has side effects. They can include breast tenderness, cramping, bloating, spotting, or a return of regular periods.

In addition, several large research studies found that MHT increases the risk of heart disease, stroke, blood clots, and breast cancer in some women. The risk of dementia in women who start MHT after age 65 also may be elevated.

Women should talk with their healthcare provider to decide if MHT is right for them. If MHT is causing side effects, the healthcare provider may change the type or dosage to decrease the side effects.

Can Herbs or Other Alternative Remedies Help Relieve Symptoms of Menopause?

Some women use herbal supplements or other alternative remedies to relieve symptoms of menopause. Some supplements may relieve symptoms in some women, but more research is needed to prove which ones work and which do not. In some cases, herbal supplements and alternative therapies pose additional risks.

A woman eating a lot of soy or using herbal supplements in an effort to control symptoms should tell her healthcare provider, because these remedies can affect how prescription drugs work. In addition, it is important to keep in mind that herbal supplements are not as closely regulated by the government as prescription drugs.

Some of the commonly discussed nontraditional treatments are listed below.

Phytoestrogens are estrogen-like substances found in some vegetables, legumes (such as soy), herbs, and grains that may relieve some symptoms of menopause. However, this hasn't been proven yet.

Black cohosh has not been proven to reduce hot flashes, but some women say it's helped them. Black cohosh has had a good safety record.

Red clover, which some women claim reduces hot flashes, was not proven in five controlled studies to be effective. However, few side effects and no serious health problems have been reported.

Ginseng may help with menopausal symptoms such as mood swings and sleep disturbances, but it has not been proven effective for hot flashes.

Evening primrose oil appears to have no effect on menopausal symptoms. Side effects include stomach upset and headache.

How Can I Stay Healthy during and after Menopause?

In general, everything that you would otherwise do to stay in good physical shape can help you stay healthy during and after menopause:

- Be physically active most days of the week for at least 60 minutes.

- Eat a low-fat, low-cholesterol diet with a lot of vegetables, fruits, and whole grains

- Get regular checkups.

- Get a flu shot every fall.

- Avoid stress.

Are There Disorders or Conditions Associated with Menopause?

Menopause is associated with a higher risk of other health conditions, but the risks can be minimized by taking appropriate precautions under a healthcare provider's advice.

- Osteoporosis is the thinning of bone tissue and loss of bone density. In menopausal women, estrogen loss is the leading cause of osteoporosis. It can be prevented through regular weight-bearing exercise, the consumption of calcium and vitamin D, the use of bone-strengthening drugs and, possibly, menopause replacement therapy.

- Heart disease can be aggravated or precipitated by the loss of estrogen or by the use of menopausal hormone therapy in women at risk for heart disease. Women who have high blood pressure, cholesterol abnormalities, or a family history of heart disease, or who are overweight, are at a higher risk for heart disease.

- Pelvic floor disorders occur when supportive tissue in the pelvic cavity weakens and organs supported by that tissue fall out of place. As a result, the uterus, bladder, or walls of the vagina can fall into the vaginal opening. Prolapse and other disorders of the pelvic floor can be caused by the lack of estrogen in menopause.

Section 4.6

Effects of Aging on Other Body Parts

This section includes text excerpted from "8 Areas of Age-Related Change," MedlinePlus, National Institutes of Health (NIH), 2007. Reviewed September 2017.

Bones and Joints

The weight-bearing bones and the movable joints take much wear and tear as the body ages. The most common age-related conditions are:

Osteoporosis(OA): Osteoporosis is a disease that weakens bones to the point where they break easily—most often bones in the hip, backbone (spine), and wrist—and most often in women. As people enter their 40s and 50s, bones begin to weaken. The outer shell of the bones also gets thinner.

Arthritis: There are different kinds of arthritis, each with different symptoms and treatments. Arthritis can attack joints in almost any part of the body. Millions of adults and half of all people age 65 and older are troubled by this disease. OA is the most common type of arthritis in older people. OA starts when cartilage begins to become ragged and wears away. At OA's worst, all of the cartilage in a joint wear away, leaving bones that rub against each other. Rheumatoid arthritis (RA) is an autoimmune disease. In RA, that means your body attacks the lining of a joint just as it would if it were trying to protect you from injury or disease. RA leads to inflammation in your joints. This inflammation causes pain, swelling, and stiffness that can last for hours.

Eyes and Ears

About the age of 40, eyesight weakens, and at around 60, cataracts and macular degeneration may develop. Hearing also declines with age.

Sight

Presbyopia is a slow loss of ability to see close objects or small print. It is a normal process that happens as you get older. Holding the newspaper at arm's length is a sign of presbyopia. Reading glasses usually fix the problem.

Cataracts are cloudy areas in the eye's lens causing loss of eyesight. Cataracts often form slowly without any symptoms. Some stay small and don't change eyesight very much. Others may become large or dense and harm vision. Cataract surgery can help. Cataract surgery is safe and is one of the most common surgeries done in the United States.

Glaucoma comes from too much pressure from fluid inside the eye. Over time, the pressure can hurt the optic nerve. This leads to vision loss and blindness. Most people with glaucoma have no early symptoms or pain from the extra pressure. You can protect yourself by having annual eye exams that include dilation of the pupils.

Retinal disorders are a leading cause of blindness in the United States. The most common is age-related macular degeneration (AMD). AMD affects the part of the retina (the macula) that gives you sharp central vision. Photodynamic therapy uses a drug and strong light to slow the progress of AMD. Another treatment uses injections. Ask your eye care professional if you have signs of AMD. Approximately 4.1 million U.S. adults 40 years and older have diabetic retinopathy, a degenerative disease affecting vision. Proper medical care, lifestyle changes, and frequent follow-ups can help reduce this alarming statistic.

Hearing

About one-third of Americans between the ages of 65 and 74 have hearing problems. About half the people who are 85 and older have hearing loss.

Presbycusis is age-related hearing loss. It becomes more common in people as they get older. The decline is slow.

Tinnitus accompanies many forms of hearing loss, including those that sometimes come with aging. People with tinnitus may hear a ringing, roaring, or some other noise inside their ears. Tinnitus may be caused by loud noise, hearing loss, certain medicines, and other health problems, such as allergies and problems in the heart and blood vessels.

Digestive and Metabolic

As we grow older, the prevalence of gastrointestinal problems increases. Gastroesophageal reflux disease, or GERD, occurs when the lower esophageal sphincter (LES) does not close properly and stomach contents leak back, or reflux, into the esophagus. Heartburn that occurs more than twice a week may be considered GERD, and it can eventually lead to more serious health problems. About 40 percent of adults ages 40 to 74—or 41 million people—have prediabetes, a condition that raises a person's risk for developing type 2 diabetes, heart disease, and stroke.

Urogenital

Incontinence: Loss of bladder control is called urinary incontinence. It can happen to anyone, but is very common in older people. At least 1 in 10 people age 65 or older has this problem. Symptoms can range from mild leaking to uncontrollable wetting. Women are more likely than men to have incontinence. Aging alone does not cause incontinence. It can occur for many reasons: Urinary tract infections, vaginal infection or irritation, constipation, and certain medicines can cause bladder control problems that last a short time. In most cases urinary incontinence can be treated and controlled, if not cured. If you are having bladder control problems, don't suffer in silence. Talk to your doctor.

Benign Prostatic Hypertrophy (BPH): The prostate gland surrounds the tube (urethra) that passes urine. This can be a source of problems as a man ages because the prostate tends to grow bigger with age and may squeeze the urethra. A tumor can also make the prostate bigger. These changes, or an infection, can cause problems passing urine. Sometimes men in their 30s and 40s may begin to have these urinary symptoms and need medical attention. For others, symptoms aren't noticed until much later in life.

Prostate Cancer: Prostate cancer is the second most common type of cancer among men in this country. Only skin cancer is more common. Out of every three men who are diagnosed with cancer each year, one is diagnosed with prostate cancer.

Dental—Gingivitis, Periodontitis, Loss of Teeth

Tooth decay is not just a problem for children. It can happen as long as you have natural teeth in your mouth. Tooth decay ruins the enamel that covers and protects your teeth. When you don't take good care of your mouth, bacteria can cling to your teeth and form a sticky, colorless film called dental plaque. This plaque can lead to tooth decay and cavities. Gum disease can also cause your teeth to decay. Fluoride is just as helpful for adults as it is for children. Using a fluoride toothpaste and mouth rinse can help protect your teeth.

Gum diseases (sometimes called periodontal or gingival diseases) are infections that harm the gum and bone that hold teeth in place. When plaque stays on your teeth too long, it forms a hard, harmful covering, called tartar, that brushing doesn't clean. The longer the plaque and tartar stay on your teeth, the more damage they cause. This is called gingivitis. If gingivitis is not treated, over time it can make your gums pull away from your teeth and form pockets that can get infected. This is called periodontitis. If not treated, this infection can ruin the bones, gums, and tissue that support your teeth. In time, it can cause loose teeth that your dentist may have to remove.

Skin

The simplest and cheapest way to keep your skin healthy and young looking is to stay out of the sun. Sunlight is a major cause of the skin changes we think of as aging—changes such as wrinkles, dryness, and age spots. Your skin does change with age. For example, you sweat less, leading to increased dryness. As your skin ages, it becomes thinner and loses fat, so it looks less plump and smooth. It's never too late to protect yourself from the harmful effects of the sun. People who smoke tend to have more wrinkles than nonsmokers of the same age, complexion, and history of sun exposure. It may be because smoking also plays a role in damaging elastin proteins. Facial wrinkling increases with the number of cigarettes and number of years a person has smoked.

- **Dry Skin** affects many older people, particularly on their lower legs, elbows, and forearms. The skin feels rough and scaly and often is accompanied by a distressing, intense itchiness. Low humidity—caused by overheating during the winter and air conditioning during the summer—contributes to dryness and itching. The loss of sweat and oil glands as you age also may worsen dry skin. Anything that further dries your skin—such as overuse of soaps, antiperspirants, perfumes, or hot baths—will make the problem worse. Dehydration, sun exposure, smoking, and stress also may cause dry skin.

- **Skin cancer** is the most common type of cancer in the United States. According to current estimates, 40 to 50 percent of Americans who live to age 65 will have skin cancer at least once. There are three common types of skin cancers. Basal cell carcinomas are the most common, accounting for more than 90 percent of all skin cancers in the United States. They are slow-growing cancers that seldom spread to other parts of the body. Squamous cell carcinomas also rarely spread, but they do so more often than basal cell carcinomas. The most dangerous of all cancers that occur in the skin is melanoma. Melanoma can spread to other organs, and when it does, it often is fatal.

- **Shingles** is a disease that affects nerves and causes pain and blisters in adults. It is caused by the same varicella-zoster virus that causes chickenpox. After you recover from chickenpox, the virus does not leave your body, but continues to live in some nerve cells. For reasons that aren't totally understood, the virus can become active instead of remaining inactive. When it's activated, it produces shingles.

Just like chickenpox, people with shingles will feel sick and have a rash on their body or face. The major difference is that chickenpox is a childhood illness, while shingles targets older people. Most adults live with the virus in their body and never get shingles. But about one in five people who have had chickenpox will get shingles later in life—usually after the age of 50.

Functional Abilities

As we age, falls become an increasingly common reason for injuries. Just ask any of the thousands of older men and women who fall each year and break a bone. Falls can come as a result of other changes in the body: Sight, hearing, muscle strength, coordination, and reflexes aren't what they once were as we age. Balance can be affected by diabetes and heart disease, or by problems with your circulation or nervous system. Some medicines can cause dizziness. Any of these things can make a fall more likely.

The more you take care of your overall health and well-being, the more likely you'll be to lower your chances of falling. Ask your doctor about a special test—called a bone mineral density test—that tells how strong your bones are. If need be, your doctor can prescribe new medications that will help make your bones stronger and harder to break.

Chapter 5

Can You Lengthen Your Life?

Want the secret to living a longer and healthier life? Scientists have found ways to prolong the healthy lifespans of worms, mice, and even monkeys. Their work has revealed exciting new clues about the biology of aging. But solid evidence still shows that the best way to boost the chance of living a long and active life is to follow the advice you likely heard from your parents: eat well, exercise regularly, get plenty of sleep, and stay away from bad habits.

Healthy and Longer Lifespan

People born in the United States today can expect to live to an average age of about 79. A century ago, life expectancy was closer to 54. "We've had a significant increase in lifespan over the last century," says Dr. Marie Bernard, deputy director of National Institutes of Health's (NIH) National Institute on Aging (NIA). "Now if you make it to age 65, the likelihood that you'll make it to 85 is very high. And

This chapter includes text excerpted from the following sources: Text in this chapter begins with excerpts from "Can You Lengthen Your Life?" *NIH News in Health*, National Institutes of Health (NIH), June 2016; Text under the heading "Take Action!" is excerpted from "Protect Your Health as You Grow Older," Office of Disease Prevention and Health Promotion (ODPHP), U.S. Department of Health and Human Services (HHS), March 31, 2017.

if you make it to 85, the likelihood that you'll make it to 92 is very high. So people are living longer, and it's happening across the globe."

Older people tend to be healthier nowadays, too. Research has shown that healthful behaviors can help you stay active and healthy into your 60s, 70s, and beyond. In fact, a long-term study of Seventh-day Adventists—a religious group with a generally healthy lifestyle—shows that they tend to remain healthier into old age. Their life expectancy is nearly 10 years longer on average than most Americans. The Adventists' age-enhancing behaviors include regular exercise, a vegetarian diet, avoiding tobacco and alcohol, and maintaining a healthy weight.

Key to Better Health and Long Life

Exercise and Physical Activity

"If I had to rank behaviors in terms of priority, I'd say that exercise is the most important thing associated with living longer and healthier," says Dr. Luigi Ferrucci, an NIH geriatrician who oversees research on aging and health. "Exercise is especially important for lengthening active life expectancy, which is life without disease, and without physical and mental/thinking disability."

Natural changes to the body as we age can lead to a gradual loss of muscle, reduced energy, and achy joints. These changes may make it tempting to move less and sit more. But doing that can raise your risk for disease, disability, and even death. It's important to work with a doctor to find the types of physical activity that can help you maintain your health and mobility.

Even frail older adults can benefit from regular physical activity. One NIH-funded study included over 600 adults, ages 70 to 89, who were at risk for disability. They were randomly placed in either a moderate exercise program or a comparison group without structured exercise. The exercise group gradually worked up to 150 minutes of weekly activity. This included brisk walking, strength and balance training, and flexibility exercises.

"After more than 2 years, the physical activity group had less disability, and if they became disabled, they were disabled for a shorter time than those in the comparison group," Bernard explains. "The combination of different types of exercise—aerobic, strength and balance training, and flexibility—is important to healthy aging." NIH's Go4Life website has tips to help older adults get and stay active.

Shed Excess Weight

Another sure way to improve your chances for a longer, healthier life is to shed excess weight. "Being obese—with a body mass index (BMI) higher than 30—is a risk factor for early death, and it shortens your active life expectancy," Ferrucci says. BMI is an estimate of your body fat based on your weight and height. Studies in animals have found that certain types of dietary changes—such as extremely low-calorie diets—can lead to longer, healthier lives. These studies offer clues to the biological processes that affect healthy aging. But to date, calorie-restricted diets and other dietary changes have had mixed results in extending the healthy lives of people.

"We have indirect evidence that nutritional adjustments can improve active longevity in people, but this is still an area of intense research," Ferrucci says. "So far, we don't really have solid evidence about caloric restriction and whether it may have a positive effect on human aging." Researchers are now studying potential drugs or other approaches that might mimic benefits of calorie restriction.

Stop Smoking

Not smoking is another pathway to a longer, healthier life. "There's no question that smoking is a hard habit to break. But data suggest that from the moment you stop smoking, there are health benefits. So it's worthwhile making that effort," Bernard says.

Genetic Factors

You might think you need good genes to live longer. But genes are only part of the equation for most of us, says Dr. Thomas Perls, an aging expert and director of the New England Centenarian Study at the Boston University School of Medicine (BUSM). "Research shows that genes account for less than one-third of your chances of surviving to age 85. The vast majority of variation in how old we live to be is due to our health behaviors," Perls says. "Our genes could get most of us close to the remarkable age of 90 if we lead a healthy lifestyle."

The influence of genes is stronger, though, for people who live to older ages, such as beyond 95. Perls has been studying people who live to age 100 and up (centenarians) and their families to learn more about the biological, psychological, and social factors that promote healthy aging.

"It seems there's not a single gene that imparts a strong effect on the ability to get to these older ages," Perls says. "Instead, it's the combined effects of probably hundreds of genes, each with weak effects individually, but having the right combination can lead to a very strong effect, especially for living to the oldest ages we study."

It's a good idea to be skeptical of claims for a quick fix to aging-related problems. Perls cautions against marketed "antiaging" measures such as "hormone replacement therapy," which has little proven benefit for healthy aging and can have severe side effects.

Lead an Active Life

"People used to say, 'the older you get the sicker you get.' But with common sense, healthy habits such as regular exercise, a healthy weight, avoiding red meat, not smoking, and managing stress, it can be 'the older you get, the healthier you've been,'" Perls says.

The key to healthy aging is to engage fully in life—mentally, physically, and socially. "Transitioning to older years isn't about sitting in a rocking chair and letting the days slip by," Bernard says. "Older adults have unique experiences, intellectual capital, and emotional involvement that can be shared with younger generations. This engagement is really key to helping our society move forward."

Take Action!

Keep Your Body Active

Staying active as you get older is one of the best things you can do for your health. Keep in mind that if you haven't been active in the past, it's not too late to start!

- Do moderate aerobic activities—like walking, swimming, or raking leaves. Aim for 2 hours and 30 minutes a week.

- To get the most health benefits, do aerobic activity for at least 10 minutes at a time and then work your way up.

- If it's hard for you to be active for more than 10 minutes at once, do 10 minutes of activity a few times during the day.

It's also important to:

- Do strengthening activities 2 or more days a week.

- Do exercises to help your balance, especially if you are at risk of falling.

Get Ideas for Eating Healthy

Eating healthy is always important, no matter how old you are. It's never too late to make healthy changes to your diet.
Try these tips:

- Choose lots of vegetables and fruits in different colors.
- Make sure most of your grains are whole grains, like brown rice and whole wheat.
- Drink low-fat or fat-free milk, and eat other low-fat dairy products.
- Choose healthy sources of protein like seafood, lean meats and poultry, eggs, beans, and nuts.
- Stay away from trans fats, saturated fats, and added sugars.
- Limit the amount of salt you eat.

If You Smoke, Quit

Quitting smoking is one of the most important things you can do for your health. Call 1-800-QUIT-NOW (1-800-784-8669) for free help with quitting.

Take Steps to Prevent Falls

Older adults are at greater risk for serious injuries from falls. Do these 3 things to lower your risk of falling:

- Do exercises to improve your balance and leg strength.
- Ask your doctor or pharmacist to review your medicines. Some medicines can make you dizzy or sleepy.
- Get your vision checked often. Update your glasses or contact lenses when your vision changes.

Make Sure You Have Smoke Alarms in Your Home

Older people are at a higher risk of home fires. To stay safe, put smoke alarms on every floor of your home.

Use long-life smoke alarms if possible. These alarms use lithium batteries and last longer than regular smoke alarms. They also have a "hush button" so you can stop the alarm quickly if there's a false alarm.

If you use regular smoke alarms, replace the batteries every year. (Tip: Change smoke alarm batteries when you change your clock back from daylight saving time in the fall.)

Follow these other tips on smoke alarms:

- Test your smoke alarms once a month by pushing the test button.

- Put smoke alarms on every floor of your home and near places where people sleep.

- Don't forget to put a smoke alarm in the basement.

- Replace your smoke alarm if it doesn't work when tested or if it's more than 10 years old.

- Dust or vacuum smoke alarms when you change the batteries.

Watch for Changes That May Affect Your Driving

Getting older doesn't make you a bad driver. But changes that come with aging can make it harder for you to drive safely. You may have trouble seeing at night or find it harder to react quickly to avoid an accident.

Take these steps to stay safe:

- Get your vision and hearing checked regularly.

- Always wear your seat belt.

- Never use your phone while driving.

- Plan your route and drive on streets you know.

Keep Your Mind Sharp

Just like physical activity is good for your body, activities that challenge your mind can help prevent memory loss and keep your brain healthy.

As you grow older, it's important to:

- **Learn new things**—take a class or challenge yourself to read a section of the newspaper that you normally skip.

- **Connect with other people**—try sharing meals with a friend or volunteering at a local school.

If you are forgetting things more often than usual and it's getting in the way of doing everyday things, talk with your doctor or nurse.

Get Support If You Are a Caregiver

A caregiver is someone who helps a family member, friend, or neighbor who is sick or has a disability.

Caregiving can be stressful. It's important to get support if you are a caregiver—and be sure to make time to care for yourself, too.

Part Two

Healthy Aging

Chapter 6

Quality of Life

There are many things you can do to help yourself age well: exercise and be physically active, make healthy food choices, and don't smoke. But did you know that participating in activities you enjoy may also help support healthy aging?

As people get older, they often find themselves spending more and more time at home alone. The isolation can lead to depression and is not good for your health. If you find yourself spending a lot of time alone, try adding a volunteer or social activity to your routine.

Benefits of an Active Lifestyle

Engaging in social and productive activities you enjoy, like taking an art class or becoming a volunteer in your community or at your place of worship, may help to maintain your well-being.

Research tells us that older people with an active lifestyle:

- **Are less likely to develop certain diseases.** Participating in hobbies and other social and leisure pursuits may lower risk for developing some health problems, including dementia.

- **Have a longer lifespan.** One study showed that older adults who reported taking part in social activities (such as playing

This chapter includes text excerpted from "Participating in Activities You Enjoy," National Institute on Aging (NIA), National Institutes of Health (NIH), August 21, 2017.

games, belonging to social groups, or traveling) or meaningful, productive activities (such as having a paid or unpaid job, or gardening) lived longer than people who did not. Researchers are further exploring this connection.

- **Are more happy and less depressed.** Studies suggest that older adults who participate in what they believe are meaningful activities, like volunteering in their communities, say they feel happier and more healthy. One study placed older adults from an urban community in their neighborhood public elementary schools to tutor children 15 hours a week. Volunteers reported personal satisfaction from the experience. The researchers found it improved the volunteers' cognitive and physical health, as well as the children's school success. They think it might also have long-term benefits, lowering the older adults' risk of developing disability, dependency, and dementia in later life.

- **Are better prepared to cope with loss.** Studies suggest that volunteering can help with stress and depression from the death of a spouse. Among people who experienced a loss, those who took part in volunteer activities felt more positive about their own abilities (reported greater self-efficacy).

- **May be able to improve their thinking abilities.** Another line of research is exploring how participating in creative arts might help people age well. For example, studies have shown that older adults' memory, comprehension, creativity, and problem-solving abilities improved after an intensive, 4-week (8-session) acting course. Other studies are providing new information about ways that creative activities like music or dance can help older adults.

Activities to Consider

Would you like to get more involved in your community or be more socially active? There are plenty of places to look for opportunities, depending on your interests. Here are some ideas:

Get out and about

- Join a senior center and take part in its events and activities
- Play cards or other games with friends
- Go to the theater, a movie, or a sporting event

- Travel with a group of older adults, such as a retiree group
- Visit friends and family
- Try different restaurants
- Join a group interested in a hobby like knitting, hiking, painting, or wood carving

Learn Something New

- Take a cooking, art, or computer class
- Form or join a book club
- Try yoga, tai chi, or another new physical activity
- Learn (or relearn) how to play a musical instrument

Become More Active in Your Community

- Serve meals or organize clothing donations at a place for homeless people
- Help an organization send care packages to soldiers stationed overseas
- Care for dogs and cats at an animal shelter
- Volunteer to run errands for people with disabilities
- Join a committee or volunteer for an activity at your place of worship
- Volunteer at a school, library, or hospital
- Help with gardening at a community garden or park
- Organize a park clean-up through your local recreation center or community association
- Sing in a community choral group, or play in a local band or orchestra
- Take part in a local theater troupe
- Get a part-time job

Be Physically Active

- Garden or do yard work

- Take an exercise class or do exercises at home
- Go dancing
- Walk or bicycle with a friend or neighbor
- Swim or take a swimming class
- Play with your grandchildren

Find the Right Balance

Everyone has different limits to the amount of time they can spend on social or other activities. What is perfect for one person might be too much for another. Be careful not to take on too much at once. You might start by adding one or two activities to your routine and see how you feel. You can always add more. Remember—participating in activities you enjoy should be fun, not stressful.

Chapter 7

Exercise and Physical Activity

Chapter Contents

Section 7.1

Fit for Life

This section includes text excerpted from "Exercise and Physical
Activity: Getting Fit for Life," National Institute on Aging (NIA),
National Institutes of Health (NIH), August 21, 2017.

Exercise and physical activity are good for you, no matter how old
you are. In fact, staying active can help you:

- Keep and improve your strength so you can stay independent

- Have more energy to do the things you want to do

- Improve your balance

- Prevent or delay some diseases like heart disease, diabetes, and
osteoporosis

- Perk up your mood and reduce depression

You don't need to buy special clothes or belong to a gym to become
more active. Physical activity can and should be part of your everyday
life. Find things you like to do. Go for brisk walks. Ride a bike. Dance.
Work around the house. Garden. Climb stairs. Swim. Rake leaves. Try
different kinds of activities that keep you moving. Look for new ways
to build physical activity into your daily routine.

Four Ways to Be Active

To get all of the benefits of physical activity, try all four types of
exercise:

1. Try to build up to at least 30 minutes of activity that makes
    you breathe hard on most or all days of the week. Every day
    is best. That's called an **endurance** activity because it builds
    your energy or "staying power." You don't have to be active
    for 30 minutes all at once. Ten minutes at a time is fine. How
    hard do you need to push yourself? If you can talk without any
    trouble at all, you are not working hard enough. If you can't
    talk at all, it's too hard.

2. Keep using your muscles. **Strength** exercises build muscles. When you have strong muscles, you can get up from a chair by yourself, you can lift your grandchildren, and you can walk through the park. Keeping your muscles in shape helps prevent falls that cause problems like broken hips. You are less likely to fall when your leg and hip muscles are strong.

3. Do things to help your **balance.** Try standing on one foot, then the other. If you can, don't hold on to anything for support. Get up from a chair without using your hands or arms. Every now and then walk heel-to-toe. As you walk, put the heel of one foot just in front of the toes of your other foot. Your heel and toes should touch or almost touch.

4. Stretching can improve your **flexibility.** Moving more freely will make it easier for you to reach down to tie your shoes or look over your shoulder when you back the car out of your driveway. Stretch when your muscles are warmed up. Don't stretch so far that it hurts.

Who Should Exercise?

Almost anyone, at any age, can do some type of physical activity. You can still exercise even if you have a health condition like heart disease or diabetes. In fact, physical activity may help. For most older adults, brisk walking, riding a bike, swimming, weight lifting, and gardening are safe, especially if you build up slowly. But, check with your doctor if you are over 50 and you aren't used to energetic activity. Other reasons to check with your doctor before you exercise include:

- Any new symptom you haven't discussed with your doctor
- Dizziness or shortness of breath
- Chest pain or pressure or the feeling that your heart is skipping, racing, or fluttering
- Blood clots
- An infection or fever with muscle aches
- Unplanned weight loss
- Foot or ankle sores that won't heal
- Joint swelling
- A bleeding or detached retina, eye surgery, or laser treatment

- A hernia

- Recent hip or back surgery

Safety Tips

Here are some things you can do to make sure you are exercising safely:

- Start slowly, especially if you haven't been active for a long time. Little by little, build up your activities and how hard you work at them.

- Don't hold your breath during strength exercises. That could cause changes in your blood pressure. It may seem strange at first, but you should breathe out as you lift something and breathe in as you relax.

- Use safety equipment. For example, wear a helmet for bike riding or the right shoes for walking or jogging.

- Unless your doctor has asked you to limit fluids, be sure to drink plenty of fluids when you are doing activities. Many older adults don't feel thirsty even if their body needs fluids.

- Always bend forward from the hips, not the waist. If you keep your back straight, you're probably bending the right way. If your back "humps," that's probably wrong.

- Warm-up your muscles before you stretch. Try walking and light arm pumping first.

Exercise should not hurt or make you feel really tired. You might feel some soreness, a little discomfort, or a bit weary, but you should not feel pain. In fact, in many ways, being active will probably make you feel better.

Frequently Asked Questions

What Are the Best Balance Exercises for Seniors?

You can do balance exercises anytime, anywhere. Good balance can help you prevent falls.

I Find It Hard to Make Myself Exercise. What Can I Do?

You're more likely to keep going if you choose exercises you enjoy. Also, many people find that having a firm goal in mind motivates them to move ahead.

I Have Arthritis. What Workout Routines Are Safe for Me?

Exercise is safe for almost everyone. You can exercise even if you have a long-term condition, like heart disease, diabetes, or arthritis.

Section 7.2

Exercise Basics for Seniors

This section includes text excerpted from "How Much Physical Activity Do Older Adults Need?" Centers for Disease Control and Prevention (CDC), June 4, 2015.

As an older adult, regular physical activity is one of the most important things you can do for your health. It can prevent many of the health problems that seem to come with age. It also helps your muscles grow stronger so you can keep doing your day-to-day activities without becoming dependent on others.

Not doing any physical activity can be bad for you, no matter your age or health condition. Keep in mind, some physical activity is better than none at all. Your health benefits will also increase with the more physical activity that you do.

If you're 65 years of age or older, are generally fit, and have no limiting health conditions you can follow the guidelines listed below.

For Important Health Benefits

Older adults need at least:

- 2 hours and 30 minutes (150 minutes) of moderate-intensity aerobic activity (i.e., brisk walking) every week **and**

- muscle-strengthening activities on 2 or more days a week that work all major muscle groups (legs, hips, back, abdomen, chest, shoulders, and arms).

OR

- 1 hour and 15 minutes (75 minutes) of vigorous-intensity aerobic activity (i.e., jogging or running) every week **and**

- muscle-strengthening activities on 2 or more days a week that work all major muscle groups (legs, hips, back, abdomen, chest, shoulders, and arms).

OR

- An equivalent mix of moderate- and vigorous-intensity aerobic activity **and**

- muscle-strengthening activities on 2 or more days a week that work all major muscle groups (legs, hips, back, abdomen, chest, shoulders, and arms).

For Even Greater Health Benefits

Older adults should increase their activity to:

- 5 hours (300 minutes) each week of moderate-intensity aerobic activity **and**

- muscle-strengthening activities on 2 or more days a week that work all major muscle groups (legs, hips, back, abdomen, chest, shoulders, and arms).

OR

- 2 hours and 30 minutes (150 minutes) each week of vigorous-intensity aerobic activity **and**

- muscle-strengthening activities on 2 or more days a week that work all major muscle groups (legs, hips, back, abdomen, chest, shoulders, and arms).

OR

- An equivalent mix of moderate- and vigorous-intensity aerobic activity **and**

- muscle-strengthening activities on 2 or more days a week that work all major muscle groups (legs, hips, back, abdomen, chest, shoulders, and arms).

Aerobic Activity—What Counts?

Aerobic activity or "cardio" gets you breathing harder and your heart beating faster. From pushing a lawn mower, to taking a dance class, to biking to the store—ll types of activities count. As long as you're doing them at a moderate or vigorous intensity for **at least 10 minutes at a time.** Even something as simple as walking is a great way to get the aerobic activity you need, as long as it's at a moderately intense pace.

Intensity is how hard your body is working during aerobic activity.

How Do You Know If You're Doing Moderate or Vigorous Aerobic Activity?

On a 10-point scale, where sitting is 0 and working as hard as you can is 10, **moderate-intensity aerobic activity is a 5 or 6**. It will make you breathe harder and your heart beat faster. You'll also notice that you'll be able to talk, but not sing the words to your favorite song.

Vigorous-intensity activity is a 7 or 8 on this scale. Your heart rate will increase quite a bit and you'll be breathing hard enough so that you won't be able to say more than a few words without stopping to catch your breath.

You can do moderate- or vigorous-intensity aerobic activity, or a mix of the two each week. Intensity is how hard your body is working during aerobic activity. A rule of thumb is that **1 minute of vigorous-intensity activity is about the same as 2 minutes of moderate-intensity activity.**

Everyone's fitness level is different. This means that walking may feel like a moderately intense activity to you, but for others, it may feel vigorous. It all depends on you—the shape you're in, what you feel comfortable doing, and your health condition. What's important is that you do physical activities that are right for you and your abilities.

Muscle-Strengthening Activities—What Counts?

Besides aerobic activity, you need to do things to make your muscles stronger at least 2 days a week. These types of activities will help keep you from losing muscle as you get older.

To gain health benefits, muscle-strengthening activities need to be done to the point where it's hard for you to do another repetition without help. A **repetition** is one complete movement of an activity, like lifting a weight or doing one sit-up. Try to do 8–12 repetitions per activity that count as **1 set**. Try to do at least 1 set of muscle-strengthening activities, but to gain even more benefits, do 2 or 3 sets.

There are many ways you can strengthen your muscles, whether it's at home or the gym. The activities you choose should work all the major muscle groups of your body (legs, hips, back, chest, abdomen, shoulders, and arms). You may want to try:

- Lifting weights

- Working with resistance bands

- Doing exercises that use your body weight for resistance (push ups, sit ups)

- Heavy gardening (digging, shoveling)

- Yoga

Section 7.3

Activities for Older Adults

This section includes text excerpted from "Making Physical Activity a Part of an Older Adult's Life," Centers for Disease Control and Prevention (CDC), November 9, 2011. Reviewed September 2017.

When it comes to getting the physical activity you need each week, it's important to pick activities you enjoy and that match your abilities. This will help ensure that you stick with them.

Things to Keep in Mind

- Try to do a variety of activities. This can make physical activity more enjoyable and reduce your risk of injury.

- Regular physical activity is still safe and beneficial even if you have problems doing normal daily activities, such as climbing stairs or walking.

- If you have to take a break from your regular workout routine due to an illness such as the flu, be sure to start again at a lower level and slowly work back up to your usual level of activity.

- To get to and stay at a healthy weight, start by doing the equivalent of 150 minutes of moderate- intensity aerobic activity each week. Keep in mind that you may need to do more activity or reduce the number of calories you eat to get to your desired weight.

Improving Your Balance

Are you at risk for falling because you've fallen in the past or have trouble walking? Older adults who are at risk for falling should do exercises that help them with balance. Try to do balance training on at least 3 days a week and do standardized exercises from a program that's been proven to reduce falls. These exercises might include backward walking, sideways walking, heel walking, toe walking, and practicing standing from a sitting position. Tai chi, a form of martial arts developed in China, may also help with balance.

What If You Have a Chronic Condition?

If you have a health condition such as arthritis, diabetes, or heart disease it doesn't mean you can't be active. In fact, it's just the opposite. Regular physical activity can improve your quality of life and even reduce your risk of developing other conditions.

Talk with your doctor to find out if your health condition limits, in any way, your ability to be active. Then, work with your doctor to come up with a physical activity plan that matches your abilities. If your condition stops you from meeting the minimum *Guidelines* (*2008 Physical Activity Guidelines for Americans*), try to do as much as you can. What's important is that you avoid being inactive. Even 60 minutes a week of moderate-intensity aerobic activity is good for you.

What If You Have a Disability?

If you are an older adult with a disability, regular physical activity can provide you with important health benefits, like a stronger heart, lungs and muscles, improved mental health and a better ability to do everyday tasks. It's best to talk with your healthcare provider before you begin a physical activity routine. Try to get advice from a professional with experience in physical activity and disability. They can tell you more about the amounts and types of physical activity that are appropriate for you and your abilities.

When to Check with Your Doctor

Doing activity that requires moderate effort is safe for most people, but if you have a health condition such as heart disease, arthritis, or diabetes be sure to talk with your doctor about the types and amounts of physical activity that are right for you.

Chapter 8

Sleep

Getting enough sleep helps you stay healthy and alert. But, many older people don't sleep well. If you're always sleepy or you find it hard to get enough sleep at night, it may be time to see a doctor. Waking up every day feeling tired is a sign that you are not getting the rest you need.

Sleep and Aging

Older adults need about the same amount of sleep as all adults—7 to 9 hours each night. But, older people tend to go to sleep earlier and get up earlier than they did when they were younger.

There are many reasons why older people may not get enough sleep at night. Feeling sick or being in pain can make it hard to sleep. Some medicines can keep you awake. No matter the reason, if you don't get a good night's sleep, the next day you may:

- Be irritable

- Have memory problems or be forgetful

- Feel depressed

- Have more falls or accidents

This chapter includes text excerpted from "A Good Night's Sleep," National Institute on Aging (NIA), National Institutes of Health (NIH), July 14, 2017.

Get a Good Night's Sleep

Being older doesn't mean you have to be tired all the time. You can do many things to help you get a good night's sleep. Here are some ideas:

- **Follow a regular sleep schedule.** Go to sleep and get up at the same time each day, even on weekends or when you are traveling.

- **Avoid napping in the late afternoon or evening,** if you can. Naps may keep you awake at night.

- **Develop a bedtime routine.** Take time to relax before bedtime each night. Some people read a book, listen to soothing music, or soak in a warm bath.

- **Try not to watch television or use your computer, cell phone, or tablet in the bedroom.** The light from these devices may make it difficult for you to fall asleep. And alarming or unsettling shows or movies, like horror movies, may keep you awake.

- **Keep your bedroom at a comfortable temperature,** not too hot or too cold, and as quiet as possible.

- **Use low lighting in the evenings** and as you prepare for bed.

- **Exercise at regular times each day** but not within 3 hours of your bedtime.

- **Avoid eating large meals close to bedtime**—they can keep you awake.

- **Stay away from caffeine late in the day.** Caffeine (found in coffee, tea, soda, and chocolate) can keep you awake.

- **Remember—alcohol won't help you sleep.** Even small amounts make it harder to stay asleep.

Insomnia Is Common in Older Adults

Insomnia is the most common sleep problem in adults age 60 and older. People with this condition have trouble falling asleep and staying asleep. Insomnia can last for days, months, and even years. Having trouble sleeping can mean you:

- Take a long time to fall asleep

- Wake up many times in the night
- Wake up early and are unable to get back to sleep
- Wake up tired
- Feel very sleepy during the day

Often, being unable to sleep becomes a habit. Some people worry about not sleeping even before they get into bed. This may make it harder to fall asleep and stay asleep.

Some older adults who have trouble sleeping may use over-the-counter sleep aids. Others may use prescription medicines to help them sleep. These medicines may help when used for a short time. But remember, medicines aren't a cure for insomnia. Developing healthy habits at bedtime may help you get a good night's sleep.

Sleep Apnea

People with sleep apnea have short pauses in breathing while they are asleep. These pauses may happen many times during the night. If not treated, sleep apnea can lead to other problems, such as high blood pressure, stroke, or memory loss.

You can have sleep apnea and not even know it. Feeling sleepy during the day and being told you are snoring loudly at night could be signs that you have sleep apnea. If you think you have sleep apnea, see a doctor who can treat this sleep problem. You may need to learn to sleep in a position that keeps your airways open. Treatment using a continuous positive airway pressure (CPAP) device almost always helps people with sleep apnea. A dental device or surgery may also help.

Movement Disorders and Sleep

Restless legs syndrome, periodic limb movement disorder, and rapid eye movement sleep behavior disorder are common in older adults. These movement disorders can rob you of needed sleep.

People with restless legs syndrome, or RLS, feel like there is tingling, crawling, or pins and needles in one or both legs. This feeling is worse at night. See your doctor for more information about medicines to treat RLS.

Periodic limb movement disorder, or PLMD, causes people to jerk and kick their legs every 20 to 40 seconds during sleep. Medication, warm baths, exercise, and relaxation exercises can help.

Rapid eye movement, or REM, sleep behavior disorder is another condition that may make it harder to get a good night's sleep. During normal REM sleep, your muscles cannot move, so your body stays still. But, if you have REM sleep behavior disorder, your muscles can move and your sleep is disrupted.

Alzheimer Disease and Sleep—a Special Problem

Alzheimer disease often changes a person's sleeping habits. Some people with Alzheimer disease sleep too much; others don't sleep enough. Some people wake up many times during the night; others wander or yell at night. The person with Alzheimer disease isn't the only one who loses sleep. Caregivers may have sleepless nights, leaving them tired for the challenges they face.

If you're caring for someone with Alzheimer disease, take these steps to make him or her safer and help you sleep better at night:

- Make sure the floor is clear of objects.
- Lock up any medicines.
- Attach grab bars in the bathroom.
- Place a gate across the stairs.

Safe Sleep for Older Adults

Try to set up a safe and restful place to sleep. Make sure you have smoke alarms on each floor of your home. Before going to bed, lock all windows and doors that lead outside. Other ideas for a safe night's sleep are:

- Keep a telephone with emergency phone numbers by your bed.
- Have a lamp within reach that is easy to turn on.
- Put a glass of water next to the bed in case you wake up thirsty.
- Don't smoke, especially in bed.
- Remove area rugs so you won't trip if you get out of bed during the night.

Tips to Help You Fall Asleep

You may have heard about some tricks to help you fall asleep. You don't really have to count sheep—you could try counting slowly to 100.

Some people find that playing mental games makes them sleepy. For example, tell yourself it is 5 minutes before you have to get up, and you're just trying to get a little bit more sleep.

Some people find that relaxing their bodies puts them to sleep. One way to do this is to imagine your toes are completely relaxed, then your feet, and then your ankles are completely relaxed. Work your way up the rest of your body, section by section. You may drift off to sleep before getting to the top of your head.

Use your bedroom only for sleeping. After turning off the light, give yourself about 20 minutes to fall asleep. If you're still awake and not drowsy, get out of bed. When you feel sleepy, go back to bed. If you feel tired and unable to do your activities for more than 2 or 3 weeks, you may have a sleep problem. Talk with your doctor about changes you can make to get a better night's sleep.

Chapter 9

Skin Care and Aging

Your skin changes with age. It becomes thinner, loses fat, and no longer looks as plump and smooth as it once did. Your veins and bones can be seen more easily. Scratches, cuts, or bumps can take longer to heal. Years of sun tanning or being out in the sunlight for a long time may lead to wrinkles, dryness, age spots, and even cancer. But, there are things you can do to protect your skin and to make it feel and look better.

Dry Skin and Itching[1]

Many older people suffer from dry spots on their skin, often on their lower legs, elbows, and lower arms. Dry skin patches feel rough and scaly. There are many possible reasons for dry skin, such as:

- Not drinking enough liquids
- Spending too much time in the sun or sun tanning
- Being in very dry air
- Smoking
- Feeling stress

This chapter includes text excerpted from documents published by two public domain sources. Text under heading marked 1 is excerpted from "Skin Care and Aging," National Institute on Aging (NIA), National Institutes of Health (NIH), August 21, 2017; Text under heading marked 2 is excerpted from "Skin Infections," MedlinePlus, National Institutes of Health (NIH), January 2, 2017.

- Losing sweat and oil glands, which is common with age

Dry skin also can be caused by health problems, such as diabetes or kidney disease. Using too much soap, antiperspirant, or perfume, and taking hot baths can make dry skin worse.

Some medicines can make skin itchy. Because older people have thinner skin, scratching can cause bleeding that may lead to infection. Here are some ways to help dry, itchy skin:

- Use moisturizers, like lotions, creams, or ointments, every day.

- Take fewer baths and use milder soap. Warm water is less drying than hot water. Don't add bath oil to your water. It can make the tub too slippery.

- Try using a humidifier, an appliance that adds moisture to a room.

Bruises[1]

Older people may bruise more easily than younger people. It can take longer for these bruises to heal. Some medicines or illnesses may also cause bruising. Talk to your doctor if you see bruises and don't know how you got them, especially on parts of your body usually covered by clothing.

Wrinkles[1]

Over time, skin begins to wrinkle. Things in the environment, like ultraviolet (UV) light from the sun, can make the skin less elastic. Gravity can cause skin to sag and wrinkle. Certain habits, like smoking, also can wrinkle the skin.

A lot of claims are made about how to make wrinkles go away. Many of them don't work. Some methods can be painful or even dangerous, and many must be done by a doctor. Talk with a doctor specially trained in skin problems, called a dermatologist, or your regular doctor if you are worried about wrinkles.

Age Spots and Skin Tags[1]

Age spots, once called "liver spots," are flat, brown spots often caused by years in the sun. They are bigger than freckles and commonly show up on areas like the face, hands, arms, back, and feet. Using a broad-spectrum sunscreen that helps protect against two types of the sun's rays may prevent more age spots.

Skin tags are small, usually flesh-colored growths of skin that have a raised surface. They become common as people age, especially for women. They are most often found on the eyelids, neck, and body folds such as the armpit, chest, and groin.

Age spots and skin tags are harmless, although sometimes skin tags can become irritated. If your age spots or skin tags bother you, talk to your doctor about having them removed.

Skin Cancer[1]

Skin cancer is a very common type of cancer in the United States. The main cause of skin cancer is the sun. Sunlamps and tanning booths can also cause skin cancer. Anyone, of any skin color, can get skin cancer. People with fair skin that freckles easily are at greatest risk. Skin cancer may be cured if it is found before it spreads to other parts of the body.

There are three types of skin cancers. Two types, basal cell carcinoma and squamous cell carcinoma, grow slowly and rarely spread to other parts of the body. These types of cancer are found mostly on parts of the skin exposed to the sun, like the head, face, neck, hands, and arms. But they can happen anywhere on your body. The third and most dangerous type of skin cancer is melanoma. It is rarer than the other types, but it can spread to other organs and be deadly.

Check your skin once a month for things that may be cancer. Skin cancer is rarely painful. Look for changes such as a new growth, a sore that doesn't heal, or a bleeding mole.

Check Moles, Birthmarks, or Other Parts of the Skin for the "ABCDE's"[1]

A = **A**symmetry (one half of the growth looks different from the other half)

B = **B**orders that are irregular

C = **C**olor changes or more than one color

D = **D**iameter greater than the size of a pencil eraser

E = **E**volving; this means the growth changes in size, shape, symptoms (itching, tenderness), surface (especially bleeding), or shades of color

See your doctor right away if you have any of these signs to make sure it is not skin cancer.

91

Common Skin Infections[1]

Your skin helps protect you from germs, but sometimes it can get infected by them. Some common types of skin infections are:

- Bacterial: Cellulitis and impetigo. Staphylococcal infections can also affect the skin
- Viral: Shingles, warts, and herpes simplex
- Fungal: Athlete's foot and yeast infections
- Parasitic: Body lice, head lice, and scabies

Treatment of skin infections depends on the cause.

Keep Your Skin Healthy[1]

Some sun can be good for you, but to keep your skin healthy, be careful:

- **Limit time in the sun.** It's okay to go out during the day, but try to avoid being in sun during peak times when the sun's rays are strongest. For example, during the summer try to stay out of the sun between 10 a.m. and 4 p.m. Don't be fooled by cloudy skies. The sun's rays can go through clouds. You can also get sunburned if you are in water, so be careful when you are in a pool, lake, or the ocean.

- **Use sunscreen.** Look for sunscreen with an SPF (sun protection factor) number of 30 or higher. It's best to choose sunscreens with "broad spectrum" on the label. Put the sunscreen on 15 to 30 minutes before you go outside. Sunscreen should be reapplied at least every 2 hours. You need to put sunscreen on more often if you are swimming, sweating, or rubbing your skin with a towel.

- **Wear protective clothing.** A hat with a wide brim can shade your neck, ears, eyes, and head. Look for sunglasses that block 99 to 100 percent of the sun's rays. If you have to be in the sun, wear loose, lightweight, long-sleeved shirts and long pants or long skirts.

- **Avoid tanning.** Don't use sunlamps or tanning beds. Tanning pills are not approved by the U.S. Food and Drug Administration (FDA) and might not be safe.

Your skin may change with age. But remember, there are things you can do to help. Check your skin often. If you find any changes that worry you, see your doctor.

Chapter 10

Nutrition and Aging

Chapter Contents

Section 10.1

Smell and Taste: Spice of Life

This section includes text excerpted from "How Smell and Taste Change as You Age," National Institute of Aging (NIA), National Institutes of Health (NIH), August 21, 2017.

Did you know that your sense of smell and taste are connected? As you get older, these senses can change, and you may find that certain foods aren't as flavorful as they used to be. Changes in smell or taste can also be a sign of a larger problem.

Your Sense of Smell

Smell is an important sense. Certain smells, like your dad's cologne, can help you recall a memory. Other smells, like smoke from a fire, can alert you to danger. When you can't smell things you enjoy, like your morning coffee or spring flowers, life may seem dull.

As you get older, your sense of smell may fade. Your sense of smell is closely related to your sense of taste. When you can't smell, food may taste bland. You may even lose interest in eating.

What Causes Loss of Smell?

Many problems cause a loss of smell that lasts for a short time. This temporary loss of smell may be due to:

- **A cold or flu that causes a stuffy nose.** The ability to smell will come back when you're better.

- **Allergies.** Try to stay away from things you're allergic to, like pollen and pets. Talk to your doctor about how to manage your allergies.

- **A harmless growth (called a polyp) in the nose or sinuses that gives you a runny nose.** Having the growth removed may help.

- **Some medications like antibiotics or blood pressure medicine.** Ask your doctor if there is another medicine you can take.

- **Radiation, chemotherapy, and other cancer treatments.**
Your sense of smell may return when treatment stops.

Some things can cause a long-lasting loss of smell. A head injury, for example, can damage the nerves related to smell.

Sometimes, losing your sense of smell may be a sign of a more serious disorder, such as Parkinson disease or Alzheimer disease. Be sure to tell your doctor about any change in your sense of smell.

Smells Can Keep You Safe

It's important to be aware of odors around you. You need to be able to smell:

- **Smoke**—check your smoke detectors once a year to make sure they work.

- **Gas leaks**—make sure you have a gas detector in your home.

- **Spoiled food**—throw out food that's been in the refrigerator too long.

- **Household chemicals**—make sure there is fresh air where you live and work.

Your Sense of Taste

There are tiny taste buds inside your mouth—on your tongue, in your throat, even on the roof of your mouth. What we call "flavor" is based on five basic tastes: sweet, salty, bitter, sour, and savory. Along with how it tastes, how food smells is also part of what makes up its flavor.

When food tastes bland, many people try to improve the flavor by adding more salt or sugar. This may not be healthy for older people, especially if you have medical problems like high blood pressure or diabetes (high blood sugar).

People who have lost some of their sense of taste may not eat the foods they need to stay healthy. This can lead to other issues such as:

- Weight loss

- Malnutrition (not getting the calories, protein, carbohydrates, vitamins, and minerals you need from the food)

- Social isolation

- Depression

Eating food that is good for you is important to your health. If you have a problem with how food tastes, be sure to talk with your doctor.

What Causes Loss of Taste?

Many things can cause you to lose your sense of taste. Most of the time there are ways to help with the problem.

Medications, like antibiotics and pills to lower cholesterol and blood pressure, can sometimes change how food tastes. Some medicines can make your mouth dry. Having a dry mouth can cause food to taste funny and also make it hard to swallow. Talk to your doctor if you think a medicine is affecting your sense of taste. There may be different medicines that you can try. Do not stop taking your medicine.

Gum disease, an infection in your mouth, or issues with your dentures can leave a bad taste in your mouth that changes the way food tastes. Brushing your teeth, flossing, and using mouthwash can help prevent these problems. Talk to your dentist if you have a bad taste in your mouth that won't go away.

Alcohol can alter how food tastes. Cutting back or stopping drinking may help. Smoking can also reduce your sense of taste. Quitting may help.

Cancer Treatments and Taste

People who are having cancer treatments might have a problem with taste. Your sense of taste will often return once treatments stop.

Cancer treatments can make food taste bad or "off." Some say that food tastes metallic. This funny taste may keep some people from eating healthy food. If this happens to you, try to:

- Eat four or five small meals during the day instead of three large meals.

- Eat cold food, including yogurt, pudding, and gelatin dessert. Cold food may taste better than hot food.

- Eat fresh, uncooked vegetables. Cooked vegetables can have strong odors that may not be appealing.

- Drink lots of fluids, including water, weak tea, juice, and ginger ale.

- Test new foods to find ones you like.

- Brush your teeth before and after eating.

- Use plastic forks and spoons if food tastes metallic.

Colors and Spices Can Help

If you're having trouble smelling and tasting your food, try adding color and texture to make your food more interesting. For example, try eating brightly colored vegetables like carrots, sweet potatoes, broccoli, and tomatoes. Also, if your diet allows, flavor your food with a little butter, olive oil, cheese, nuts, or fresh herbs like sage, thyme, or rosemary. To put some zing in your food, add mustard, hot pepper, onions, garlic, ginger, different spices, or lemon or lime juice. Choose foods that look good to you.

Special Doctor for Smell and Taste, an Otolaryngologist

If the foods you enjoy don't smell or taste the way you think they should, talk to your doctor. He or she might suggest you see a specialist who treats people with smell and taste problems. This kind of doctor is called an otolaryngologist, also known as an ENT (which stands for ear, nose, and throat). An otolaryngologist works on problems related to the ear, nose, and throat, as well as the larynx (voice box), mouth, and parts of the neck and face. The doctor may ask:

- Can you smell anything at all?
- Can you taste any food?
- When did you first notice the problem?
- Is the problem getting worse?
- Have you been told that you have allergies or chronic sinus problems?
- What medicines do you take?

There are likely ways to help fix the problem. If not, the doctor can help you cope with the changes in smell and taste.

Section 10.2

Choosing Healthy Meals as You Get Older

This section includes text excerpted "Choosing Healthy
Meals as You Get Older," National Institute on Aging (NIA),
National Institutes of Health (NIH), July 23, 2017.

Choosing Healthy Meals as You Get Older: 10 Healthy Eating Tips for People Age 65+

Making healthy food choices is a smart thing to do—no matter how old you are! Your body changes through your 60s, 70s, 80s, and beyond. Food provides nutrients you need as you age. Use these tips to choose foods for better health at each stage of life.

1. **Drink plenty of liquids.** With age, you may lose some of your sense of thirst. Drink water often. Low-fat or fat-free milk or 100 percent juice also helps you stay hydrated. Limit beverages that have lots of added sugars or salt. Learn which liquids are better choices.

2. **Make eating a social event.** Meals are more enjoyable when you eat with others. Invite a friend to join you or take part in a potluck at least twice a week. A senior center or place of worship may offer meals that are shared with others. There are many ways to make mealtimes pleasing.

3. **Plan healthy meals.** Find trusted nutrition information from ChooseMyPlate.gov and the National Institute on Aging (NIA). Get advice on what to eat, how much to eat, and which foods to choose, all based on the *Dietary Guidelines for Americans*. Find sensible, flexible ways to choose, and prepare tasty meals so you can eat foods you need.

4. **Know how much to eat.** Learn to recognize how much to eat so you can control portion size. My Plate's SuperTracker (www.supertracker.usda.gov) shows amounts of food you need. When eating out, pack part of your meal to eat later. One restaurant dish might be enough for two meals or more.

5   **Vary your vegetables.** Include a variety of different colored vegetables to brighten your plate. Most vegetables are a low-calorie source of nutrients. Vegetables are also a good source of fiber.

6.   **Eat for your teeth and gums.** Many people find that their teeth and gums change as they age. People with dental problems sometimes find it hard to chew fruits, vegetables, or meats. Don't miss out on needed nutrients! Eating softer foods can help. Try cooked or canned foods like unsweetened fruit, low-sodium soups, or canned tuna.

7.   **Use herbs and spices.** Foods may seem to lose their flavor as you age. If favorite dishes taste different, it may not be the cook! Maybe your sense of smell, sense of taste, or both have changed. Medicines may also change how foods taste. Add flavor to your meals with herbs and spices.

8.   **Keep food safe.** Don't take a chance with your health. A food-related illness can be life threatening for an older person. Throw out food that might not be safe. Avoid certain foods that are always risky for an older person, such as unpasteurized dairy foods. Other foods can be harmful to you when they are raw or undercooked, such as eggs, sprouts, fish, shellfish, meat, or poultry.

9.   **Read the nutrition facts label.** Make the right choices when buying food. Pay attention to important nutrients to know as well as calories, fats, sodium, and the rest of the Nutrition Facts label. Ask your doctor if there are ingredients and nutrients you might need to limit or to increase.

10. **Ask your doctor about vitamins or supplements.** Food is the best way to get nutrients you need. Should you take vitamins or other pills or powders with herbs and minerals? These are called dietary supplements. Your doctor will know if you need them. More may not be better. Some can interfere with your medicines or affect your medical conditions.

HARPER COLLEGE LIBRARY
PALATINE, ILLINOIS 60067

Section 10.3

Healthy Eating after 50

This section includes text excerpted from "Healthy Eating—Smart
Food Choices for Healthy Aging," National Institute on Aging (NIA),
National Institutes of Health (NIH), July 23, 2017.

Smart Food Choices for Healthy Aging

If you and your healthcare provider are worried about weight gain,
you should choose nutrient-dense foods. These foods give you lots of
nutrients without a lot of extra calories.

On the other hand, foods that are high in calories for the amount
of food are called calorie dense. They may or may not have nutrients.
High-calorie foods with little nutritional value, like potato chips, sug-
ar-sweetened drinks, candy, baked goods, and alcoholic beverages, are
sometimes called "empty calories."

One way to think about the idea of nutrient-dense and calorie-dense
foods is to look at a variety of foods that all provide the same calories.
Let's say that you wanted to have a snack that contained about 100
calories. You might choose one of these:

- 7- or 8-inch banana
- two ounces baked chicken breast with no skin
- three cups low-fat popcorn
- two regular chocolate-sandwich cookies
- half cup low-fat ice cream
- one scrambled large egg cooked with fat
- 20 peanuts
- half of the average-size candy bar

Which would make a better snack for you? Although these examples
all have about 100 calories, there are some big differences:

- banana, chicken, peanuts, or egg are more nutrient dense

100

- popcorn or chicken are likely to help you feel more satisfied
- chicken, peanuts, or egg have more protein
- cookies, candy, and ice cream have more added sugars

How Many Calories Do You Need?

If you are over age 50 and you want to stay at the weight you are now—not lose and not gain, how many calories do you need to eat each day? The *Dietary Guidelines* suggest:

Table 10.1. Calorie Chart

Not physically Active	Moderately Active	Active Lifestyle
	For a woman	
1,600 calories	1,800 calories	2,000–2,200 calories
	For a man	
2,000–2,200 calories	2,200–2,400 calories	2,400–2800 calories

Physical activity refers to the voluntary movements you do that burn calories. Brisk walking, dancing, and swimming are examples of moderate activity. An active lifestyle might include jogging, singles tennis, or swimming laps.

Section 10.4

Dietary Supplements

This section includes text excerpted from "Dietary Supplements," National Institute on Aging (NIA), National Institutes of Health (NIH), August 21, 2017.

What Is a Dietary Supplement?

Dietary supplements are substances you might use to add nutrients to your diet or to lower your risk of health problems, like osteoporosis or arthritis. Dietary supplements come in the form of pills, capsules, powders, gel tabs, extracts, or liquids. They might contain vitamins, minerals, fiber, amino acids, herbs or other plants, or enzymes. Sometimes, the ingredients in dietary supplements are added to foods, including drinks. A doctor's prescription is not needed to buy dietary supplements.

Should I Take a Dietary Supplement?

Do you need one? Maybe you do, but usually not. Ask yourself why you think you might want to take a dietary supplement. Are you concerned about getting enough nutrients? Is a friend, a neighbor, or someone on a commercial suggesting you take one? Some ads for dietary supplements in magazines or on TV seem to promise that these supplements will make you feel better, keep you from getting sick, or even help you live longer. Sometimes, there is little, if any, good scientific research supporting these claims. Dietary supplements may give you nutrients that might be missing from your daily diet. But eating a variety of healthy foods is the best way to get the nutrients you need. Supplements may cost a lot, could be harmful, or simply might not be helpful. Some supplements can change how medicines you may already be taking will work. You should talk to your doctor or a registered dietitian for advice.

What If I'm over 50?

People over 50 may need more of some vitamins and minerals than younger adults do. Your doctor or a dietitian can tell you whether you need to change your diet or take vitamins or minerals to get enough of these:

- **Vitamin B12.** Vitamin B12 helps keep your red blood cells and nerves healthy. Vitamin B12 is mainly found in fish, shellfish, meat, and dairy products. As people grow older, some have trouble absorbing vitamin B12 naturally found in food. They can choose foods, like fortified cereals, that have this vitamin added or use a B12 supplement.

- **Calcium.** Calcium works with vitamin D to keep bones strong at all ages. Bone loss can lead to fractures in both older women and men. Calcium is found in milk and milk products (fat-free or low-fat is best), canned fish with soft bones, dark-green leafy vegetables like kale, and foods with calcium added like breakfast cereals.

- **Vitamin D.** Some people's bodies make enough vitamin D if they are in the sun for 10 to 15 minutes at least twice a week. But, if you are older, you may not be able to get enough vitamin D that way. Try adding vitamin D-fortified milk and milk products, vitamin D-fortified cereals, and fatty fish to your diet, and/or use a vitamin D supplement.

- **Vitamin B6.** This vitamin is needed to form red blood cells. It is found in potatoes, bananas, chicken breasts, and fortified cereals.

Different Vitamin and Mineral Recommendations for People over 50

The National Academy of Sciences (NAS) recommends how much of each vitamin and mineral men and women of different ages need. Sometimes, the Academy also tells us how much of a vitamin or mineral is too much.

- **Vitamin B12**—2.4 mcg (micrograms) each day (if you are taking medicine for acid reflux, you might need a different form, which your healthcare provider can give you)

- **Calcium**—Women over 50 need 1,200 mg (milligrams) each day, and men need 1,000 mg between age 51 and 70, and 1,200 mg after 70, but not more than 2,000 mg a day.

- **Vitamin D**—600 IU (International Units) for people age 51 to 70 and 800 IU for those over 70, but not more than 4,000 IU each day

- **Vitamin B6**—1.7 mg for men and 1.5 mg for women each day

When thinking about whether you need more of a vitamin or mineral, think about how much of each nutrient you get from food and drinks, as well as from any supplements you take. Check with a doctor or dietitian to learn whether you need to supplement your diet.

What Are Antioxidants?

You might hear about antioxidants in the news. These are natural substances found in food that might help protect you from some diseases. Here are some common sources of antioxidants that you should be sure to include in your diet:

- **Beta-carotene**—fruits and vegetables that are either dark green or dark orange
- **Selenium**—seafood, liver, meat, and grains
- **Vitamin C**—citrus fruits, peppers, tomatoes, and berries
- **Vitamin E**—wheat germ, nuts, sesame seeds, and canola, olive, and peanut oils.

Right now, research results suggest that large doses of supplements with antioxidants will not prevent chronic diseases such as heart disease or diabetes. In fact, some studies have shown that taking large doses of some antioxidants could be harmful. Again, it is best to check with your doctor before taking a dietary supplement.

What about Herbal Supplements?

Herbal supplements are dietary supplements that come from plants. A few that you may have heard of are gingko biloba, ginseng, echinacea, and black cohosh. Researchers are looking at using herbal supplements to prevent or treat some health problems. It's too soon to know if herbal supplements are both safe and useful. But, studies of some have not shown benefits.

Are Dietary Supplements Safe?

Scientists are still working to answer this question. The U.S. Food and Drug Administration (FDA) checks prescription medicines, such as antibiotics or blood pressure medicines, to make sure they are safe and do what they promise. The same is true for over-the-counter drugs like pain and cold medicines. But, the FDA does not consider dietary supplements to be medicines. The FDA does not watch over dietary supplements in the same way it does prescription medicines. The Federal Government does not regularly test what is in dietary supplements. So, just because you see a dietary supplement on a store shelf does not mean it is safe, that it does what the label says it will, or that it contains what the label says it contains.

If the FDA receives reports of possible problems with a supplement, it will issue warnings about products that are clearly unsafe. The FDA may also take these supplements off the market. The Federal Trade Commission (FTC) looks into reports of ads that might misrepresent what dietary supplements do.

A few private groups, such as the U.S. Pharmacopeia (USP), NSF International, ConsumerLab.com, and the Natural Products Association (NPA), have their own "seals of approval" for dietary supplements. To get such a seal, products must be made by following good manufacturing procedures, must contain what is listed on the label, and must not have harmful levels of things that don't belong there, like lead.

What's Best for Me?

If you are thinking about using dietary supplements:

- **Learn.** Find out as much as you can about any dietary supplement you might take. Talk to your doctor, your pharmacist, or a registered dietitian. A supplement that seemed to help your neighbor might not work for you. If you are reading fact sheets or checking websites, be aware of the source of the information. Could the writer or group profit from the sale of a particular supplement?

- **Remember.** Just because something is said to be "natural" doesn't also mean it is either safe or good for you. It could have side effects. It might make a medicine your doctor prescribed for you either weaker or stronger.

- **Tell your doctor.** He or she needs to know if you decide to go ahead and use a dietary supplement. Do not diagnose or treat your health condition without first checking with your doctor.

- **Buy wisely.** Choose brands that your doctor, dietitian, or pharmacist says are trustworthy. Don't buy dietary supplements with ingredients you don't need. Don't assume that more is better. It is possible to waste money on unneeded supplements.

- **Check the science.** Make sure any claim made about a dietary supplement is based on scientific proof. The company making the dietary supplement should be able to send you information on the safety and/or effectiveness of the ingredients in a product, which you can then discuss with your doctor. Remember that if something sounds too good to be true, it probably is.

Section 10.5

Overcoming Roadblocks to Eating

This section includes text excerpted from "Overcoming Roadblocks
to Healthy Eating," National Institute on Aging (NIA), National
Institutes of Health (NIH), July 23, 2017.

Some common problems, like those listed below, can make it harder
for older people to follow through on smart food choices. Here are some
problem-solving suggestions.

Tired of Cooking or Eating Alone?

Maybe you are tired of planning and cooking dinners every night.
Have you considered some potluck meals? If everyone brings one part
of the meal, cooking is a lot easier, and there might be leftovers to
share. Or try cooking with a friend to make a meal you can enjoy
together. Also look into having some meals at a nearby senior center,
community center, or religious facility. Not only will you enjoy a free
or low-cost meal, but you will have some company while you eat.

Give Cooking a Try

It's never too late to learn some cooking skills—or refresh those you
might not have used in a while. You can go online to find information
on basic cooking techniques and recipes for one person. Borrow simple
cookbooks from your local library, or try an adult education cooking
course. TV cooking shows might be helpful—they often show you step-
by-step how to prepare and cook foods. Some grocery stores are even
beginning to have cooking coaches available to answer your cooking
questions.

Problems Chewing Food?

Do you avoid some foods because they are hard to chew? People who
have problems with their teeth or dentures often avoid eating meat,
fruits, or vegetables and might miss out on important nutrients. If you

are having trouble chewing, see your dentist to check for problems. If you wear dentures, the dentist can check how they fit.

Sometimes Hard to Swallow Your Food?

If food seems to get stuck in your throat, it might be that less saliva in your mouth is making it hard for you to swallow your food. Drinking plenty of liquids with your meal might help. There may be other reasons you are having trouble swallowing your food, including problems with the muscles or nerves in your throat, problems with your esophagus, or gastroesophageal reflux disease (GERD). Talk to your doctor about what might be causing the problem.

Food Tastes Different?

Are foods not as tasty as they used to be? It might not be the cook's fault! Maybe your sense of taste, smell, or both has changed. Growing older can cause your senses to change, but so can a variety of other things such as dental problems or medication side effects. Taste and smell are important for healthy appetite and eating.

Feeling Sad and Don't Want to Eat?

Feeling blue now and then is normal, but if you continue to feel sad, ask your doctor for help. Being unhappy can cause a loss of appetite. Help might be available. For example, you might need to talk with someone trained to work with people who are depressed.

Just Not Hungry?

- Maybe you are not sad, but just can't eat very much. Changes to your body as you age can cause some people to feel full sooner than they did when younger. Or lack of appetite might be the side effect of a medicine you are taking—your doctor might be able to suggest a different drug.

- Try being more physically active. In addition to all the other benefits of exercise and physical activity, it may make you hungrier.

- If you aren't hungry because food just isn't appealing, there are ways to make it more interesting. Make sure your foods are seasoned well, but not with extra salt. Try using lemon juice, vinegar, or herbs to boost the flavor of your food.

- Vary the shape, color, and texture of foods you eat. When you go shopping, look for a new vegetable, fruit, or seafood you haven't tried before or one you haven't eaten in a while. Sometimes grocery stores have recipe cards near items. Or ask the produce staff or meat or seafood department staff for suggestions about preparing the new food. Find recipes online. Type the name of a food and the word "recipes" into a search window to look for ideas.

- Foods that are overcooked tend to have less flavor. Try cooking or steaming your vegetables for a shorter time, and see if that gives them a crunch that will help spark your interest. Spices, herbs, and lemon juice add flavor to your food, without adding salt.

Trouble Getting Enough Calories?

- If you aren't eating enough, add snacks throughout the day to help you get more nutrients and calories. Snacks can be healthy—for example, raw vegetables with a low-fat dip or hummus, low-fat cheese and whole-grain crackers, or a piece of fruit. Unsalted nuts or nut butters are nutrient-dense snacks that give you added protein. You could try putting shredded low-fat cheese on your soup or popcorn or sprinkling nuts or wheat germ on yogurt or cereal.

- If you are eating so little that you are losing weight but don't need to, your doctor might suggest protein and energy supplements. Sometimes these supplements help undernourished people gain a little weight. If so, they should be used as snacks between meals or after dinner, not in place of a meal and not right before one. Ask your doctor how to choose a supplement.

Physical Problems Making It Hard to Eat?

- Sometimes illnesses like Parkinson disease, stroke, or arthritis can make it harder for you to cook or feed yourself. Your doctor might recommend an occupational therapist. He or she might suggest rearranging things in your kitchen, make a custom splint for your hand, or give you special exercises to strengthen your muscles.

- Devices like special utensils and plates might make meal time easier or help with food preparation. You can search the U.S. Department of Education's (ED) AbleData assistive technology website (www.abledata.com) for information on products designed to make it easier for people to do things on their own. Or call 1-800-227-0216 to learn more.

Can Foods and Medicines Interact?

Medicines can change how food tastes, make your mouth dry, or take away your appetite. In turn, some foods can change how certain medicines work. You might have heard that grapefruit juice is a common culprit when used with any of several drugs. Chocolate, licorice, and alcohol are some of the others. Whenever your doctor prescribes a new drug for you, be sure to ask about any food/drug interactions.

Lactose Intolerant?

Some older people believe they are lactose intolerant because they have uncomfortable stomach and intestinal symptoms when they have dairy products. Your doctor can do tests to learn whether or not you do indeed need to limit or avoid dairy foods when you eat. If so, talk to your healthcare practitioner about how to meet your calcium and vitamin D needs. Even lactose-intolerant people might be able to have small amounts of milk when taken with food. There are nondairy food sources of calcium, lactose-free milk and milk products, calcium- and vitamin D-fortified foods, and supplements.

Weight Issues Adding to Frailty?

- Older people who don't get enough of the right nutrients can be too thin or too heavy. Some may be too thin because they don't get enough food. But others might be overweight partly because they get too much of the wrong types of foods. Keeping track of what you are eating could help you see which foods you should eat less of, more of, or not at all.

- Obesity is a growing problem in the United States, and the number of older people who are overweight or obese is also increasing. But frailty is also a problem, and not just in thin people. As you grow older, you can lose muscle strength, but you also get more fat tissue. This can make you frail, and in time, you might have problems getting around and taking care of yourself. Being overweight puts you more at risk for frailty and disability.

- But, just losing weight is not necessarily the answer. That's because sometimes when older people lose weight, they lose even more muscle than they already have lost. That puts them at greater risk for becoming frail and falling. They also might lose bone strength and be at more risk for a broken bone after a fall. Exercise helps you keep muscle and bone. Also, for some people, a few extra pounds late in life can act as a safety net should they get a serious illness that limits how much they can eat for a while.

- The *2010 Dietary Guidelines* encourage people 65 and older who are overweight to try to avoid gaining more weight. But, those who are very overweight (obese) might be helped by intentional weight loss, especially if they are at risk for heart disease, suggest the Guidelines. So, if you think you weigh too much, check with your doctor before starting a diet. He or she can decide whether or not losing a few pounds will be good for you and how you can safely lose weight.

Chapter 11

Older Adults and Cognitive Health

Chapter Contents

111

Section 11.1

What's Normal, What's Not

This section includes text excerpted from "Memory and Thinking: What's Normal and What's Not?" National Institute on Aging (NIA), National Institutes of Health (NIH), July 23, 2017.

Many older people worry about their memory and other thinking abilities. For example, they might be concerned about taking longer than before to learn new things, or they might sometimes forget to pay a bill. These changes are usually signs of mild forgetfulness—often a normal part of aging—not serious memory problems.

Talk with your doctor to determine if memory and other thinking problems are normal or not, and what is causing them.

What's Normal and What's Not?

What's the difference between normal, age-related forgetfulness, and a serious memory problem? Serious memory problems make it hard to do everyday things like driving and shopping. Signs may include:

- Asking the same questions over and over again

- Getting lost in familiar places

- Not being able to follow instructions

- Becoming confused about time, people, and places

Mild Cognitive Impairment

Some older adults have a condition called mild cognitive impairment, or MCI, in which they have more memory or other thinking problems than other people their age. People with MCI can take care of themselves and do their normal activities. MCI may be an early sign of Alzheimer, but not everyone with MCI will develop Alzheimer disease.

Signs of MCI include:

- Losing things often

- Forgetting to go to important events and appointments
- Having more trouble coming up with desired words than other people of the same age

If you have MCI, visit your doctor every 6 to 12 months to see if you have any changes in memory or thinking skills over time. There may be things you can do to maintain your memory and mental skills. No medications have been approved to treat MCI.

Dementia

Dementia is the loss of cognitive functioning—thinking, remembering, learning and reasoning—and behavioral abilities to such an extent that it interferes with daily life and activities. Memory loss, though common, is not the only sign. A person may also have problems with language skills, visual perception, or paying attention. Some people have personality changes. Dementia is not a normal part of aging.

There are different forms of dementia. Alzheimer disease is the most common form in people over age 65. Table 11.1 below explains some differences between normal signs of aging and Alzheimer disease.

Table 11.1. Differences between Normal Aging and Alzheimer Disease

Normal Aging	Alzheimer Disease
Making a bad decision once in a while	Making poor judgments and decisions a lot of the time
Missing a monthly payment	Problems taking care of monthly bills
Forgetting which day it is and remembering it later	Losing track of the date or time of year
Sometimes forgetting which word to use	Trouble having a conversation
Losing things from time to time	Misplacing things often and being unable to find them

When to Visit the Doctor

If you, a family member, or friend has problems remembering recent events or thinking clearly, talk with a doctor. He or she may suggest a thorough checkup to see what might be causing the symptoms.

The annual Medicare wellness visit includes an assessment for cognitive impairment. This visit is covered by Medicare for patients who have had Medicare Part B insurance for at least 1 year.

Memory and other thinking problems have many possible causes, including depression, an infection, or a medication side effect. Sometimes, the problem can be treated, and the thinking problems disappear. Other times, the problem is a brain disorder, such as Alzheimer disease, which cannot be reversed. Finding the cause of the problems is important to determine the best course of action.

A note about unproven treatments: Some people are tempted by untried or unproven "cures" that claim to make the brain sharper or prevent dementia. Check with your doctor before trying pills, supplements or other products that promise to improve memory or prevent brain disorders. These "treatments" might be unsafe, a waste of money, or both. They might even interfere with other medical treatments. Currently there is no drug or treatment that prevents Alzheimer disease or other dementias.

Section 11.2

Cognitive Health and Older Adults

This section includes text excerpted from "Cognitive Health and Older Adults," National Institute on Aging (NIA), National Institutes of Health (NIH), August 21, 2017.

Cognitive health—the ability to clearly think, learn, and remember—is an important component of brain health. Others include:

- **Motor function**—how well you make and control movements

- **Emotional function**—how well you interpret and respond to emotions

- **Sensory function**—how well you feel and respond to sensations of touch, including pressure, pain, and temperature

Tips to Maintain Your Cognitive Health

The following steps can help you function every day and stay independent—and they have been linked to cognitive health, too.

Take Care of Your Health

Taking care of your physical health may help your cognitive health. You can:

- Get recommended health screenings.

- Manage chronic health problems like diabetes, high blood pressure, depression, and high cholesterol.

- Consult with your healthcare provider about the medicines you take and possible side effects on memory, sleep, and brain function.

- Reduce risk for brain injuries due to falls and other accidents.

- Limit use of alcohol (some medicines can be dangerous when mixed with alcohol).

- Quit smoking, if you smoke.

- Get enough sleep, generally 7–8 hours each night.

Eat Healthy Foods

A healthy diet can help reduce the risk of many chronic diseases, such as heart disease or diabetes. It may also help keep your brain healthy.

In general, a healthy diet consists of fruits and vegetables; whole grains; lean meats, fish, and poultry; and low-fat or nonfat dairy products. You should also limit solid fats, sugar, and salt. Be sure to control portion sizes and drink enough water and other fluids.

Researchers are looking at whether a healthy diet can help preserve cognitive function or reduce the risk of Alzheimer disease. For example, there is some evidence that people who eat a "Mediterranean diet" have a lower risk of developing mild cognitive impairment.

Researchers have developed and are testing another diet, called MIND (Mediterranean-DASH Intervention for Neurodegenerative Delay), a combination of the Mediterranean and DASH (Dietary Approaches to Stop Hypertension) diets. One study suggests that MIND may affect the risk of Alzheimer disease.

Be Physically Active

Being physically active—through regular exercise, household chores, or other activities—has many benefits. It can help you:

- Keep and improve your strength

- Have more energy

- Improve your balance

- Prevent or delay heart disease, diabetes, and other diseases

- Perk up your mood and reduce depression

Studies link ongoing physical activity with benefits for the brain, too. In one study, exercise stimulated the human brain's ability to maintain old network connections and make new ones that are vital to cognitive health. Other studies have shown that exercise increased the size of a brain structure important to memory and learning, improving spatial memory.

Aerobic exercise, such as brisk walking, is thought to be more beneficial to cognitive health than nonaerobic stretching and toning exercise. Studies are ongoing.

Federal guidelines recommend that all adults get at least 150 minutes of physical activity each week. Aim to move about 30 minutes on most days. Walking is a good start. You can also join programs that teach you to move safely and prevent falls, which can lead to brain and other injuries. Check with your healthcare provider if you haven't been active and want to start a vigorous exercise program.

Keep Your Mind Active

Being intellectually engaged may benefit the brain. People who engage in meaningful activities, like volunteering or hobbies, say they feel happier and healthier. Learning new skills may improve your thinking ability, too. For example, one study found that older adults who learned quilting or digital photography had more memory improvement than those who only socialized or did less cognitively demanding activities.

Lots of activities can keep your mind active. For example, read books and magazines. Play games. Take or teach a class. Learn a new skill or hobby. Work or volunteer. These types of mentally stimulating activities have not been proven to prevent serious cognitive impairment or Alzheimer disease, but they can be fun!

Scientists think that such activities may protect the brain by establishing "cognitive reserve." They may help the brain become more adaptable in some mental functions, so it can compensate for age–related brain changes and health conditions that affect the brain.

Formal cognitive training also seems to have benefits. In the Advanced Cognitive Training for Independent and Vital Elderly (ACTIVE) trial, healthy adults 65 and older participated in 10 sessions of memory training, reasoning training, or processing–speed training. The sessions improved participants' mental skills in the area in which they were trained. Most of these improvements persisted 10 years after the training was completed.

Be wary of claims that playing certain computer and online games can improve your memory and other types of thinking. Evidence to back up such claims is evolving. National Institute on Aging (NIA) and others are supporting research to determine if different types of cognitive training have lasting effects.

Stay Connected

Connecting with other people through social activities and community programs can keep your brain active and help you feel less isolated and more engaged with the world around you. Participating in social activities may lower the risk for some health problems and improve well-being.

So, visit with family and friends. Join programs through your Area Agency on Aging, senior center, or other community organizations.

It's not known for sure yet if any of these actions can prevent or delay Alzheimer disease and age-related cognitive decline. But some of them have been associated with reduced risk of cognitive impairment and dementia.

Section 11.3

Memory Problems among Older Adults

This section includes text excerpted from "Healthy Living— Memory and Healthy Aging," Centers for Disease Control and Prevention (CDC), September 22, 2015.

Some declines in cognition and memory with age are normal, but sometimes they can signal problems. Learn the signs and symptoms of dementia and cognitive impairments so you can help the older adults in your life seek treatment at the right time.

Physical activity, social engagement, and a healthy diet help prevent chronic conditions and increase the longevity and quality of life of older adults, but despite engaging in these healthy activities, some adults may develop memory loss or dementia. Some declines in memory are a normal part of aging, but sometimes they can signal a problem. Learn how to tell the difference.

What Cognitive Decline Means

Cognition is a combination of mental processes that include intuition, judgment, language, remembering, and the ability to learn new things. When cognition is impaired (referred to as cognitive impairment or decline), a person has trouble with these processes that begins to affect the things he or she can do in everyday life.

The decline of cognitive health—from mild cognitive decline to dementia—can have profound implications for an individual's health and well-being. Older adults and others experiencing cognitive decline may be unable to care for themselves or conduct necessary activities of daily living, such as meal preparation and money management, cooccurring medical conditions, and the inability to effectively manage medications are particular concerns when an individual's memory is impaired.

Forgetfulness or Something More?

Forgetfulness can be a normal part of aging. Some people may notice that it takes longer to learn new things, they don't remember information as well as they did, or they lose things like their glasses. These usually are signs of mild forgetfulness, not a serious memory problem.

Some memory problems are related to health issues that may be treatable. For example, medication side effects, vitamin B 12 deficiency, chronic alcoholism, tumors or infections in the brain, or blood clots in the brain can cause memory loss or possibly dementia. Some thyroid, kidney, or liver disorders also can lead to memory loss. A doctor should treat serious medical conditions like these as soon as possible.

For some older people, memory problems are a sign of a serious problem, such as mild cognitive impairment, dementia, or Alzheimer disease. People who are worried about memory problems should see a doctor. The doctor might conduct or order a thorough physical and mental health evaluation to reach a diagnosis. Often, these evaluations are conducted by a neurologist, a physician who specializes in problems related to the brain and central nervous system.

Treatment

A person with dementia should be under a doctor's care. The doctor might be a neurologist, family doctor, internist, geriatrician, or psychiatrist. He or she can treat the patient's physical and behavioral problems (such as aggression, agitation, or wandering) and answer the many questions that the person or family may have. At this time, however, there are no effective treatments to slow the progression, or to cure dementia or Alzheimer disease.

Family members and friends can help people in the early stages of dementia to continue their daily routines, physical activities, and social contacts. People with dementia should be kept up to date about the details of their lives, such as the time of day, where they live, and what is happening at home or in the world. Memory aids may help. Some families find that a big calendar, a list of daily plans, notes about simple safety measures, and written directions describing how to use common household items are useful aids.

Caring for a Person with Dementia or Memory Loss

According to a study published in a March 2015 release of Centers for Disease Control and Prevention (CDC)'s journal *Preventing Chronic Disease*, a total of 12.6 percent of households reported at least one adult who experienced increased confusion or memory loss, and in nearly 6 percent of households all adults experienced increased confusion or memory loss. Based on these results, an estimated 4 million households in the 13 U.S. states included in the study have a family member with increased confusion or memory loss, potentially affecting more than 10 million people. This leaves many people who are left with the task of caring for someone suffering from a memory problem.

Many caregivers of older adults express satisfaction with the care they are able to provide, but they often face challenges, especially when caring for people with chronic diseases such as dementia. The day-to-day tasks may seem endless: arranging doctor's appointments and transportation, moving the person safely around, ensuring proper nutrition, and much more. Difficult situations, such as hospitalization and making decisions about long-term care, also arise. The National

Institute on Aging (NIA) at the National Institute of Health (NIH) has information that can help caregivers approach many of these issues.

If you're concerned that you or someone you know has a serious memory problem, talk with your doctor. He or she may be able to diagnose the problem or refer you to a specialist, such as a neurologist or geriatric psychiatrist. Healthcare professionals who specialize in Alzheimer disease and other dementias can recommend ways to manage the problem or suggest treatment or services that might help.

Chapter 12

Sexuality and Aging

Chapter Contents

Section 12.1

Sexuality Later in Life

This section includes text excerpted from "Sexuality in Later Life," National Institute on Aging (NIA), National Institutes of Health (NIH), July 19, 2017.

What Are Normal Changes?

Normal aging brings physical changes in both men and women. These changes sometimes affect the ability to have and enjoy sex. A woman may notice changes in her vagina. As a woman ages, her vagina can shorten and narrow. Her vaginal walls can become thinner and also a little stiffer. Most women will have less vaginal lubrication. These changes could affect sexual function and/or pleasure. Talk with your doctor about these problems.

As men get older, impotence (also called erectile dysfunction–ED) becomes more common. ED is the loss of ability to have and keep an erection for sexual intercourse. ED may cause a man to take longer to have an erection. His erection may not be as firm or as large as it used to be. The loss of erection after orgasm may happen more quickly, or it may take longer before another erection is possible. ED is not a problem if it happens every now and then, but if it occurs often, talk with your doctor.

What Causes Sexual Problems?

Some illnesses, disabilities, medicines, and surgeries can affect your ability to have and enjoy sex. Problems in your relationship can also affect your ability to enjoy sex.

Arthritis. Joint pain due to arthritis can make sexual contact uncomfortable. Exercise, drugs, and possibly joint replacement surgery may relieve this pain. Rest, warm baths, and changing the position or timing of sexual activity can be helpful.

Chronic pain. Any constant pain can interfere with intimacy between older people. Chronic pain does not have to be part of growing older and can often be treated. But, some pain medicines can interfere with sexual function. You should always talk with your doctor if you have unwanted side effects from any medication.

Dementia. Some people with dementia show increased interest in sex and physical closeness, but they may not be able to judge what is appropriate sexual behavior. Those with severe dementia may not recognize their spouse but still seek sexual contact. This can be a confusing problem for the spouse. A doctor, nurse, or social worker with training in dementia care may be helpful.

Diabetes. This is one of the illnesses that can cause ED in some men. In most cases, medical treatment can help. Less is known about how diabetes affects sexuality in older women. Women with diabetes are more likely to have vaginal yeast infections, which can cause itching and irritation and make sex uncomfortable or undesirable. Yeast infections can be treated.

Heart disease. Narrowing and hardening of the arteries can change blood vessels so that blood does not flow freely. As a result, men and women may have problems with orgasms, and men may have trouble with erections. People who have had a heart attack, or their partners, may be afraid that having sex will cause another attack. Even though sexual activity is generally safe, always follow your doctor's advice. If your heart problems get worse and you have chest pain or shortness of breath even while resting, talk to your doctor. He or she may want to change your treatment plan.

Incontinence. Loss of bladder control or leaking of urine is more common as we grow older, especially in women. Extra pressure on the belly during sex can cause loss of urine, which may result in some people avoiding sex. This can be helped by a change in positions. The good news is that incontinence can usually be treated.

Stroke. The ability to have sex is sometimes affected by a stroke. A change in positions or medical devices may help people with ongoing weakness or paralysis to have sex. Some people with paralysis from the waist down are still able to experience orgasm and pleasure.

Depression. Lack of interest in activities you used to enjoy, such as intimacy and sexual activity, can be a symptom of depression. It's sometimes hard to know if you're depressed. Talk with your doctor. Depression can be treated.

What Else May Cause Sexuality Problems?

Surgery. Many of us worry about having any kind of surgery—it may be even more troubling when the breasts or genital area are involved. Most people do return to the kind of sex life they enjoyed before surgery.

Hysterectomy is surgery to remove a woman's uterus. Often, when an older woman has a hysterectomy, the ovaries are also removed. The surgery can leave both women and men worried about their sex lives. If you're afraid that a hysterectomy will change your sex life, talk with your gynecologist or surgeon.

Mastectomy is surgery to remove all or part of a woman's breast. This surgery may cause some women to lose their sexual interest or their sense of being desired or feeling feminine. In addition to talking with your doctor, sometimes it is useful to talk with other women who have had this surgery. If you want your breast rebuilt (reconstruction), talk to your cancer doctor or surgeon.

Prostatectomy is surgery that removes all or part of a man's prostate because of cancer or an enlarged prostate. It may cause urinary incontinence or ED. If removal of the prostate gland is needed, talk to your doctor before surgery about your concerns.

Medications. Some drugs can cause sexual problems. These include some blood pressure medicines, antihistamines, antidepressants, tranquilizers, appetite suppressants, drugs for mental problems, and ulcer drugs. Some can lead to ED or make it hard for men to ejaculate. Some drugs can reduce a woman's sexual desire or cause vaginal dryness or difficulty with arousal and orgasm. Check with your doctor to see if there is a different drug without this side effect.

Alcohol. Too much alcohol can cause erection problems in men and delay orgasm in women.

Am I Too Old to Worry about Safe Sex?

Age does not protect you from sexually transmitted diseases. Older people who are sexually active may be at risk for diseases such as syphilis, gonorrhea, chlamydial infection, genital herpes, hepatitis B, genital warts, and trichomoniasis.

Almost anyone who is sexually active is also at risk of being infected with human immunodeficiency virus (HIV), the virus that causes acquired immunodeficiency syndrome (AIDS). The number of older people with HIV/AIDS is growing. You are at risk for HIV/AIDS if you or your partner has more than one sexual partner or if you are having unprotected sex. To protect yourself, always use a condom during sex. For women with vaginal dryness, lubricated condoms or a water-based lubricating jelly with condoms may be more comfortable. A man needs to have a full erection before putting on a condom.

Talk with your doctor about ways to protect yourself from all sexually transmitted diseases. Go for regular checkups and testing. Talk with your partner. You are never too old to be at risk.

Can Emotions Play a Part?

Sexuality is often a delicate balance of emotional and physical issues. How you feel may affect what you are able to do. Many older couples find greater satisfaction in their sex life than they did when they were younger. They have fewer distractions, more time and privacy, no worries about getting pregnant, and greater intimacy with a lifelong partner.

Some older people are concerned about sex as they age. A woman who is unhappy about how her looks are changing as she ages may think her partner will no longer find her attractive. This focus on youthful physical beauty may get in the way of her enjoyment of sex. Men may fear that ED will become a more common problem as they age. Most men have a problem with ED once in awhile. But, if you worry too much about that happening, you can cause enough stress to trigger ED.

Older couples face the same daily stresses that affect people of any age. They may also have the added concerns of age, illness, retirement, and other lifestyle changes, all of which may lead to sexual difficulties. Try not to blame yourself or your partner. You may find it helpful to talk to a therapist. Some therapists have special training in helping with sexual problems. If your male partner is troubled by ED or your female partner seems less interested in sex, don't assume he or she is no longer interested in you or in sex. Many of the things that cause these problems can be helped.

What Can I Do?

There are things you can do on your own for an active sexual life. Make your partner a high priority. Take time to enjoy each other and to understand the changes you both are facing. Try different positions and new times, like having sex in the morning when you both may be well-rested. Don't hurry—you or your partner may need to spend more time touching to become fully aroused. Masturbation is a sexual activity that many older people, with and without a partner, find satisfying.

Don't be afraid to talk with your doctor if you have a problem that affects your sex life. He or she may be able to suggest a treatment. For example, the most common sexual difficulty of older women is painful intercourse caused by vaginal dryness. Your doctor or a pharmacist can suggest over-the-counter vaginal lubricants or moisturizers to use. Water-based lubricants are helpful when needed to make sex more comfortable. Moisturizers are used on a regular basis, every 2 or 3 days. Or, your doctor might suggest a form of vaginal estrogen.

If ED is the problem, it can often be managed and perhaps even reversed. There are pills that can help. They should not be used by men taking medicines containing nitrates, such as nitroglycerin. The pills do have possible side effects. Other available treatments include vacuum devices, self-injection of a drug, or penile implants.

Physical problems can change your sex life as you get older. But, you and your partner may discover you have a new closeness. Talk to your partner about your needs. You may find that affection—hugging, kissing, touching, and spending time together—can make a good beginning.

Section 12.2

Sexuality and Menopause

This section includes text excerpted from "Menopause and Sexuality," Office on Women's Health (OWH), U.S. Department of Health and Human Services (HHS), September 22, 2010. Reviewed September 2017.

Sexual Issues and Menopause

In the years around menopause, you may experience changes in your sexual life. Some women say they enjoy sex more after they don't have to worry about getting pregnant. Other women find that they think about sex less often or don't enjoy it as much.

Changes in sexuality at this time of life have several possible causes, including:

- Decreased hormones can make vaginal tissues drier and thinner, which can make sex uncomfortable.

- Decreased hormones may reduce sex drive.

- Night sweats can disturb a woman's sleep and make her too tired for sex.

- Emotional changes can make a woman feel too stressed for sex.

Keep in mind that being less interested in sex as you get older is not a medical condition that needs treatment. But if you are upset about sexual changes, you can get help. Don't be shy about talking with your doctor or nurse. They certainly have talked with many women about these issues before.

Lifestyle Changes

Some simple steps may help with sexual issues you face at this time:

- **Get treated for any medical problems.** Your overall health can affect your sexual health. For example, you need healthy arteries to supply blood to your vagina.

- **Try to exercise.** Physical activity can increase your energy, lift your mood, and improve your body image—all of which can help with sexual interest.

- **Don't smoke.** Cigarette smoking can reduce both the blood flow to the vagina and the effects of estrogen, which are important to sexual health.

- **Avoid drugs and alcohol.** They can slow down how your body responds.

- **Try to have sex more often.** Sex can increase blood flow to your vagina and help keep tissues healthy.

- **Allow time to become aroused during sex.** Moisture from being aroused protects tissues. Also, avoid sex if you have any vaginal irritation.

- **Practice pelvic floor exercises.** These can increase blood flow to the vagina and strengthen the muscles involved in orgasm.

- **Avoid products that irritate your vagina.** Bubble bath and strong soaps might cause irritation. Don't douche. If you're experiencing vaginal dryness, allergy and cold medicines may add to the problem.

Treatment Options

Discuss your symptoms and personal health issues with your doctor to decide whether one or more treatment options are right for you.

If vaginal dryness is an issue:

- Using an over-the-counter, water-based vaginal lubricant like K-Y Jelly or Astroglide when you have sex can lessen discomfort.

- An over-the-counter vaginal moisturizer like Replens can help put moisture back in vaginal tissues. You may need to use it every few days.

- Prescription medicines that are put into a woman's vagina may increase moisture and sensation. These include estrogen creams, tablets, or rings. If you have severe vaginal dryness, the most effective treatment may be menopausal hormone therapy.

If sexual interest is an issue:

- Treating vaginal dryness may help. Talking with your partner or making lifestyle changes also may help. Learn about lifestyle changes on the Natural/alternative treatments and lifestyle changes page.

- You may wonder about Viagra. This medication has helped men with erection problems, but it has not proven effective in increasing women's sexual interest.

- Some women try products like pills or creams that contain the male hormone testosterone or similar products. The U.S. Food and Drug Administration (FDA) has not approved these products for treating reduced female sex drive because there is not enough research proving them safe and effective.

- The FDA has approved menopausal hormone therapy (MHT) for symptoms like hot flashes, but research has not proven that MHT increases sex drive.

Talking with Your Partner

Talking with your partner about your sexual changes can be very helpful. Some possible topics to discuss include:

- What feels good and what doesn't

- Times that you may feel more relaxed

- Which positions are more comfortable

- Whether you need more time to get aroused than you used to

- Concerns you have about the way your appearance may be changing

- Ways to enjoy physical connection other than intercourse, like massage

Talking with your partner can strengthen your sexual relationship and your overall connection. If you need help, consider meeting with a therapist or sex counselor for individual or couples therapy.

Section 12.3

Male Menopause

"Male Menopause," © 2018 Omnigraphics.
Reviewed September 2017.

What Is Male Menopause?

Male menopause refers to a decline in male hormone levels that occurs due to the aging process. Since men aged 50 or older often undergo a drop in testosterone production, this condition is also known as androgen (testosterone) decline, andropause, or simply low testosterone.

Testosterone is a hormone that is found in both men and women. In men, it is produced in the testes and is responsible for the development of male sex organs before birth, brings about changes during puberty, plays a role in sex drive and sperm production, fuels physical and mental energy, and helps maintain muscle mass.

Although menopause affects men at about the same age as women, it is not the same as female menopause. In women, menopause occurs as ovulation ends and hormone production drops off quickly. In men, however, hormone production declines at a slower rate, and this may lead to only slight changes in the way the testes function.

What Are Its Symptoms?

Male menopause can lead to physical, sexual, and psychological problems that may worsen as the person ages.
These problems can include:

- lack of energy

- decreased muscle mass

- feelings of physical weakness

- insomnia or other sleep disorders

- increased body fat

- decreased libido

- erectile dysfunction

- infertility

- lowered self-confidence

- decreased motivation

- difficulty concentrating

- depression

Other less common symptoms may include reduced testicle size, tender or enlarged breasts, hot flashes, loss of body hair, and in rare cases osteoporosis.

How Is It Diagnosed?

A doctor will generally diagnose male menopause by asking about symptoms and performing a physical examination. During this conversation, it is vital that the patient inform the doctor fully about issues like sexual problems. Blood tests may be ordered to measure testosterone levels, and in some cases other tests may be required to rule out medical issues that may contribute to this condition.

How Is It Treated?

Symptoms of male menopause are commonly treated through lifestyle changes, such as eating a healthier diet, getting more sleep and regular exercise, and reducing stress. Antidepressants and therapy may be prescribed if the individual is suffering from depression.

Testosterone replacement therapy may also be suggested to help alleviate such symptoms as fatigue, decreased libido, and depression. Much like hormone replacement therapy for women, treatment using synthetic hormones is controversial and comes with potential risks and side effects. For instance, in an individual with prostate cancer, synthetic hormones may cause an increase in the growth of cancer cells. If a doctor suggests hormone replacement therapy, it is advisable to consider both the positives and negatives of this treatment option thoroughly before making a decision.

References

1. Krans, Brian. "What Is Male Menopause?" Healthline Media, March 8, 2016.

2. Derrer, David T. "Male Menopause," WebMD, LLC, August 17, 2014.

Section 12.4

Intimacy and Alzheimer Disease

This section includes text excerpted from "Changes in Intimacy and Sexuality in Alzheimer's Disease," National Institute on Aging (NIA), National Institutes of Health (NIH), July 13, 2017.

Alzheimer disease (AD) can cause changes in intimacy and sexuality in both a person with the disease and the caregiver. The person with AD may be stressed by the changes in his or her memory and behaviors. Fear, worry, depression, anger, and low self-esteem (how much the person likes himself or herself) are common. The person may become dependent and cling to you. He or she may not remember your life together and feelings toward one another. The person may even fall in love with someone else.

You, the caregiver, may pull away from the person in both an emotional and physical sense. You may be upset by the demands of caregiving. You also may feel frustrated by the person's constant forgetfulness, repeated questions, and other bothersome behaviors.

Most caregivers learn how to cope with these challenges, but it takes time. Some learn to live with the illness and find new meaning in their relationships with people who have Alzheimer disease.

How to Cope with Changes in Intimacy

Most people with Alzheimer disease need to feel that someone loves and cares about them. They also need to spend time with other people as well as you. Your efforts to take care of these needs can help the person with AD to feel happy and safe. It's important to reassure the person that:

- You love him or her.

- You will keep him or her safe.

- Others also care about him or her.

The following tips may help you cope with your own needs:

- Talk with a doctor, social worker, or clergy member about these changes. It may feel awkward to talk about such personal issues, but it can help.

- Talk about your concerns in a support group.

- Think more about the positive parts of the relationship.

How to Cope with Changes in Sexuality

The well spouse/partner or the person with Alzheimer disease may lose interest in having sex. This change can make you feel lonely or frustrated. You may feel that:

- It's not okay to have sex with someone who has AD.

- The person with AD seems like a stranger.

- The person with AD seems to forget that the spouse/partner is there or how to make love.

A person with Alzheimer disease may have side effects from medications that affect his or her sexual interest. He or she may also have memory loss, changes in the brain, or depression that affect his or her interest in sex.

Here are some tips for coping with changes in sexuality:

- Explore new ways of spending time together.

- Focus on other ways to show affection, such as snuggling or holding hands.

- Try other nonsexual forms of touching, such as massage, hugging, and dancing.

- Consider other ways to meet your sexual needs. Some caregivers report that they masturbate.

Hypersexuality

Sometimes, people with Alzheimer disease are overly interested in sex. This is called hypersexuality. The person may masturbate a lot and try to seduce others. These behaviors are symptoms of the disease and don't always mean that the person wants to have sex.

To cope with hypersexuality, try giving the person more attention and reassurance. You might gently touch, hug, or use other kinds of affection to meet his or her emotional needs. Some people with this problem need medicine to control their behaviors. Talk to the doctor about what steps to take.

Chapter 13

Mental and Emotional Health

Chapter Contents

Section 13.1

Mental Health and Older Adults

This section contains text excerpted from the following sources:
Text under the heading "Why Is Mental Health a Public Health
Issue?" is excerpted from "The State of Mental Health and Aging in
America," Centers for Disease Control and Prevention (CDC), 2008.
Reviewed September 2017; Text under the heading "Warning Signs"
is excerpted from "Older Adults and Mental Health," National
Institute of Mental Health (NIMH), October 2016.

Why Is Mental Health a Public Health Issue?

The World Health Organization (WHO) defines health as "a state
of complete physical, mental, and social well-being and not merely the
absence of disease or infirmity." Because mental health is essential to
overall health and well-being, it must be recognized and treated in all
Americans, including older adults, with the same urgency as physical
health. For this reason, mental health is becoming an increasingly
important part of the public health mission.

Mental Health Problems in Older Adults

People age 55 years or older experience some type of mental health
concern. The most common conditions include anxiety, severe cognitive
impairment, and mood disorders (such as depression or bipolar disorder). Mental health issues are often implicated as a factor in cases
of suicide. Older men have the highest suicide rate of any age group.

The Significance of Depression

Depression, a type of mood disorder, is the most prevalent mental health problem among older adults. It is associated with distress
and suffering. It also can lead to impairments in physical, mental,
and social functioning. The presence of depressive disorders often
adversely affects the course and complicates the treatment of other
chronic diseases. Older adults with depression visit the doctor and
emergency room more often, use more medication, incur higher outpatient charges, and stay longer in the hospital.

Although the rate of older adults with depressive symptoms tends to increase with age, depression is not a normal part of growing older. Rather, in 80 percent of cases it is a treatable condition. Unfortunately, depressive disorders are a widely under-recognized condition and often are untreated or undertreated among older adults.

Social and Emotional Support

* Social support serves major support functions, including emotional support (e.g., sharing problems or venting emotions), informational support (e.g., advice and guidance), and instrumental support (e.g., providing rides or assisting with housekeeping).

* Adequate social and emotional support is associated with reduced risk of mental illness, physical illness, and mortality.

* The majority of adults age 50 or older indicated that they received adequate amounts of support.

* Adults age 65 or older were more likely than adults age 50–64 to report that they "rarely" or "never" received the social and emotional support they needed.

* Among adults age 50 or older, men were more likely than women to report they "rarely" or "never" received the support they needed.

Life Satisfaction

* Life satisfaction is the self-evaluation of one's life as a whole, and is influenced by socioeconomic, health, and environmental factors.

* Life dissatisfaction is associated with obesity and risky health behaviors such as smoking, physical inactivity, and heavy drinking.

* Nearly 95 percent of adults age 50 or older reported being "satisfied" or "very satisfied" with their lives, with approximately 5 percent indicating that they were "dissatisfied" or "very dissatisfied" with their lives.

* Adults age 50–64 were more likely than adults age 65 or older to report that they were "dissatisfied" or "very dissatisfied" with their lives.

- Men and women age 50 or older reported similar rates of life satisfaction.

Frequent Mental Distress

- Frequent mental distress (FMD) may interfere with major life activities, such as eating well, maintaining a household, working, or sustaining personal relationships.

- FMD can also affect physical health. Older adults with FMD were more likely to engage in behaviors that can contribute to poor health, such as smoking, not getting recommend amounts of exercise, or eating a diet with few fruits and vegetables.

- Women aged 50–64 and 65 or older reported more FMD than men in the same age groups.

Depression

- Depression is more than just a passing mood. Rather, it is a condition in which one may experience persistent sadness, withdrawal from previously enjoyed activities, difficulty sleeping, physical discomforts, and feeling "slowed down."

- Risk factors for late-onset depression included widowhood, physical illness, low educational attainment (less than high school), impaired functional status, and heavy alcohol consumption.

- Depression is one of the most successfully treated illnesses. There are highly effective treatments for depression in late life, and most depressed older adults can improve dramatically from treatment.

Anxiety Disorder

- Anxiety, like depression, is among the most prevalent mental health problems among older adults. The two conditions often go hand in hand, with almost half of older adults who are diagnosed with a major depression also meeting the criteria for anxiety.

- Late-life anxiety is not well understood, but is believed to be as common in older adults as in younger age groups (although how and when it appears is distinctly different in older adults). Anxiety in this age group may be underestimated because older adults are less likely to report psychiatric symptoms and more likely to emphasize physical complaints.

- Adults age 50–64 reported a lifetime diagnosis of an existing anxiety disorder more than adults age 65 or older.

- Women age 50–64 years report a lifetime diagnosis of an anxiety disorder more often than men in this age group.

Warning Signs

- Noticeable changes in mood, energy level, or appetite
- Feeling flat or having trouble feeling positive emotions
- Difficulty sleeping or sleeping too much
- Difficulty concentrating, feeling restless, or on edge
- Increased worry or feeling stressed
- Anger, irritability or aggressiveness
- Ongoing headaches, digestive issues, or pain
- A need for alcohol or drugs
- Sadness or hopelessness
- Suicidal thoughts
- Engaging in high-risk activities
- Obsessive thinking or compulsive behavior
- Thoughts or behaviors that interfere with work, family, or social life
- Unusual thinking or behaviors that concern other people

Section 13.2

Expanding Circles—Preventing Loneliness as You Age

This section includes text excerpted from "Expand Your Circles Prevent Isolation and Loneliness as You Age," Eldercare Locator, U.S. Administration on Aging (AOA), May 2016.

As we age, circumstances in our lives often change. We retire from a job, friends move away or health issues convince us to eliminate or restrict driving. When changes like these occur, we may not fully realize how they will affect our ability to stay connected and engaged and how much they can impact our overall health and well-being.

We need social connection to thrive—no matter our age—but research shows that the negative health consequences of chronic isolation and loneliness may be especially harmful for older adults. The good news is that with greater awareness, we can take steps to maintain and strengthen our ties to family and friends, expand our social circles and become more involved in the community around us.

Having a social network that meets our needs means different things to each of us. Evaluate your situation and, if needed, take action to strengthen the relationships that matter the most to you. And don't forget—when you open up your world to new people, sharing your time, talents and wisdom, it's a win-win for you and your entire community.

How Widespread Is the Problem of Social Isolation?

- An estimated one in five adults over age 50—at least 8 million—are affected by isolation.

- Prolonged isolation can be as bad for your health as smoking 15 cigarettes a day.

What Are the Factors That Put You at Greater Risk?

- Living alone

- Mobility or sensory impairment

- Major life transitions or losses
- Low income or limited financial resources
- Being a caregiver for someone with a serious condition
- Psychological or cognitive challenges
- Inadequate social support
- Rural, unsafe and/or inaccessible neighborhood
- Transportation access challenges
- Language barriers
- Age, racial, ethnic, sexual orientation and/or gender identity barriers

Caregivers: These risk factors may also provide you with clues to what to look for should you have a family member or neighbor who is isolated or lonely.

Negative Health Effects of Isolation and Loneliness

Associated with higher rates of:

- Chronic health conditions, including heart disease
- Weakened immune system
- Depression and anxiety
- Dementia, including Alzheimer
- Admission to nursing homes or use of emergency services
- Death

What Steps Can You Take to Stay Connected and Engaged?

Sometimes it takes effort to stay connected. You may have noticed that your social engagements have decreased or that you have gone days or weeks without speaking to or interacting with others. It never hurts to take stock of your network of activities and friends and to evaluate what you can do to make more connections.

Here are some actions you may want to consider taking to help you stay ahead of the "Connection Curve:"

- Nurture and strengthen existing relationships; invite people over for coffee or call them to suggest a trip to a museum or to see a movie.

- Schedule a time each day to call a friend or visit someone.

- Meet your neighbors—young and old.

- Don't let being a nondriver stop you from staying active. Find out about your transportation options.

- Use social media like Facebook to stay in touch with long-distance friends or write an old-fashioned letter.

- Stay physically active and include group exercise in the mix, like joining a walking club.

- Take a class to learn something new and, at the same time, expand your circle of friends.

- Revisit an old hobby you've set aside and connect with others who share your interests.

- Volunteer to deepen your sense of purpose and help others.

- Visit your local community wellness or senior center and become involved in a wide range of interesting programs.

- Check out faith-based organizations for spiritual engagement, as well as to participate in activities and events.

- Get involved in your community by taking on a cause, such as making your community more age-friendly.

Section 13.3

Mourning the Death of a Spouse

This section includes text excerpted from "Mourning the Death of a Spouse," National Institute on Aging (NIA), National Institutes of Health (NIH), August 21, 2017.

When your spouse dies, your world changes. You are in mourning—feeling grief and sorrow at the loss. You may feel numb, shocked, and fearful. You may feel guilty for being the one who is still alive. At some point, you may even feel angry at your spouse for leaving you. All of these feelings are normal. There are no rules about how you should feel. There is no right or wrong way to mourn.

When you grieve, you can feel both physical and emotional pain. People who are grieving often cry easily and can have:

- Trouble sleeping

- Little interest in food

- Problems with concentration

- A hard time making decisions

In addition to dealing with feelings of loss, you also may need to put your own life back together. This can be hard work. Some people feel better sooner than they expect. Others may take longer. Family, friends, and faith may be sources of support. Grief counseling or grief therapy also is helpful to some people.

As time passes, you may still miss your spouse. But for most people, the intense pain will lessen. There will be good and bad days. You will know you are feeling better when there are more good days than bad. Don't feel guilty if you laugh at a joke or enjoy a visit with a friend.

For some people, mourning can go on so long that it becomes unhealthy. This can be a sign of serious depression and anxiety. Talk with your doctor if sadness keeps you from carrying on with your day-to-day life. Support may be available until you can manage the grief on your own.

What Can You Do?

In the beginning, you may find that taking care of details and keeping busy helps. For a while, family and friends may be around to assist you. But, there comes a time when you will have to face the change in your life.

Here are some ideas to keep in mind:

- **Take care of yourself.** Grief can be hard on your health. Exercise regularly, eat healthy food, and get enough sleep. Bad habits, such as drinking too much alcohol or smoking, can put your health at risk.

- **Try to eat right.** Some widowed people lose interest in cooking and eating. It may help to have lunch with friends. Sometimes, eating at home alone feels too quiet. Turning on the radio or TV during meals can help. For information on nutrition and cooking for one, look for helpful books at your local library or bookstore or online.

- **Talk with caring friends.** Let family and friends know when you want to talk about your spouse. They may be grieving too and may welcome the chance to share memories. Accept their offers of help and company, when possible.

- **Join a grief support group.** Sometimes, it helps to talk with people who also are grieving. Check with hospitals, religious communities, and local agencies to find out about support groups. Choose a support group where you feel comfortable sharing your feelings and concerns. Members of support groups often have helpful ideas or know of useful resources based on their own experiences. Online support groups make it possible to get help without leaving home.

- **Visit with members of your religious community.** Many people who are grieving find comfort in their faith. Praying, talking with others of your faith, reading religious or spiritual texts, or listening to uplifting music also may bring comfort.

- **Try not to make any major changes right away.** It's a good idea to wait for a while before making big decisions, like moving or changing jobs.

- **See your doctor.** Keep up with your usual visits to your healthcare provider. If it has been awhile, schedule a physical and bring your doctor up to date on any pre-existing medical conditions. Talk about any new health issues that may be of concern. Be sure to let your healthcare provider know if you are having trouble taking care of your everyday activities, like getting dressed or fixing meals.

- **Don't be afraid to seek professional help.** Sometimes, short-term talk therapy with a counselor can help.

- **Remember that your children are grieving, too.** It will take time for the whole family to adjust to life without your spouse. You may find that your relationship with your children and their relationships with each other have changed. Open, honest communication is important.

- **Mourning takes time.** It's common to have rollercoaster emotions for a while.

Does Everyone Feel the Same Way?

Men and women share many of the same feelings when a spouse dies. Both may deal with the pain of loss, and both may worry about the future. But, there also can be differences.

Many married couples divide up their household tasks. One person may pay bills and handle car repairs. The other person may cook meals and mow the lawn. Splitting up jobs often works well until there is only one person who has to do it all. Learning to manage new tasks—from chores to household repairs to finances—takes time, but it can be done.

Being alone can increase concerns about safety. It's a good idea to make sure there are working locks on the doors and windows. If you need help, ask your family or friends.

Facing the future without a husband or wife can be scary. Many men and women have never lived alone. Those who are both widowed and retired may feel very lonely and become depressed. Talk with your doctor about how you are feeling.

Take Charge of Your Life

After years of being part of a couple, it can be upsetting to be alone. Many people find it helps to have things to do every day. Whether you are still working or are retired, write down your weekly plans. You might:

- Take a walk with a friend.
- Visit the library.
- Volunteer.
- Try an exercise class.
- Join a singing group.
- Join a bowling league.
- Offer to watch your grandchildren.
- Consider adopting a pet.
- Take a class at a nearby senior center, college, or recreation center.
- Stay in touch with family and friends, either in person or online.

Is There More to Do?

When you feel stronger, you should think about getting your legal and financial affairs in order. For example, you might need to:

- Write a new will and advance directive.

- Look into a durable power of attorney for legal matters and healthcare, in case you are unable to make your own medical decisions in the future.

- Put joint property (such as a house or car) in your name.

- Check on changes you might need to make to your health insurance as well as your life, car, and homeowner's insurance.

- Sign up for Medicare by your 65th birthday.

- Make a list of bills you will need to pay in the next few months: for instance, state and federal taxes and your rent or mortgage.

When you are ready, go through your husband's or wife's clothes and other personal items. It may be hard to give away these belongings. Instead of parting with everything at once, you might make three piles: one to keep, one to give away, and one "not sure." Ask your children or others to help. Think about setting aside items like a special piece of clothing, watch, favorite book, or picture to give to your children or grandchildren as personal reminders of your spouse.

What about Going Out?

Having a social life on your own can be tough. It may be hard to think about going to parties or other social events by yourself. It can be hard to think about coming home alone. You may be anxious about dating. Many people miss the feeling of closeness that marriage brings. After time, some are ready to have a social life again.

Here are some things to remember:

- Go at a comfortable pace. There's no rush.

- It's okay to make the first move when it comes to planning things to do.

- Try group activities. Invite friends for a potluck dinner or go to a senior center.

- With married friends, think about informal outings like walks, picnics, or movies rather than couple's events that remind you of the past.

- Find an activity you like. You may have fun and meet people who like to do the same thing.

- You can develop meaningful relationships with friends and family members of all ages.

- Many people find that pets provide important companionship.

Chapter 14

Immunizations

Older adults need to get shots (vaccines) to prevent serious diseases. Protect your health by getting all your shots on schedule.

If you are age 60 or older:

- Get a shot to prevent shingles. Shingles causes a rash and can lead to pain that lasts for months.

If you are age 65 or older:

- Get shots to prevent pneumococcal disease. Pneumococcal disease can include pneumonia, meningitis, and blood infections.

Need for Shots

Shots help protect you against diseases that can be serious and sometimes deadly. Many of these diseases are common.

Even if you have always gotten your shots on schedule, you still need to get some shots as an older adult. This is because:

- Older adults are more likely to get certain diseases.

This chapter contains text excerpted from the following sources: Text in this chapter begins with excerpts from "Get Shots to Protect Your Health (for Older Adults)," Office of Disease Prevention and Health Promotion (ODPHP), U.S. Department of Health and Human Services (HHS), January 31, 2017; Text beginning with the heading "Shots Recommended for Senior Adults" is excerpted from "Shots for Safety," National Institute on Aging (NIA), National Institutes of Health (NIH), July 6, 2017.

149

- Older adults are more at risk for serious complications from infections.

- The protection from some shots can wear off over time.

Getting Your Shots Protects Other People

When you get shots, you don't just protect yourself–you also protect others. This is especially important if you spend time around anyone with a long-term health problem or a weak immune system (the system in the body that fights infections).

Protect yourself and those around you by staying up to date on your shots.

When to Take Shots

You may need other shots if you:

- Didn't get all of your shots as a child

- Have a health condition that weakens your immune system (like cancer or human immunodeficiency virus (HIV))

- Have a chronic (long-term) health problem like diabetes or heart, lung, or liver disease

- Are a man who has sex with men

- Smoke

- Spend time with infants or young children

- Work or spend time in a school, hospital, prison, or health clinic

- Travel outside the United States

Ask your doctor or nurse if you need any other shots.

Take Action!

Talk with a doctor, nurse, or pharmacist about getting up to date on your shots.

Make a Plan to Get Your Shots

Schedule an appointment with your doctor or nurse to get the shots you need. You may also be able to get shots at your local pharmacy.

Get a Seasonal Flu Shot Every Year

Remember, everyone—6 months and older—needs to get the seasonal flu vaccine every year.

What about Cost?

Under the Affordable Care Act (ACA), the healthcare reform law passed in 2010, most private insurance plans must cover recommended shots for adults. Depending on your insurance plan, you may be able to get your shots at no cost to you.

Medicare also covers most recommended shots for older adults, depending on your plan.

If you don't have insurance, you still may be able to get free shots.

- Call your state health department to find a free or low-cost vaccination program.

- Find a health center near you and ask about affordable vaccine services.

Keep a Copy of Your Vaccination Record

Ask your doctor to print out a record of all the shots you've had. Keep this record in a safe place. You may need it for certain jobs or if you travel outside the United States.

If you aren't sure which shots you've had, try finding old vaccination records. If you still can't find a record of your shots, talk with your doctor about getting some shots again.

Shots Recommended for Senior Adults

As you get older, your doctor may recommend vaccinations—shots—to help prevent certain illnesses and to keep you healthy.

Talk with your doctor about which of the following shots you need. And, make sure to protect yourself by keeping your vaccinations up to date.

Flu

Flu—short for influenza—is a virus that can cause fever, chills, sore throat, stuffy nose, headache, and muscle aches. Flu is very serious when it gets in your lungs.

The flu is easy to pass from person to person. The virus also changes over time, which means you can get it over and over again. That's why most people (age 6 months and older) should get the flu shot each year.

Get your shot between September and November. Then, you may be protected when the winter flu season starts.

Pneumococcal Disease

Pneumococcal disease is a serious infection that spreads from person to person by air. It often causes pneumonia in the lungs, and it can affect other parts of the body.

Most people age 65 and older should get a pneumococcal shot to help prevent getting the disease. It's generally safe and can be given at the same time as the flu shot. Usually, people only need the shot once. But, if you were younger than age 65 when you had the shot, you may need a second one to stay protected.

Tetanus and Diphtheria

Tetanus (sometimes called lockjaw) is caused by bacteria found in soil, dust, and manure. It enters the body through cuts in the skin.

Diphtheria is also caused by bacteria. It is a serious illness that can affect the tonsils, throat, nose, or skin. It can spread from person to person.

Both tetanus and diphtheria can lead to death.

Getting a shot is the best way to keep from getting tetanus and diphtheria. Most people get their first shots as children. For adults, a booster shot every 10 years will keep you protected. Ask your doctor if and when you need a booster shot.

Measles, Mumps, and Rubella

Measles, mumps, and rubella are viruses that cause several flu-like symptoms, but may lead to much more serious, long-term health problems, especially in adults.

The vaccine given to children to prevent measles, mumps, and rubella has made these diseases rare. If you don't know if you've had the diseases or the shot, you can still get the vaccine.

Shots for Travel

Check with your doctor or local health department about shots you will need if traveling to other countries. Sometimes, a series of shots is needed. It's best to get them at least 2 weeks before you travel.

Side Effects of Shots

Common side effects for all these shots are mild and include pain, swelling, or redness where the shot was given.

Before getting any vaccine, make sure it's safe for you. Talk with your doctor about your health history, including past illnesses and treatments, as well as any allergies.

It's a good idea to keep your own shot record, listing the types and dates of your shots, along with any side effects or problems.

Part Three

Aging-Associated Diseases and Medical Conditions

Chapter 15

Aging-Associated Cancers

Chapter Contents

Section 15.1

Aging and Cancer

This section contains text excerpted from the following sources:
Text beginning with the heading "What Is Cancer?" is excerpted
from "Understanding Cancer—What Is Cancer?" National Cancer
Institute (NCI), February 9, 2015; Text under the heading "Aging—
An Important Risk Factor" is excerpted from "About Cancer—Causes
and Prevention—Risk Factors," National Cancer Institute (NCI),
April 29, 2015.

What Is Cancer?

Cancer is the name given to a collection of related diseases. In all
types of cancer, some of the body's cells begin to divide without stopping and spread into surrounding tissues.

Cancer can start almost anywhere in the human body, which is
made up of trillions of cells. Normally, human cells grow and divide to
form new cells as the body needs them. When cells grow old or become
damaged, they die, and new cells take their place.

When cancer develops, however, this orderly process breaks down.
As cells become more and more abnormal, old or damaged cells survive
when they should die, and new cells form when they are not needed.
These extra cells can divide without stopping and may form growths
called tumors.

Many cancers form solid tumors, which are masses of tissue.
Cancers of the blood, such as leukemias, generally do not form solid
tumors.

Cancerous tumors are malignant, which means they can spread
into, or invade, nearby tissues. In addition, as these tumors grow,
some cancer cells can break off and travel to distant places in the body
through the blood, or the lymph system, and form new tumors far from
the original tumor.

Unlike malignant tumors, benign tumors do not spread into, or
invade, nearby tissues. Benign tumors can sometimes be quite large,
however. When removed, they usually don't grow back, whereas malignant tumors sometimes do. Unlike most benign tumors elsewhere in
the body, benign brain tumors can be life threatening.

Types of Cancer

There are more than 100 types of cancer. Types of cancer are usually named for the organs or tissues where the cancers form. For example, lung cancer starts in cells of the lung, and brain cancer starts in cells of the brain. Cancers also may be described by the type of cell that formed them, such as an epithelial cell or a squamous cell.

Aging—An Important Risk Factor

Advancing age is the most important risk factor for cancer overall, and for many individual cancer types. According to statistical data from National Cancer Institute's (NCI) Surveillance, Epidemiology, and End Results (SEER) program, the median age of a cancer diagnosis is 66 years. This means that half of cancer cases occur in people below this age and half in people above this age. One-quarter of new cancer cases are diagnosed in people aged 65 to 74.

A similar pattern is seen for many common cancer types. For example, the median age at diagnosis is 61 years for breast cancer, 68 years for colorectal cancer, 70 years for lung cancer, and 66 years for prostate cancer.

But the disease can occur at any age. For example, bone cancer is most frequently diagnosed among people under age 20, with more than one-fourth of cases occurring in this age group. And 10 percent of leukemias are diagnosed in children and adolescents under 20 years of age, whereas only 1 percent of cancer overall is diagnosed in that age group. Some types of cancer, such as neuroblastoma, are more common in children or adolescents than in adults.

Section 15.2

Breast Cancer

This section includes text excerpted from "Breast
Cancer—Basic Information," Centers for Disease
Control and Prevention (CDC), April 4, 2016.

What Is Breast Cancer?

Breast cancer is a disease in which cells in the breast grow out of
control. There are different kinds of breast cancer. The kind of breast
cancer depends on which cells in the breast turn into cancer.

Breast cancer can begin in different parts of the breast. A breast
is made up of three main parts: lobules, ducts, and connective tissue.
The lobules are the glands that produce milk. The ducts are tubes
that carry milk to the nipple. The connective tissue (which consists
of fibrous and fatty tissue) surrounds and holds everything together.
Most breast cancers begin in the ducts or lobules.

Breast cancer can spread outside the breast through blood vessels
and lymph vessels. When breast cancer spreads to other parts of the
body, it is said to have metastasized.

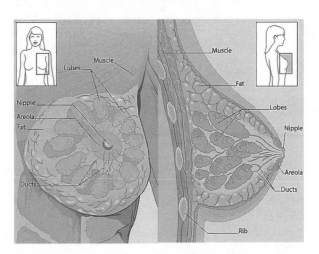

Figure 15.1. *Anterior and Cross-Section View of Breast*

Kinds of Breast Cancer

The most common kinds of breast cancer are:

- **Invasive ductal carcinoma.** The cancer cells grow outside the ducts into other parts of the breast tissue. Invasive cancer cells can also spread, or metastasize, to other parts of the body.

- **Invasive lobular carcinoma.** Cancer cells spread from the lobules to the breast tissues that are close by. These invasive cancer cells can also spread to other parts of the body.

There are several other less common kinds of breast cancer, such as Paget disease, medullary, mucinous, and inflammatory breast cancer.

Ductal carcinoma in situ (DCIS) is a breast disease that may lead to breast cancer. The cancer cells are only in the lining of the ducts, and have not spread to other tissues in the breast.

What Are the Symptoms of Breast Cancer?

Different people have different symptoms of breast cancer. Some people do not have any signs or symptoms at all. A person may find out they have breast cancer after a routine mammogram.

Some warning signs of breast cancer are:

- New lump in the breast or underarm (armpit)

- Thickening or swelling of part of the breast

- Irritation or dimpling of breast skin

- Redness or flaky skin in the nipple area or the breast

- Pulling in of the nipple or pain in the nipple area

- Nipple discharge other than breast milk, including blood

- Any change in the size or the shape of the breast

- Pain in any area of the breast

Keep in mind that these symptoms can happen with other conditions that are not cancer. If you have any signs or symptoms that worry you, be sure to see your doctor right away.

What Is a Normal Breast?

No breast is typical. What is normal for you may not be normal for another woman. Most women say their breasts feel lumpy or uneven.

The way your breasts look and feel can be affected by getting your period, having children, losing or gaining weight, and taking certain medications. Breasts also tend to change as you age.

What Do Lumps in My Breast Mean?

Many conditions can cause lumps in the breast, including cancer. But most breast lumps are caused by other medical conditions. The two most common causes of breast lumps are fibrocystic breast condition and cysts. Fibrocystic condition causes noncancerous changes in the breast that can make them lumpy, tender, and sore. Cysts are small fluid-filled sacs that can develop in the breast.

What Are the Risk Factors for Breast Cancer?

Studies have shown that your risk for breast cancer is due to a combination of factors. The main factors that influence your risk include being a woman and getting older. Most breast cancers are found in women who are 50 years old or older.

Some women will get breast cancer even without any other risk factors that they know of. Having a risk factor does not mean you will get the disease, and not all risk factors have the same effect. Most women have some risk factors, but most women do not get breast cancer. If you have breast cancer risk factors, talk with your doctor about ways you can lower your risk, and about screening for breast cancer.

Your risk of getting breast cancer increases as you get older. Most breast cancers are diagnosed after age 50.

Other risk factors include having:

- **Genetic mutations.** Inherited changes (mutations) to certain genes, such as *BRCA1* and *BRCA2*. Women who have inherited these genetic changes are at higher risk of breast and ovarian cancer.

- **Early menstrual period.** Women who start their periods before age 12 are exposed to hormones longer, raising the risk for breast cancer by a small amount.

- **Late or no pregnancy.** Having the first pregnancy after age 30 and never having a full-term pregnancy can raise breast cancer risk.

- **Starting menopause after age 55.** Like starting one's period early, being exposed to estrogen hormones for a longer time later in life also raises the risk of breast cancer.

- **Not being physically active.** Women who are not physically active have a higher risk of getting breast cancer.

- **Being overweight or obese after menopause.** Older women who are overweight or obese have a higher risk of getting breast cancer than those at a normal weight.

- **Having dense breasts.** Dense breasts have more connective tissue than fatty tissue, which can sometimes make it hard to see tumors on a mammogram. Women with dense breasts are more likely to get breast cancer.

- **Using combination hormone therapy.** Taking hormones to replace missing estrogen and progesterone in menopause for more than five years raises the risk for breast cancer. The hormones that have been shown to increase risk are estrogen and progestin when taken together.

- **Taking oral contraceptives (birth control pills).** Certain forms of oral contraceptive pills have been found to raise breast cancer risk.

- **Personal history of breast cancer.** Women who have had breast cancer are more likely to get breast cancer a second time.

- **Personal history of certain noncancerous breast diseases.** Some noncancerous breast diseases such as atypical hyperplasia or lobular carcinoma in situ are associated with a higher risk of getting breast cancer.

- **Family history of breast cancer.** A woman's risk for breast cancer is higher if she has a mother, sister, or daughter (first-degree relative) or multiple family members on either her mother's or father's side of the family who have had breast cancer. Having a first-degree male relative with breast cancer also raises a woman's risk.

- **Previous treatment using radiation therapy.** Women who had radiation therapy to the chest or breasts (like for treatment of Hodgkin lymphoma) before age 30 have a higher risk of getting breast cancer later in life.

- **Women who took the drug diethylstilbestrol (DES),** which was given to some pregnant women in the United States between 1940 and 1971 to prevent miscarriage, have a higher risk. Women whose mothers took DES while pregnant with them are also at risk.

• **Drinking alcohol.** Studies show that a woman's risk for breast cancer increases with the more alcohol she drinks.

Research suggests that other factors such as smoking, being exposed to chemicals that can cause cancer, and night shift working also may increase breast cancer risk.

What Is Breast Cancer Screening?

Breast cancer screening means checking a woman's breasts for cancer before there are signs or symptoms of the disease. All women need to be informed by their healthcare provider about the best screening options for them. When you are told about the benefits and risks, and decide with your healthcare provider what screening test, if any, is right for you, this is called informed and shared decision-making. Although breast cancer screening cannot prevent breast cancer, it can help find breast cancer early, when it is easier to treat. Talk to your doctor about which breast cancer screening tests are right for you, and when you should have them.

Breast Cancer Screening Recommendations

The United States Preventive Services Task Force (USPSTF) recommends that women who are 50 to 74 years old, and are at average risk for breast cancer, get mammogram every two years. Women who are 40 to 49 years old should talk to their doctor or other healthcare professional about when to start and how often to get a mammogram. Women should weigh the benefits and risks of screening tests when deciding whether to begin getting mammograms at age 40.

Breast Cancer Screening Tests

Mammogram

A mammogram is an X-ray of the breast. Mammograms are the best way to find breast cancer early, when it is easier to treat, and before it is big enough to feel or cause symptoms. Having regular mammograms can lower the risk of dying from breast cancer.

Breast Magnetic Resonance Imaging (MRI)

A breast MRI uses magnets and radio waves to take pictures of the breast. MRI is used along with mammograms to screen women who are at high risk for getting breast cancer. Because breast MRIs may appear abnormal even when there is no cancer, it is not used for women at average risk.

Where Can I Go to Get Screened?

You can get screened for breast cancer at a clinic, hospital, or doctor's office. If you want to be screened for breast cancer, call your doctor's office. They can help you schedule an appointment. Most health insurance plans are required to cover mammograms every one to two years for women beginning at age 40 with no out-of-pocket cost (like a copay, deductible, or coinsurance).

Other Exams

At this time, the best way to find breast cancer is with a mammogram.

Clinical Breast Exam

A clinical breast exam is an examination by a doctor or nurse, who uses his or her hands to feel for lumps or other changes.

Breast Self-Awareness

Being familiar with how your breasts look and feel can help you notice symptoms such as lumps, pain, or changes in size that may be of concern. These could include changes found during a breast self-exam. You should report any changes that you notice to your doctor or healthcare provider. Having a clinical breast exam or doing a breast self-exam has not been found to lower the risk of dying from breast cancer.

How Is Breast Cancer Diagnosed?

Doctors often use additional tests to find or diagnose breast cancer. They may refer women to a breast specialist or a surgeon. This does not mean that she has cancer or that she needs surgery. These doctors are experts in diagnosing breast problems.

- **Breast ultrasound.** A machine that uses sound waves to make detailed pictures, called sonograms, of areas inside the breast.

- **Diagnostic mammogram.** If you have a problem in your breast, such as lumps, or if an area of the breast looks abnormal on a screening mammogram, doctors may have you get a diagnostic mammogram. This is a more detailed X-ray of the breast.

- **MRI.** A kind of body scan that uses a magnet linked to a computer. The MRI scan will make detailed pictures of areas inside the breast.

- **Biopsy.** This is a test that removes tissue or fluid from the breast to be looked at under a microscope and do more testing. There are different kinds of biopsies (for example, fine-needle aspiration, core biopsy, or open biopsy).

Staging

If breast cancer is diagnosed, other tests are done to find out if cancer cells have spread within the breast or to other parts of the body. This process is called staging. Whether the cancer is only in the breast, is found in lymph nodes under your arm, or has spread outside the breast determines your stage of breast cancer. The type and stage of breast cancer tells doctors what kind of treatment you need.

How Is Breast Cancer Treated?

Breast cancer is treated in several ways. It depends on the kind of breast cancer and how far it has spread. People with breast cancer often get more than one kind of treatment.

- **Surgery.** An operation where doctors cut out cancer tissue.

- **Chemotherapy.** Using special medicines to shrink or kill the cancer cells. The drugs can be pills you take or medicines given in your veins, or sometimes both.

- **Hormonal therapy.** Blocks cancer cells from getting the hormones they need to grow.

- **Biological therapy.** Works with your body's immune system to help it fight cancer cells or to control side effects from other cancer treatments.

- **Radiation therapy.** Using high-energy rays (similar to X-rays) to kill the cancer cells.

Doctors from different specialties often work together to treat breast cancer. Surgeons are doctors who perform operations. Medical oncologists are doctors who treat cancer with medicine. Radiation oncologists are doctors who treat cancer with radiation.

Complementary and Alternative Medicine

Complementary and alternative medicine are medicines and health practices that are not standard cancer treatments. Complementary medicine is used in addition to standard treatments, and alternative medicine is used instead of standard treatments. Meditation, yoga, and supplements like vitamins and herbs are some examples. Many kinds of complementary and alternative medicine have not been tested scientifically and may not be safe. Talk to your doctor about the risks and benefits before you start any kind of complementary or alternative medicine.

Section 15.3

Colorectal Cancer

This section contains text excerpted from the following sources: Text beginning with the heading "What Is Colorectal Cancer?" is excerpted from "Colorectal Cancer—Basic Information," Centers for Disease Control and Prevention (CDC), April 25, 2016; Text under the heading "How Is Colon Cancer Treated?" is excerpted from "Colon Cancer Treatment (PDQ®)—Patient Version," National Cancer Institute (NCI), February 27, 2017; Text under the heading "How Is Rectal Cancer Treated?" is excerpted from "Rectal Cancer Treatment (PDQ®)—Patient Version," National Cancer Institute (NCI), May 19, 2017.

What Is Colorectal Cancer?

Colorectal cancer is cancer that occurs in the colon or rectum. Sometimes it is called colon cancer, for short. As the drawing shows, the colon is the large intestine or large bowel. The rectum is the passageway that connects the colon to the anus.

Sometimes abnormal growths, called polyps, form in the colon or rectum. Over time, some polyps may turn into cancer. Screening tests can find polyps so they can be removed before turning into cancer. Screening also helps find colorectal cancer at an early stage, when treatment often leads to a cure.

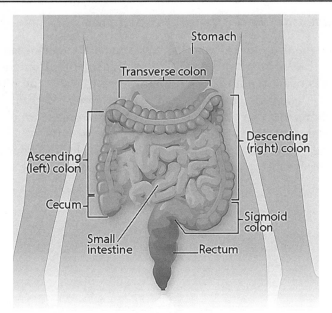

Figure 15.2. *The Colon and Rectum*

What Are the Risk Factors for Colorectal Cancer?

Your risk of getting colorectal cancer increases as you get older. More than 90 percent of cases occur in people who are 50 years old or older.

Other risk factors include having:

- Inflammatory bowel disease such as Crohn's disease or ulcerative colitis

- A personal or family history of colorectal cancer or colorectal polyps

- A genetic syndrome such as familial adenomatous polyposis (FAP) or hereditary nonpolyposis colorectal cancer (Lynch syndrome)

Lifestyle factors that may contribute to an increased risk of colorectal cancer include:

- Lack of regular physical activity

- A diet low in fruit and vegetables

- A low-fiber and high-fat diet

168

- Overweight and obesity

- Alcohol consumption

- Tobacco use

What Are the Symptoms of Colorectal Cancer?

Colorectal polyps and colorectal cancer don't always cause symptoms, especially at first. Someone could have polyps or colorectal cancer and not know it. That is why getting screened regularly for colorectal cancer is so important.

If you have symptoms, they may include:

- Blood in or on your stool (bowel movement)

- Stomach pain, aches, or cramps that don't go away

- Losing weight and you don't know why

If you have any of these symptoms, talk to your doctor. They may be caused by something other than cancer. The only way to know what is causing them is to see your doctor.

What Is Colorectal Cancer Screening?

A screening test is used to look for a disease when a person doesn't have symptoms. (When a person has symptoms, diagnostic tests are used to find out the cause of the symptoms.)

Colorectal cancer almost always develops from precancerous polyps (abnormal growths) in the colon or rectum. Screening tests can find precancerous polyps, so that they can be removed before they turn into cancer. Screening tests can also find colorectal cancer early, when treatment works best.

The United States Preventive Services Task Force (USPSTF) recommends that adults age 50 to 75 be screened for colorectal cancer. The decision to be screened after age 75 should be made on an individual basis. If you are older than 75, ask your doctor if you should be screened. People at an increased risk of developing colorectal cancer should talk to their doctors about when to begin screening, which test is right for them, and how often to get tested.

Several screening tests can be used to find polyps or colorectal cancer. The Task Force outlines the following colorectal cancer screening strategies. Talk to your doctor about which of the following tests are right for you.

Stool Tests

- The **guaiac-based fecal occult blood test (gFOBT)** uses the chemical guaiac to detect blood in the stool. It is done once a year. For this test, you receive a test kit from your health-care provider. At home, you use a stick or brush to obtain a small amount of stool. You return the test kit to the doctor or a lab, where the stool samples are checked for the presence of blood.

- The **fecal immunochemical test (FIT)** uses antibodies to detect blood in the stool. It is also done once a year in the same way as a gFOBT.

- The **FIT- Deoxyribonucleic acid (DNA) test** (also referred to as the stool DNA test) combines the FIT with a test that detects altered DNA in the stool. For this test, you collect an entire bowel movement and send it to a lab to be checked for cancer cells. It is done once every one or three years.

Flexible Sigmoidoscopy

For this test, the doctor puts a short, thin, flexible, lighted tube into your rectum. The doctor checks for polyps or cancer inside the rectum and lower third of the colon.

How often: Every 5 years, or every 10 years with a FIT every year.

Colonoscopy

This is similar to flexible sigmoidoscopy, except the doctor uses a longer, thin, flexible, lighted tube to check for polyps or cancer inside the rectum and the entire colon. During the test, the doctor can find and remove most polyps and some cancers. Colonoscopy also is used as a follow-up test if anything unusual is found during one of the other screening tests.

How often: Every 10 years.

CT Colonography (Virtual Colonoscopy)

Computed tomography (CT) colonography, also called a virtual colonoscopy, uses X-rays and computers to produce images of the entire colon, which are displayed on a computer screen for the doctor to analyze.

How often: Every 5 years.

How Do I Know Which Screening Test Is Right for Me?

There is no single "best test" for any person. Each test has advantages and disadvantages. Talk to your doctor about the pros and cons of each test, and how often to be tested. Which test to use depends on:

- Your preferences

- Your medical condition

- The likelihood that you will get the test

- The resources available for testing and follow-up

How Is Colon Cancer Treated?

Six types of standard treatment are used:

1. **Surgery**

   Surgery (removing the cancer in an operation) is the most common treatment for all stages of colon cancer. A doctor may remove the cancer using one of the following types of surgery:

   - Local excision

   - Resection of the colon with anastomosis

   - Resection of the colon with colostomy

2. **Radiofrequency ablation**

   Radiofrequency ablation is the use of a special probe with tiny electrodes that kill cancer cells.

3. **Cryosurgery**

   Cryosurgery is a treatment that uses an instrument to freeze and destroy abnormal tissue. This type of treatment is also called cryotherapy.

4. **Chemotherapy**

   Chemotherapy is a cancer treatment that uses drugs to stop the growth of cancer cells, either by killing the cells or by stopping them from dividing. When chemotherapy is taken by mouth or injected into a vein or muscle, the drugs enter the bloodstream and can reach cancer cells throughout the body (systemic chemotherapy).

5. Radiation therapy

Radiation therapy is a cancer treatment that uses high-energy X-rays or other types of radiation to kill cancer cells or keep them from growing. There are two types of radiation therapy:

- External radiation therapy
- Internal radiation therapy

6. Targeted therapy

Targeted therapy is a type of treatment that uses drugs or other substances to identify and attack specific cancer cells without harming normal cells. Types of targeted therapies used in the treatment of colon cancer include the following:

- Monoclonal antibodies
- Angiogenesis inhibitors

How Is Rectal Cancer Treated?

Five types of standard treatment are used:

1. Surgery

Surgery is the most common treatment for all stages of rectal cancer. The cancer is removed using one of the following types of surgery:

- Polypectomy
- Local excision
- Resection
- Radiofrequency ablation
- Cryosurgery
- Pelvic exenteration

2. Radiation therapy

Radiation therapy is a cancer treatment that uses high-energy X-rays or other types of radiation to kill cancer cells or keep them from growing. There are two types of radiation therapy:

- External radiation therapy
- Internal radiation therapy

3. Chemotherapy

Chemotherapy is a cancer treatment that uses drugs to stop the growth of cancer cells, either by killing the cells or by stopping the cells from dividing. When chemotherapy is taken by mouth or injected into a vein or muscle, the drugs enter the bloodstream and can reach cancer cells throughout the body (systemic chemotherapy.)

4. Active surveillance

Active surveillance is closely following a patient's condition without giving any treatment unless there are changes in test results. It is used to find early signs that the condition is getting worse. In active surveillance, patients are given certain exams and tests to check if the cancer is growing. When the cancer begins to grow, treatment is given to cure the cancer.

5. Targeted therapy

Targeted therapy is a type of treatment that uses drugs or other substances to identify and attack specific cancer cells without harming normal cells. Types of targeted therapies used in the treatment of rectal cancer include the following:

- Monoclonal antibodies

- Angiogenesis inhibitors

Section 15.4

Prostate Cancer

This section includes text excerpted from "Prostate Cancer,"
Centers for Disease Control and Prevention (CDC),
February 27, 2017.

Prostate cancer is the most common nonskin cancer among American men. Prostate cancers usually grow slowly. Most men with prostate cancer are older than 65 years and do not die from the disease.

What Is Prostate Cancer?

When cancer starts in the prostate, it is called prostate cancer. Except for skin cancer, prostate cancer is the most common cancer in American men.

What Is the Prostate?

The prostate is a part of the male reproductive system, which includes the penis, prostate, and testicles. The prostate is located just below the bladder and in front of the rectum. It is about the size of a walnut and surrounds the urethra (the tube that empties urine from the bladder). It produces fluid that makes up a part of semen.

As a man ages, the prostate tends to increase in size. This can cause the urethra to narrow and decrease urine flow. This is called benign prostatic hyperplasia, and it is not the same as prostate cancer. Men may also have other prostate changes that are not cancer.

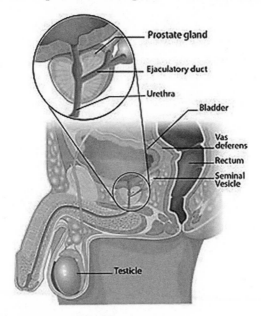

Figure 15.3. *Male Reproductive System*

What Are the Risk Factors?

The older a man is, the greater his risk for getting prostate cancer. Research has found other risk factors that increase your chances of getting prostate cancer.

These risk factors include:

- **Family history:** Certain genes (passed from parent to child) that you inherited from your parents may affect your prostate cancer risk. Currently, no single gene is sure to raise or lower your risk of getting prostate cancer. However, a man with a father, brother, or son who has had prostate cancer is two to three times more likely to develop the disease himself.

- **Race:** Prostate cancer is more common in African-American men. It tends to start at younger ages and grow faster than in other racial or ethnic groups, but medical experts do not know why.

Researchers are trying to determine the causes of prostate cancer and whether it can be prevented. They do not yet agree on the factors that can influence a man's risk of developing the disease, either positively or negatively.

What Screening Tests Are There for Prostate Cancer?

Cancer screening means looking for cancer before it causes symptoms. However, most prostate cancers grow slowly or not at all. Two tests are commonly used to screen for prostate cancer:

- **Digital rectal exam (DRE):** A doctor or nurse inserts a gloved, lubricated finger into the rectum to estimate the size of the prostate and feel for lumps or other abnormalities.

- **Prostate specific antigen (PSA) test:** Measures the level of PSA in the blood. PSA is a substance made by the prostate. The levels of PSA in the blood can be higher in men who have prostate cancer. The PSA level may also be elevated in other conditions that affect the prostate.

As a rule, the higher the PSA level in the blood, the more likely a prostate problem is present. But many factors, such as age and race, can affect PSA levels. Some prostate glands make more PSA than others. PSA levels also can be affected by:

- Certain medical procedures
- Certain medications
- An enlarged prostate
- A prostate infection

Because many factors can affect PSA levels, your doctor is the best person to interpret your PSA test results. Only a biopsy can diagnose prostate cancer for sure.

How Is Prostate Cancer Diagnosed?

If your PSA test or DRE is abnormal, doctors may do more tests to find or diagnose prostate cancer.

A biopsy is when a small piece of tissue is removed from the prostate and looked at under a microscope to see if there are cancer cells.

A Gleason score is determined when the biopsy is looked at under the microscope. If there is a cancer, the score indicates how likely it is to spread. The score ranges from 2 to 10. The lower the score, the less likely it is that the cancer will spread.

A biopsy is the main tool for diagnosing prostate cancer, but a doctor can use other tools to help make sure the biopsy is made in the right place. For example, doctors may use a transrectal ultrasound, when a probe the size of a finger is inserted into the rectum and high-energy sound waves (ultrasound) are bounced off the prostate to create a picture of the prostate called a sonogram. Doctors also may use magnetic resonance imaging (MRI) to guide the biopsy.

Staging

If prostate cancer is diagnosed, other tests are done to find out if cancer cells have spread within the prostate or to other parts of the body. This process is called staging. Whether the cancer is only in the prostate, or has spread outside the prostate, determines your stage of prostate cancer. The stage of prostate cancer tells doctors what kind of treatment you need.

How Is Prostate Cancer Treated?

Different types of treatment are available for prostate cancer. You and your doctor will decide which treatment is right for you. Some common treatments are:

- **Active surveillance.** Closely monitoring the prostate cancer by performing PSA and DRE tests regularly, and treating the cancer only if it grows or causes symptoms.

- **Surgery.** A prostatectomy is an operation where doctors remove the prostate. Radical prostatectomy removes the prostate as well as the surrounding tissue.

- **Radiation therapy.** Using high-energy rays (similar to X-rays) to kill the cancer. There are two types of radiation therapy:

- **External radiation therapy.** A machine outside the body directs radiation at the cancer cells.

- **Internal radiation therapy (Brachytherapy).** Radioactive seeds or pellets are surgically placed into or near the cancer to destroy the cancer cells.

- **Hormone therapy.** Blocks cancer cells from getting the hormones they need to grow.

Other therapies used in the treatment of prostate cancer that are still under investigation include:

- **Cryotherapy.** Placing a special probe inside or near the prostate cancer to freeze and kill the cancer cells.

- **Chemotherapy.** Using special drugs to shrink or kill the cancer. The drugs can be pills you take or medicines given through your veins, or, sometimes, both.

- **Biological therapy.** Works with your body's immune system to help it fight cancer or to control side effects from other cancer treatments. Side effects are how your body reacts to drugs or other treatments.

- **High-intensity focused ultrasound.** This therapy directs high-energy sound waves (ultrasound) at the cancer to kill cancer cells.

Chapter 16

Vascular Disorders

Chapter Contents

Section 16.1

Atherosclerosis

This section includes text excerpted from "Atherosclerosis,"
National Heart, Lung, and Blood Institute (NHLBI), June 22, 2016.

What Is Atherosclerosis?

Atherosclerosis is a disease in which plaque builds up inside your arteries. Arteries are blood vessels that carry oxygen-rich blood to your heart and other parts of your body. Plaque is made up of fat, cholesterol, calcium, and other substances found in the blood. Over time, plaque hardens and narrows your arteries. This limits the flow of oxygen-rich blood to your organs and other parts of your body. Atherosclerosis can lead to serious problems, including heart attack, stroke, or even death.

Atherosclerosis-Related Diseases

Atherosclerosis can affect any artery in the body, including arteries in the heart, brain, arms, legs, pelvis, and kidneys. As a result, different diseases may develop based on which arteries are affected.

Coronary Heart Disease (CHD)

CHD, also called coronary artery disease, occurs when plaque builds up in the coronary arteries. These arteries supply oxygen-rich blood to your heart. Plaque narrows the coronary arteries and reduces blood flow to your heart muscle. Plaque buildup also makes it more likely that blood clots will form in your arteries. Blood clots can partially or completely block blood flow. If blood flow to your heart muscle is reduced or blocked, you may have angina (chest pain or discomfort) or a heart attack. Plaque also can form in the heart's smallest arteries. This disease is called coronary microvascular disease (MVD). In coronary MVD, plaque doesn't cause blockages in the arteries as it does in CHD.

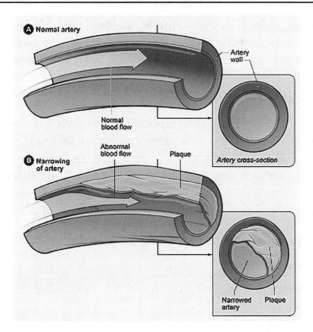

Figure 16.1. *Atherosclerosis*

Figure A shows a normal artery with normal blood flow. The inset image shows a cross-section of a normal artery. Figure B shows an artery with plaque buildup. The inset image shows a cross-section of an artery with plaque buildup.

Carotid Artery Disease

Carotid artery disease occurs if plaque builds up in the arteries on each side of your neck (the carotid arteries). These arteries supply oxygen-rich blood to your brain. If blood flow to your brain is reduced or blocked, you may have a stroke.

Peripheral Artery Disease

Peripheral artery disease (P.A.D.) occurs if plaque builds up in the major arteries that supply oxygen-rich blood to your legs, arms, and pelvis. If blood flow to these parts of your body is reduced or blocked, you may have numbness, pain, and sometimes, dangerous infections.

Chronic Kidney Disease

Chronic kidney disease can occur if plaque builds up in the renal arteries. These arteries supply oxygen-rich blood to your kidneys. Over time, chronic kidney disease causes a slow loss of kidney function. The main function of the kidneys is to remove waste and extra water from the body.

What Causes Atherosclerosis?

The exact cause of atherosclerosis isn't known. However, studies show that atherosclerosis is a slow, complex disease that may start in childhood. It develops faster as you age. Atherosclerosis may start when certain factors damage the inner layers of the arteries. These factors include:

- Smoking

- High amounts of certain fats and cholesterol in the blood

- High blood pressure

- High amounts of sugar in the blood due to insulin resistance or diabetes

Plaque may begin to build up where the arteries are damaged. Over time, plaque hardens and narrows the arteries. Eventually, an area of plaque can rupture (break open). When this happens, blood cell fragments called platelets stick to the site of the injury. They may clump together to form blood clots. Clots narrow the arteries even more, limiting the flow of oxygen-rich blood to your body. Depending on which arteries are affected, blood clots can worsen angina (chest pain) or cause a heart attack or stroke. Researchers continue to look for the causes of atherosclerosis. They hope to find answers to questions such as:

- Why and how do the arteries become damaged?

- How does plaque develop and change over time?

- Why does plaque rupture and lead to blood clots?

Who Is at Risk for Atherosclerosis?

The exact cause of atherosclerosis isn't known. However, certain traits, conditions, or habits may raise your risk for the disease. These conditions are known as risk factors. The more risk factors you have, the more likely it is that you'll develop atherosclerosis. You can control most risk factors and help prevent or delay atherosclerosis. Other risk factors can't be controlled.

Major Risk Factors

- **Older age.** As you get older, your risk for atherosclerosis increases. Genetic or lifestyle factors cause plaque to build up in your arteries as you age. By the time you're middle-aged or older, enough plaque has built up to cause signs or symptoms. In men, the risk increases after age 45. In women, the risk increases after age 55.

- **Unhealthy blood cholesterol levels.** This includes high LDL cholesterol (Low-Density Lipoprotein) (sometimes called "bad" cholesterol) and low HDL (High-Density Lipoprotein) cholesterol (sometimes called "good" cholesterol).

- **High blood pressure.** Blood pressure is considered high if it stays at or above 140/90 mmHg over time. If you have diabetes or chronic kidney disease, high blood pressure is defined as 130/80 mmHg or higher. (The mmHg is millimeters of mercury—the units used to measure blood pressure.)

- **Smoking.** Smoking can damage and tighten blood vessels, raise cholesterol levels, and raise blood pressure. Smoking also doesn't allow enough oxygen to reach the body's tissues.

- **Insulin resistance.** This condition occurs if the body can't use its insulin properly. Insulin is a hormone that helps move blood sugar into cells where it's used as an energy source. Insulin resistance may lead to diabetes.

- **Diabetes.** With this disease, the body's blood sugar level is too high because the body doesn't make enough insulin or doesn't use its insulin properly.

- **Overweight or obesity.** The terms "overweight" and "obesity" refer to body weight that's greater than what is considered healthy for a certain height.

- **Lack of physical activity.** A lack of physical activity can worsen other risk factors for atherosclerosis, such as unhealthy blood cholesterol levels, high blood pressure, diabetes, and overweight and obesity.

- **Unhealthy diet.** An unhealthy diet can raise your risk for atherosclerosis. Foods that are high in saturated and trans fats, cholesterol, sodium (salt), and sugar can worsen other atherosclerosis risk factors.

- **Family history of early heart disease.** Your risk for atherosclerosis increases if your father or a brother was diagnosed with heart disease before 55 years of age, or if your mother or a sister was diagnosed with heart disease before 65 years of age.

Although age and a family history of early heart disease are risk factors, it doesn't mean that you'll develop atherosclerosis if you have one or both. Controlling other risk factors often can lessen genetic influences and prevent atherosclerosis, even in older adults. Studies show that an increasing number of children and youth are at risk for atherosclerosis. This is due to a number of causes, including rising childhood obesity rates.

What Are the Signs and Symptoms of Atherosclerosis?

Atherosclerosis usually doesn't cause signs and symptoms until it severely narrows or totally blocks an artery. Many people don't know they have the disease until they have a medical emergency, such as a heart attack or stroke. Some people may have signs and symptoms of the disease. Signs and symptoms will depend on which arteries are affected.

Coronary Arteries

The coronary arteries supply oxygen-rich blood to your heart. If plaque narrows or blocks these arteries (a disease called coronary heart disease, or CHD), a common symptom is angina. Angina is chest pain or discomfort that occurs when your heart muscle doesn't get enough oxygen-rich blood. Angina may feel like pressure or squeezing in your chest. You also may feel it in your shoulders, arms, neck, jaw, or back. Angina pain may even feel like indigestion. The pain tends to get worse with activity and go away with rest. Emotional stress also can trigger the pain.

Other symptoms of CHD are shortness of breath and arrhythmias. Arrhythmias are problems with the rate or rhythm of the heartbeat. Plaque also can form in the heart's smallest arteries. This disease is called coronary microvascular disease (MVD). Symptoms of coronary MVD include angina, shortness of breath, sleep problems, fatigue (tiredness), and lack of energy.

Carotid Arteries

The carotid arteries supply oxygen-rich blood to your brain. If plaque narrows or blocks these arteries (a disease called carotid artery disease), you may have symptoms of a stroke. These symptoms may include:

- Sudden weakness
- Paralysis (an inability to move) or numbness of the face, arms, or legs, especially on one side of the body
- Confusion
- Trouble speaking or understanding speech
- Trouble seeing in one or both eyes
- Problems breathing
- Dizziness, trouble walking, loss of balance or coordination, and unexplained falls
- Loss of consciousness
- Sudden and severe headache

How Is Atherosclerosis Diagnosed?

Your doctor will diagnose atherosclerosis based on your medical and family histories, a physical exam, and test results.

Physical Exam

During the physical exam, your doctor may listen to your arteries for an abnormal whooshing sound called a bruit. Your doctor can hear a bruit when placing a stethoscope over an affected artery. A bruit may indicate poor blood flow due to plaque buildup. Your doctor also may check to see whether any of your pulses (for example, in the leg or foot) are weak or absent. A weak or absent pulse can be a sign of a blocked artery.

Diagnostic Tests

Your doctor may recommend one or more tests to diagnose atherosclerosis. These tests also can help your doctor learn the extent of your disease and plan the best treatment.

Blood Tests

Blood tests check the levels of certain fats, cholesterol, sugar, and proteins in your blood. Abnormal levels may be a sign that you're at risk for atherosclerosis.

Electrocardiogram (EKG)

An EKG is a simple, painless test that detects and records the heart's electrical activity. The test shows how fast the heart is beating and its rhythm (steady or irregular). An EKG also records the strength and timing of electrical signals as they pass through the heart. An EKG can show signs of heart damage caused by CHD. The test also can show signs of a previous or current heart attack.

Chest X-Ray

A chest X-ray takes pictures of the organs and structures inside your chest, such as your heart, lungs, and blood vessels. A chest X-ray can reveal signs of heart failure.

Ankle / Brachial Index

This test compares the blood pressure in your ankle with the blood pressure in your arm to see how well your blood is flowing. This test can help diagnose P.A.D.

Echocardiography

Echocardiography (echo) uses sound waves to create a moving picture of your heart. The test provides information about the size and shape of your heart and how well your heart chambers and valves are working. Echo also can identify areas of poor blood flow to the heart, areas of heart muscle that aren't contracting normally, and previous injury to the heart muscle caused by poor blood flow.

Computed Tomography (CT) Scan

A CT scan creates computer-generated pictures of the heart, brain, or other areas of the body. The test can show hardening and narrowing of large arteries. A cardiac CT scan also can show whether calcium has built up in the walls of the coronary (heart) arteries. This may be an early sign of CHD.

Stress Testing

During stress testing, you exercise to make your heart work hard and beat fast while heart tests are done. If you can't exercise, you may be given medicine to make your heart work hard and beat fast. When your heart is working hard, it needs more blood and oxygen.

Plaque-narrowed arteries can't supply enough oxygen-rich blood to meet your heart's needs. A stress test can show possible signs and symptoms of CHD, such as:

- Abnormal changes in your heart rate or blood pressure
- Shortness of breath or chest pain
- Abnormal changes in your heart rhythm or your heart's electrical activity

As part of some stress tests, pictures are taken of your heart while you exercise and while you rest. These imaging stress tests can show how well blood is flowing in various parts of your heart. They also can show how well your heart pumps blood when it beats.

Angiography

Angiography is a test that uses dye and special X-rays to show the inside of your arteries. This test can show whether plaque is blocking your arteries and how severe the blockage is. A thin, flexible tube called a catheter is put into a blood vessel in your arm, groin (upper thigh), or neck. Dye that can be seen on an X-ray picture is injected through the catheter into the arteries. By looking at the X-ray picture, your doctor can see the flow of blood through your arteries.

Other Tests

Other tests are being studied to see whether they can give a better view of plaque buildup in the arteries. Examples of these tests include MRI and positron emission tomography (PET).

How Is Atherosclerosis Treated?

Treatments for atherosclerosis may include heart-healthy lifestyle changes, medicines, and medical procedures or surgery. The goals of treatment include:

- Lowering the risk of blood clots forming
- Preventing atherosclerosis-related diseases
- Reducing risk factors in an effort to slow or stop the buildup of plaque
- Relieving symptoms
- Widening or bypassing plaque-clogged arteries

Heart-Healthy Lifestyle Changes

Your doctor may recommend heart-healthy lifestyle changes if you have atherosclerosis. Heart-healthy lifestyle changes include heart-healthy eating, aiming for a healthy weight, managing stress, physical activity, and quitting smoking.

Medicines

Sometimes lifestyle changes alone aren't enough to control your cholesterol levels. For example, you also may need statin medications to control or lower your cholesterol. By lowering your blood cholesterol level, you can decrease your chance of having a heart attack or stroke. Doctors usually prescribe statins for people who have:

- Coronary heart disease, peripheral artery disease, or had a prior stroke
- Diabetes
- High LDL cholesterol levels

Doctors may discuss beginning statin treatment with people who have an elevated risk for developing heart disease or having a stroke. Your doctor also may prescribe other medications to:

- Lower your blood pressure
- Lower your blood sugar levels
- Prevent blood clots, which can lead to heart attack and stroke
- Prevent inflammation

Take all medicines regularly, as your doctor prescribes. Don't change the amount of your medicine or skip a dose unless your doctor tells you to. You should still follow a heart healthy lifestyle, even if you take medicines to treat your atherosclerosis.

Medical Procedures and Surgery

If you have severe atherosclerosis, your doctor may recommend a medical procedure or surgery.

- **Percutaneous coronary intervention (PCI),** also known as coronary angioplasty, is a procedure that's used to open blocked or narrowed coronary (heart) arteries. PCI can improve blood flow to the heart and relieve chest pain. Sometimes a small mesh tube called a stent is placed in the artery to keep it open after the procedure.

- **Coronary artery bypass grafting (CABG)** is a type of surgery. In CABG, arteries or veins from other areas in your body are used to bypass or go around your narrowed coronary arteries. CABG can improve blood flow to your heart, relieve chest pain, and possibly prevent a heart attack.

- **Bypass grafting** also can be used for leg arteries. For this surgery, a healthy blood vessel is used to bypass a narrowed or blocked artery in one of the legs. The healthy blood vessel redirects blood around the blocked artery, improving blood flow to the leg.

- **Carotid endarterectomy** is a type of surgery to remove plaque buildup from the carotid arteries in the neck. This procedure restores blood flow to the brain, which can help prevent a stroke.

How Can Atherosclerosis Be Prevented or Delayed?

Taking action to control your risk factors can help prevent or delay atherosclerosis and its related diseases. Your risk for atherosclerosis increases with the number of risk factors you have. One step you can take is to adopt a healthy lifestyle, which can include:

- Heart-healthy eating

- Physical activity

- Quit smoking

- Weight control

Other steps that can prevent or delay atherosclerosis include knowing your family history of atherosclerosis. If you or someone in your family has an atherosclerosis-related disease, be sure to tell your doctor. If lifestyle changes aren't enough, your doctor may prescribe medicines to control your atherosclerosis risk factors. Take all of your medicines as your doctor advises.

Section 16.2

Heart Attack

This section includes text excerpted from "Heart Attack,"
National Heart, Lung, and Blood Institute (NHLBI),
January 27, 2015.

What Is a Heart Attack?

A heart attack happens when the flow of oxygen-rich blood to a section of heart muscle suddenly becomes blocked and the heart can't get oxygen. If blood flow isn't restored quickly, the section of heart muscle begins to die.

Heart attacks most often occur as a result of coronary heart disease (CHD), also called coronary artery disease. CHD is a condition in which a waxy substance called plaque builds up inside the coronary arteries. These arteries supply oxygen-rich blood to your heart.

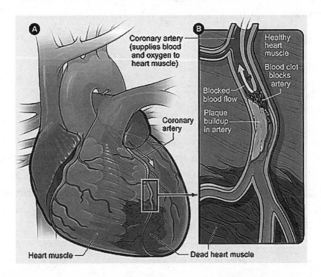

Figure 16.2. *Heart with Muscle Damage and a Blocked Artery*

Figure A is an overview of a heart and coronary artery showing damage (dead heart muscle) caused by a heart attack. Figure B is a cross-section of the coronary artery with plaque buildup and a blood clot.

A less common cause of heart attack is a severe spasm (tightening) of a coronary artery. The spasm cuts off blood flow through the artery. Spasms can occur in coronary arteries that aren't affected by atherosclerosis. Heart attacks can be associated with or lead to severe health problems, such as heart failure and life-threatening arrhythmias. Heart failure is a condition in which the heart can't pump enough blood to meet the body's needs. Arrhythmias are irregular heartbeats. Ventricular fibrillation is a life-threatening arrhythmia that can cause death if not treated right away.

Who Is at Risk for a Heart Attack?

Certain risk factors make it more likely that you'll develop CHD and have a heart attack. You can control many of these risk factors.

Risk Factors You Can't Control

Risk factors that you can't control include:

- **Age.** The risk of heart disease increases for men after age 45 and for women after age 55 (or after menopause).

- **Family history of early heart disease.** Your risk increases if your father or a brother was diagnosed with heart disease before 55 years of age, or if your mother or a sister was diagnosed with heart disease before 65 years of age.

- **Preeclampsia.** This condition can develop during pregnancy. The two main signs of preeclampsia are a rise in blood pressure and excess protein in the urine. Preeclampsia is linked to an increased lifetime risk of heart disease, including CHD, heart attack, heart failure, and high blood pressure.

Risk Factors You Can Control

The major risk factors for a heart attack that you can control include:

- Smoking

- High blood pressure

- High blood cholesterol

- Overweight and obesity

- An unhealthy diet (for example, a diet high in saturated fat, trans fat, cholesterol, and sodium)

- Lack of routine physical activity

- High blood sugar due to insulin resistance or diabetes

Some of these risk factors—such as obesity, high blood pressure, and high blood sugar—tend to occur together. When they do, it's called metabolic syndrome.

In general, a person who has metabolic syndrome is twice as likely to develop heart disease and five times as likely to develop diabetes as someone who doesn't have metabolic syndrome.

What Are the Symptoms of a Heart Attack?

Not all heart attacks begin with the sudden, crushing chest pain that often is shown on TV or in the movies. In one study, for example, one-third of the patients who had heart attacks had no chest pain. These patients were more likely to be older, female, or diabetic.

The symptoms of a heart attack can vary from person to person. Some people can have few symptoms and are surprised to learn they've had a heart attack. If you've already had a heart attack, your symptoms may not be the same for another one. It is important for you to know the most common symptoms of a heart attack and also remember these facts:

- Heart attacks can start slowly and cause only mild pain or discomfort. Symptoms can be mild or more intense and sudden. Symptoms also may come and go over several hours.

- People who have high blood sugar (diabetes) may have no symptoms or very mild ones.

- The most common symptom, in both men and women, is chest pain or discomfort.

- Women are somewhat more likely to have shortness of breath, nausea and vomiting, unusual tiredness (sometimes for days), and pain in the back, shoulders, and jaw.

Some people don't have symptoms at all. Heart attacks that occur without any symptoms or with very mild symptoms are called silent heart attacks.

Not everyone having a heart attack has typical symptoms. If you've already had a heart attack, your symptoms may not be the same for another one. However, some people may have a pattern of symptoms that recur. The more signs and symptoms you have, the more likely it is that you're having a heart attack.

How Is a Heart Attack Diagnosed?

Your doctor will diagnose a heart attack based on your signs and symptoms, your medical and family histories, and test results.

Diagnostic Tests

EKG (Electrocardiogram)

An EKG is a simple, painless test that detects and records the heart's electrical activity. The test shows how fast the heart is beating and its rhythm (steady or irregular). An EKG also records the strength and timing of electrical signals as they pass through each part of the heart. An EKG can show signs of heart damage due to CHD and signs of a previous or current heart attack.

Blood Tests

During a heart attack, heart muscle cells die and release proteins into the bloodstream. Blood tests can measure the amount of these proteins in the bloodstream. Higher than normal levels of these proteins suggest a heart attack. Commonly used blood tests include troponin tests, CK or CK–MB tests, and serum myoglobin tests. Blood tests often are repeated to check for changes over time.

Coronary Angiography

Coronary angiography is a test that uses dye and special X-rays to show the insides of your coronary arteries. This test often is done during a heart attack to help find blockages in the coronary arteries. To get the dye into your coronary arteries, your doctor will use a procedure called cardiac catheterization.

A thin, flexible tube called a catheter is put into a blood vessel in your arm, groin (upper thigh), or neck. The tube is threaded into your coronary arteries, and the dye is released into your bloodstream. Special X-rays are taken while the dye is flowing through the coronary arteries. The dye lets your doctor study the flow of blood through the heart and blood vessels.

If your doctor finds a blockage, he or she may recommend a procedure called percutaneous coronary intervention (PCI), sometimes referred to as coronary angioplasty. This procedure can help restore blood flow through a blocked artery. Sometimes a small mesh tube called a stent is placed in the artery to help prevent blockages after the procedure.

How Is a Heart Attack Treated?

Immediate Treatment

Certain treatments usually are started right away if a heart attack is suspected, even before the diagnosis is confirmed. These include:

- Aspirin to prevent further blood clotting
- Nitroglycerin to reduce your heart's workload and improve blood flow through the coronary arteries
- Oxygen therapy
- Treatment for chest pain

Once the diagnosis of a heart attack is confirmed or strongly suspected, doctors start treatments promptly to try to restore blood flow through the blood vessels supplying the heart. The two main treatments are clot-busting medicines and percutaneous coronary intervention, also known as coronary angioplasty, a procedure used to open blocked coronary arteries.

Clot-Busting Medicines

Thrombolytic medicines, also called clot busters, are used to dissolve blood clots that are blocking the coronary arteries. To work best, these medicines must be given within several hours of the start of heart attack symptoms. Ideally, the medicine should be given as soon as possible.

Percutaneous Coronary Intervention

Percutaneous coronary intervention is a nonsurgical procedure that opens blocked or narrowed coronary arteries. A thin, flexible tube (catheter) with a balloon or other device on the end is threaded through a blood vessel, usually in the groin (upper thigh), to the narrowed or blocked coronary artery. Once in place, the balloon located at the tip of the catheter is inflated to compress the plaque and related clot against the wall of the artery. This restores blood flow through the artery. During the procedure, the doctor may put a small mesh tube called a stent in the artery. The stent helps to keep the blood vessel open to prevent blockages in the artery in the months or years after the procedure.

Other Treatments for Heart Attack

Other treatments for heart attack include:

Medicines

Your doctor may prescribe one or more of the following medicines:

- **ACE inhibitors.** ACE inhibitors lower blood pressure and reduce strain on your heart. They also help slow down further weakening of the heart muscle.

- **Anticlotting medicines.** Anticlotting medicines stop platelets from clumping together and forming unwanted blood clots. Examples of anticlotting medicines include aspirin and clopidogrel.

- **Anticoagulants.** Anticoagulants, or blood thinners, prevent blood clots from forming in your arteries. These medicines also keep existing clots from getting larger.

- **Beta blockers.** Beta blockers decrease your heart's workload. These medicines also are used to relieve chest pain and discomfort and to help prevent another heart attack. Beta blockers also are used to treat arrhythmias (irregular heartbeats).

- **Statin medicines.** Statins control or lower your blood cholesterol. By lowering your blood cholesterol level, you can decrease your chance of having another heart attack or stroke.

You also may be given medicines to relieve pain and anxiety, and treat arrhythmias. Take all medicines regularly, as your doctor prescribes. Don't change the amount of your medicine or skip a dose unless your doctor tells you to.

Medical Procedures

Coronary artery bypass grafting also may be used to treat a heart attack. During coronary artery bypass grafting, a surgeon removes a healthy artery or vein from your body. The artery or vein is then connected, or grafted, to bypass the blocked section of the coronary artery. The grafted artery or vein bypasses (that is, goes around) the blocked portion of the coronary artery. This provides a new route for blood to flow to the heart muscle.

Heart-Healthy Lifestyle Changes

Treatment for a heart attack usually includes making heart-healthy lifestyle changes. Your doctor also may recommend:

- Heart-healthy eating

- Aiming for healthy weight

- Managing stress

- Physical activity

- Quitting smoking

Taking these steps can lower your chances of having another heart attack.

Cardiac Rehabilitation

Your doctor may recommend cardiac rehabilitation (cardiac rehab) to help you recover from a heart attack and to help prevent another heart attack. Nearly everyone who has had a heart attack can benefit from rehab. Cardiac rehab is a medically supervised program that may help improve the health and well-being of people who have heart problems. The cardiac rehab team may include doctors, nurses, exercise specialists, physical and occupational therapists, dietitians or nutritionists, and psychologists or other mental health specialists.

Rehab has two parts:

- **Education, counselling, and training.** This part of rehab helps you understand your heart condition and find ways to reduce your risk for future heart problems. The rehab team will help you learn how to cope with the stress of adjusting to a new lifestyle and how to deal with your fears about the future.

- **Exercise training.** This part helps you learn how to exercise safely, strengthen your muscles, and improve your stamina. Your exercise plan will be based on your personal abilities, needs, and interests.

How Can a Heart Attack Be Prevented?

Lowering your risk factors for coronary heart disease can help you prevent a heart attack. Even if you already have coronary heart disease, you still can take steps to lower your risk for a heart attack. These steps involve making heart-healthy lifestyle changes and getting ongoing medical care for related conditions that make heart attack more likely. Talk to your doctor about whether you may benefit from aspirin primary prevention, or using aspirin to help prevent your first heart attack.

Ongoing Care

Treat Related Conditions

Treating conditions that make a heart attack more likely also can help lower your risk for a heart attack. These conditions may include:

- Diabetes
- High blood cholesterol
- High blood pressure
- Chronic kidney disease
- Peripheral artery disease

Section 16.3

High Blood Pressure

This section includes text excerpted from "High Blood Pressure," National Heart, Lung, and Blood Institute (NHLBI), September 10, 2015.

What Is High Blood Pressure?

High blood pressure is a common disease in which blood flows through blood vessels (arteries) at higher than normal pressures.

Measuring Blood Pressure

Blood pressure is the force of blood pushing against the walls of the arteries as the heart pumps blood. High blood pressure, sometimes called hypertension, happens when this force is too high. Healthcare workers check blood pressure readings the same way for children, teens, and adults. They use a gauge, stethoscope or electronic sensor, and a blood pressure cuff. With this equipment, they measure:

- **Systolic Pressure:** Blood pressure when the heart beats while pumping blood

- **Diastolic Pressure:** Blood pressure when the heart is at rest between beats

Healthcare workers write blood pressure numbers with the systolic number above the diastolic number. For example: 118/76 mmHg. People read "118 over 76" millimeters of mercury.

Normal Blood Pressure

Normal blood pressure for adults is defined as a systolic pressure below 120 mmHg and a diastolic pressure below 80 mmHg. It is normal for blood pressures to change when you sleep, wake up, or are excited or nervous. When you are active, it is normal for your blood pressure to increase. However, once the activity stops, your blood pressure returns to your normal baseline range.

Blood pressure normally rises with age and body size. New born babies often have very low blood pressure numbers that are considered normal for babies, while older teens have numbers similar to adults.

Abnormal Blood Pressure

Abnormal increases in blood pressure are defined as having blood pressures higher than 120/80 mmHg. The following table outlines and defines high blood pressure severity levels.

Stages of High Blood Pressure in Adults

The ranges in the table are blood pressure guides for adults who do not have any short-term serious illnesses. People with diabetes or chronic kidney disease should keep their blood pressure below 130/80 mmHg. Although blood pressure increases seen in prehypertension are less than those used to diagnose high blood pressure, prehypertension can progress to high blood pressure and should be taken seriously.

Table 16.1. High Blood Pressure Severity Levels

Stages	Systolic (Top Number)		Diastolic (Bottom Number)
Prehypertension	120-139	OR	80-89
High blood pressure Stage 1	140-159	OR	90-99
High blood pressure Stage 2	160 or higher	OR	100 or higher

Over time, consistently high blood pressure weakens and damages your blood vessels, which can lead to complications.

Types of High Blood Pressure

There are two main types of high blood pressure: primary and secondary high blood pressure.

Primary High Blood Pressure: Primary, or essential, high blood pressure is the most common type of high blood pressure. This type of high blood pressure tends to develop over years as a person ages.

Secondary High Blood Pressure: Secondary high blood pressure is caused by another medical condition or use of certain medicines. This type usually resolves after the cause is treated or removed.

Causes of High Blood Pressure

Changes, either from genes or the environment, in the body's normal functions may cause high blood pressure, including changes to kidney fluid and salt balances, the renin-angiotensin-aldosterone system, sympathetic nervous system activity, and blood vessel structure and function.

Biology and High Blood Pressure

Researchers continue to study how various changes in normal body functions cause high blood pressure. The key functions affected in high blood pressure include:

Kidney Fluid and Salt Balances

The kidneys normally regulate the body's salt balance by retaining sodium and water and excreting potassium. Imbalances in this kidney function can expand blood volumes, which can cause high blood pressure.

Renin-Angiotensin-Aldosterone System

The renin-angiotensin-aldosterone system makes angiotensin and aldosterone hormones. Angiotensin narrows or constricts blood vessels, which can lead to an increase in blood pressure. Aldosterone controls how the kidneys balance fluid and salt levels. Increased aldosterone levels or activity may change this kidney function, leading to increased blood volumes and high blood pressure.

Sympathetic Nervous System Activity

The sympathetic nervous system has important functions in blood pressure regulation, including heart rate, blood pressure, and breathing rate. Researchers are investigating whether imbalances in this system cause high blood pressure.

Blood Vessel Structure and Function

Changes in the structure and function of small and large arteries may contribute to high blood pressure. The angiotensin pathway and the immune system may stiffen small and large arteries, which can affect blood pressure.

Genetic Causes of High Blood Pressure

Much of the understanding of the body systems involved in high blood pressure has come from genetic studies. High blood pressure often runs in families. Years of research have identified many genes and other mutations associated with high blood pressure, some in the renal salt regulatory and renin-angiotensin-aldosterone pathways. However, these known genetic factors only account for 2 to 3 percent of all cases. Emerging research suggests that certain deoxyribonucleic acid (DNA) changes during fetal development also may cause the development of high blood pressure later in life.

Environmental Causes of High Blood Pressure

Environmental causes of high blood pressure include:

Unhealthy Lifestyle Habits

Unhealthy lifestyle habits can cause high blood pressure, including:

- High dietary sodium intake and sodium sensitivity

- Drinking excess amounts of alcohol
- Lack of physical activity

Overweight and Obesity

Research studies show that being overweight or obese can increase the resistance in the blood vessels, causing the heart to work harder and leading to high blood pressure.

Medicines

Prescription medicines such as asthma or hormone therapies, including birth control pills and estrogen, and over-the-counter medicines such as cold relief medicines may cause this form of high blood pressure. This happens because medicines can change the way your body controls fluid and salt balances, cause your blood vessels to constrict, or impact the renin-angiotensin-aldosterone system leading to high blood pressure.

Other Medical Causes of High Blood Pressure

Other medical causes of high blood pressure include other medical conditions such as chronic kidney disease, sleep apnea, thyroid problems, or certain tumors. This happens because these other conditions change the way your body controls fluids, sodium, and hormones in your blood, which leads to secondary high blood pressure.

Risk Factors for High Blood Pressure

Anyone can develop high blood pressure; however, age, race or ethnicity, being overweight, gender, lifestyle habits, and a family history of high blood pressure can increase your risk for developing high blood pressure.

Age

Blood pressure tends to rise with age. About 65 percent of Americans age 60 or older have high blood pressure. However, the risk for prehypertension and high blood pressure is increasing for children and teens, possibly due to the rise in the number of overweight children and teens.

Race / Ethnicity

High blood pressure is more common in African American adults than in Caucasian or Hispanic American adults. Compared with these ethnic groups, African Americans:

- Tend to get high blood pressure earlier in life.

- Often, on average, have higher blood pressure numbers.

- Are less likely to achieve target blood pressure goals with treatment.

Overweight

You are more likely to develop prehypertension or high blood pressure if you're overweight or obese. The terms "overweight" and "obese" refer to body weight that's greater than what is considered healthy for a certain height.

Gender

Before age 55, men are more likely than women to develop high blood pressure. After age 55, women are more likely than men to develop high blood pressure.

Lifestyle Habits

Unhealthy lifestyle habits can raise your risk for high blood pressure, and they include:

- Eating too much sodium or too little potassium

- Lack of physical activity

- Drinking too much alcohol

- Stress

Family History

A family history of high blood pressure raises the risk of developing prehypertension or high blood pressure. Some people have a high sensitivity to sodium and salt, which may increase their risk for high blood pressure and may run in families. Genetic causes of this condition are why family history is a risk factor for this condition.

What Are the Signs, Symptoms, and Complications of High Blood Pressure?

Because diagnosis is based on blood pressure readings, this condition can go undetected for years, as symptoms do not usually appear until the body is damaged from chronic high blood pressure.

Complications of High Blood Pressure

When blood pressure stays high over time, it can damage the body and cause complications. Some common complications and their signs and symptoms include:

- Aneurysms
- Chronic kidney disease
- Cognitive changes
- Eye damage
- Heart attack
- Heart failure
- Peripheral artery disease
- Stroke

Diagnosis of High Blood Pressure

For most patients, healthcare providers diagnose high blood pressure when blood pressure readings are consistently 140/90 mmHg or above.

Confirming High Blood Pressure

A blood pressure test is easy and painless and can be done in a healthcare provider's office or clinic. To prepare for the test:

- Don't drink coffee or smoke cigarettes for 30 minutes prior to the test.
- Go to the bathroom before the test.
- Sit for 5 minutes before the test.

To track blood pressure readings over a period of time, the healthcare provider may ask you to come into the office on different days and at different times to take your blood pressure. The healthcare provider also may ask you to check readings at home or at other locations that have blood pressure equipment and to keep a written log of all your results.

Whenever you have an appointment with the healthcare provider, be sure to bring your log of blood pressure readings. Every time you visit the healthcare provider, he or she should tell you what your blood pressure numbers are; if he or she does not, you should ask for your readings.

Blood Pressure Severity and Type

Your healthcare provider usually takes 2–3 readings at several medical appointments to diagnose high blood pressure. Using the results of your blood pressure test, your healthcare provider will diagnose prehypertension or high blood pressure if:

- Your systolic or diastolic readings are consistently higher than 120/80 mmHg.

- Your child's blood pressure numbers are outside average numbers for children of the same age, gender, and height.

Once your healthcare provider determines the severity of your blood pressure, he or she can order additional tests to determine if your blood pressure is due to other conditions or medicines or if you have primary high blood pressure. Healthcare providers can use this information to develop your treatment plan.

Some people have "white coat hypertension." This happens when blood pressure readings are only high when taken in a healthcare provider's office compared with readings taken in any other location. Healthcare providers diagnose this type of high blood pressure by reviewing readings in the office and readings taken anywhere else. Researchers believe stress, which can occur during the medical appointment, causes white coat hypertension.

How Is High Blood Pressure Treated?

Based on your diagnosis, healthcare providers develop treatment plans for high blood pressure that include lifelong lifestyle changes and medicines to control high blood pressure; lifestyle changes such as weight loss can be highly effective in treating high blood pressure.

Treatment Plans

Healthcare providers work with you to develop a treatment plan based on whether you were diagnosed with primary or secondary high blood pressure and if there is a suspected or known cause. Treatment plans may evolve until blood pressure control is achieved.

If your healthcare provider diagnoses you with secondary high blood pressure, he or she will work to treat the other condition or change the medicine suspected of causing your high blood pressure. If high blood pressure persists or is first diagnosed as primary high blood pressure, your treatment plan will include lifestyle changes. When lifestyle changes alone do not control or lower blood pressure, your healthcare provider may change or update your treatment plan by prescribing medicines to treat the disease.

If your healthcare provider prescribes medicines as a part of your treatment plan, keep up your healthy lifestyle habits. The combination of the medicines and the healthy lifestyle habits helps control and lower your high blood pressure.

Some people develop "resistant" or uncontrolled high blood pressure. This can happen when the medications they are taking do not work well for them or another medical condition is leading to uncontrolled blood pressure. Healthcare providers treat resistant or uncontrolled high blood pressure with an intensive treatment plan that can include a different set of blood pressure medications or other special treatments.

To achieve the best control of your blood pressure, follow your treatment plan and take all medications as prescribed. Following your prescribed treatment plan is important because it can prevent or delay complications that high blood pressure can cause and can lower your risk for other related problems.

Healthy Lifestyle Changes

Healthy lifestyle habits can help you control high blood pressure. These habits include:

- Healthy eating
- Being physically active
- Maintaining a healthy weight
- Limiting alcohol intake
- Managing and coping with stress

To help make lifelong lifestyle changes, try making one healthy lifestyle change at a time and add another change when you feel that you have successfully adopted the earlier changes. When you practice several healthy lifestyle habits, you are more likely to lower your blood pressure and maintain normal blood pressure readings.

Medicines

Blood pressure medicines work in different ways to stop or slow some of the body's functions that cause high blood pressure. Medicines to lower blood pressure include:

- Diuretics (water or fluid pills)
- Beta blockers
- Angiotensin-converting enzyme (ACE) inhibitors
- Angiotensin II receptor blockers (ARBs)
- Calcium channel blockers
- Alpha blockers
- Alpha-beta blockers
- Central acting agents
- Vasodilators

To lower and control blood pressure, many people take two or more medicines. If you have side effects from your medicines, don't stop taking your medicines. Instead, talk with your healthcare provider about the side effects to see if the dose can be changed or a new medicine prescribed.

Prevention of High Blood Pressure

Healthy lifestyle habits, proper use of medicines, and regular medical care can prevent high blood pressure or its complications.

Preventing Worsening High Blood Pressure or Complications

If you have been diagnosed with high blood pressure, it is important to obtain regular medical care and to follow your prescribed treatment plan, which will include healthy lifestyle habit recommendations and possibly medicines. Not only can healthy lifestyle habits prevent high blood pressure from occurring, but they can reverse prehypertension and help control existing high blood pressure or prevent complications and long-term problems associated with this condition, such as coronary heart disease, stroke, or kidney disease.

Section 16.4

Stroke

This section contains text excerpted from the following sources:
Text beginning with the heading "What Is a Stroke?" is excerpted
from "Stroke," National Heart, Lung, and Blood Institute (NHLBI),
January 27, 2017; Text under the heading "What to Expect after a
Stroke" is excerpted from "About Stroke—Recovering from Stroke,"
Centers for Disease Control and Prevention (CDC), January 17, 2017.

What Is a Stroke?

A stroke occurs if the flow of oxygen-rich blood to a portion of the
brain is blocked. Without oxygen, brain cells start to die after a few
minutes. Sudden bleeding in the brain also can cause a stroke if it
damages brain cells.

If brain cells die or are damaged because of a stroke, symptoms
occur in the parts of the body that these brain cells control. Examples
of stroke symptoms include sudden weakness; paralysis or numbness
of the face, arms, or legs (paralysis is an inability to move); trouble
speaking or understanding speech; and trouble seeing.

A stroke is a serious medical condition that requires emergency
care. A stroke can cause lasting brain damage, long-term disability,
or even death.

Types of Stroke

Ischemic Stroke

An ischemic stroke occurs if an artery that supplies oxygen-rich
blood to the brain becomes blocked. Blood clots often cause the blockages that lead to ischemic strokes. The two types of ischemic stroke are
thrombotic and embolic. In a thrombotic stroke, a blood clot (thrombus)
forms in an artery that supplies blood to the brain.

In an embolic stroke, a blood clot or other substance (such as plaque,
a fatty material) travels through the bloodstream to an artery in the
brain. (A blood clot or piece of plaque that travels through the bloodstream is called an embolus.). With both types of ischemic stroke, the

blood clot or plaque blocks the flow of oxygen-rich blood to a portion of the brain.

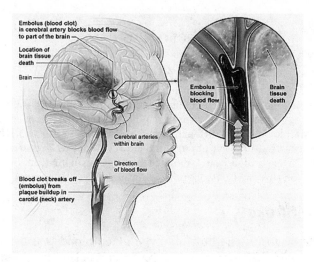

Figure 16.3. *Ischemic Stroke*

The illustration shows how an ischemic stroke can occur in the brain. If a blood clot breaks away from plaque buildup in a carotid (neck) artery, it can travel to and lodge in an artery in the brain. The clot can block blood flow to part of the brain, causing brain tissue death.

Hemorrhagic Stroke

A hemorrhagic stroke occurs if an artery in the brain leaks blood or ruptures (breaks open). The pressure from the leaked blood damages brain cells. The two types of hemorrhagic stroke are intracerebral and subarachnoid. In an intracerebral hemorrhage, a blood vessel inside the brain leaks blood or ruptures. In a subarachnoid hemorrhage, a blood vessel on the surface of the brain leaks blood or ruptures. When this happens, bleeding occurs between the inner and middle layers of the membranes that cover the brain. In both types of hemorrhagic stroke, the leaked blood causes swelling of the brain and increased pressure in the skull. The swelling and pressure damage cells and tissues in the brain.

Who Is at Risk for a Stroke?

Certain traits, conditions, and habits can raise your risk of having a stroke or TIA. These traits, conditions, and habits are known as risk factors.

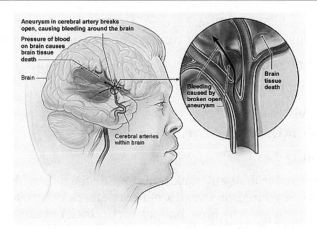

Figure 16.4. *Hemorrhagic Stroke*

The illustration shows how a hemorrhagic stroke can occur in the brain. An aneurysm in a cerebral artery breaks open, which causes bleeding in the brain. The pressure of the blood causes brain tissue death.

The more risk factors you have, the more likely you are to have a stroke. You can treat or control some risk factors, such as high blood pressure and smoking. Other risk factors, such as age and gender, you can't control.

The major risk factors for stroke include:

- High blood pressure
- Diabetes
- Heart diseases
- Smoking
- Age and gender
- Race and ethnicity
- Personal or family history of stroke or TIA
- Brain aneurysms or AVMs

Other risk factors for stroke, many of which of you can control, include:

- Alcohol and illegal drug use, including cocaine, amphetamines, and other drugs

- Certain medical conditions, such as sickle cell disease, vasculitis (inflammation of the blood vessels), and bleeding disorders
- Lack of physical activity
- Overweight and Obesity
- Stress and depression
- Unhealthy cholesterol levels
- Unhealthy diet
- Use of nonsteroidal anti-inflammatory drugs (NSAIDs), but not aspirin, may increase the risk of heart attack or stroke, particularly in patients who have had a heart attack or cardiac bypass surgery. The risk may increase the longer NSAIDs are used. Common NSAIDs include ibuprofen and naproxen.

Following a heart-healthy lifestyle can lower the risk of stroke. Some people also may need to take medicines to lower their risk. Sometimes strokes can occur in people who don't have any known risk factors.

What Are the Signs and Symptoms of a Stroke?

The signs and symptoms of a stroke often develop quickly. However, they can develop over hours or even days. The type of symptoms depends on the type of stroke and the area of the brain that's affected. How long symptoms last and how severe they are, vary among different people.

Signs and symptoms of a stroke may include:

- Sudden weakness
- Paralysis (an inability to move) or numbness of the face, arms, or legs, especially on one side of the body
- Confusion
- Trouble speaking or understanding speech
- Trouble seeing in one or both eyes
- Problems breathing
- Dizziness, trouble walking, loss of balance or coordination, and unexplained falls
- Loss of consciousness
- Sudden and severe headache

A TIA has the same signs and symptoms as a stroke. However, TIA symptoms usually last less than 1–2 hours (although they may last up to 24 hours). A TIA may occur only once in a person's lifetime or more often. At first, it may not be possible to tell whether someone is having a TIA or stroke. All stroke-like symptoms require medical care.

Stroke Complications

After you've had a stroke, you may develop other complications, such as:

- **Blood clots and muscle weakness.** Being immobile (unable to move around) for a long time can raise your risk of developing blood clots in the deep veins of the legs. Being immobile also can lead to muscle weakness and decreased muscle flexibility.

- **Problems swallowing and pneumonia.** If a stroke affects the muscles used for swallowing, you may have a hard time eating or drinking. You also may be at risk of inhaling food or drink into your lungs. If this happens, you may develop pneumonia.

- **Loss of bladder control.** Some strokes affect the muscles used to urinate. You may need a urinary catheter (a tube placed into the bladder) until you can urinate on your own. Use of these catheters can lead to urinary tract infections. Loss of bowel control or constipation also may occur after a stroke.

How Is a Stroke Diagnosed?

Your doctor will diagnose a stroke based on your signs and symptoms, your medical history, a physical exam, and test results. Your doctor will want to find out the type of stroke you've had, its cause, the part of the brain that's affected, and whether you have bleeding in the brain. If your doctor thinks you've had a TIA, he or she will look for its cause to help prevent a future stroke.

Medical History and Physical Exam

Your doctor will ask you or a family member about your risk factors for stroke. Examples of risk factors include high blood pressure, smoking, heart disease, and a personal or family history of stroke. Your doctor also will ask about your signs and symptoms and when they began.

During the physical exam, your doctor will check your mental alertness and your coordination and balance. He or she will check for numbness or weakness in your face, arms, and legs; confusion; and trouble speaking and seeing clearly.

Your doctor will look for signs of carotid artery disease, a common cause of ischemic stroke. He or she will listen to your carotid arteries with a stethoscope. A whooshing sound called a bruit may suggest changed or reduced blood flow due to plaque buildup in the carotid arteries.

Diagnostic Tests and Procedures

Your doctor may recommend one or more of the following tests to diagnose a stroke or TIA.

Brain Computed Tomography

A brain computed tomography scan, or brain CT scan, is a painless test that uses X-rays to take clear, detailed pictures of your brain. This test often is done right after a stroke is suspected. A brain CT scan can show bleeding in the brain or damage to the brain cells from a stroke. The test also can show other brain conditions that may be causing your symptoms.

Magnetic Resonance Imaging (MRI)

An MRI uses magnets and radio waves to create pictures of the organs and structures in your body. This test can detect changes in brain tissue and damage to brain cells from a stroke. An MRI may be used instead of, or in addition to, a CT scan to diagnose a stroke.

Computed Tomography Arteriogram (CTA) and Magnetic Resonance Arteriogram (MRA)

A CTA and an MRA can show the large blood vessels in the brain. These tests may give your doctor more information about the site of a blood clot and the flow of blood through your brain.

Carotid Ultrasound

Carotid ultrasound is a painless and harmless test that uses sound waves to create pictures of the insides of your carotid arteries. These arteries supply oxygen-rich blood to your brain. Carotid ultrasound shows whether plaque has narrowed or blocked your carotid arteries. Your carotid ultrasound test may include a Doppler ultrasound.

Doppler ultrasound is a special test that shows the speed and direction of blood moving through your blood vessels.

Carotid Angiography

Carotid angiography is a test that uses dye and special X-ray to show the insides of your carotid arteries. For this test, a small tube called a catheter is put into an artery, usually in the groin (upper thigh). The tube is then moved up into one of your carotid arteries. Your doctor will inject a substance (called contrast dye) into the carotid artery. The dye helps make the artery visible on X-ray pictures.

Heart Tests

Electrocardiogram (EKG)

An EKG is a simple, painless test that records the heart's electrical activity. The test shows how fast the heart is beating and its rhythm (steady or irregular). An EKG also records the strength and timing of electrical signals as they pass through each part of the heart. An EKG can help detect heart problems that may have led to a stroke. For example, the test can help diagnose atrial fibrillation or a previous heart attack.

Echocardiography

Echocardiography, or echo, is a painless test that uses sound waves to create pictures of your heart. The test gives information about the size and shape of your heart and how well your heart's chambers and valves are working. Echo can detect possible blood clots inside the heart and problems with the aorta. The aorta is the main artery that carries oxygen-rich blood from your heart to all parts of your body.

Blood Tests

Your doctor also may use blood tests to help diagnose a stroke. A blood glucose test measures the amount of glucose (sugar) in your blood. Low blood glucose levels may cause symptoms similar to those of a stroke. A platelet count measures the number of platelets in your blood. Blood platelets are cell fragments that help your blood clot. Abnormal platelet levels may be a sign of a bleeding disorder (not enough clotting) or a thrombotic disorder (too much clotting).

Your doctor also may recommend blood tests to measure how long it takes for your blood to clot. Two tests that may be used are called prothrombin time (PT) and partial thromboplastin time (PTT) tests. These tests show whether your blood is clotting normally.

How Is a Stroke Treated?

Treatment for a stroke depends on whether it is ischemic or hemorrhagic. Treatment for a TIA depends on its cause, how much time has passed since symptoms began, and whether you have other medical conditions.

Strokes and TIAs are medical emergencies. If you have stroke symptoms, call 9–1–1 right away. Do not drive to the hospital or let someone else drive you. Call an ambulance so that medical personnel can begin lifesaving treatment on the way to the emergency room. During a stroke, every minute counts. Once you receive immediate treatment, your doctor will try to treat your stroke risk factors and prevent complications by recommending heart-healthy lifestyle changes.

Treating an Ischemic Stroke or Transient Ischemic Attack (TIA)

An ischemic stroke or TIA occurs if an artery that supplies oxygen-rich blood to the brain becomes blocked. Often, blood clots cause the blockages that lead to ischemic strokes and TIAs. Treatment for an ischemic stroke or TIA may include medicines and medical procedures.

Medicines

If you have a stroke caused by a blood clot, you may be given a clot-dissolving, or clot-busting, medication called tissue plasminogen activator (tPA). A doctor will inject tPA into a vein in your arm. This type of medication must be given within 4 hours of symptom onset. Ideally, it should be given as soon as possible. The sooner treatment begins, the better your chances of recovery.

If you can't have tPA for medical reasons, your doctor may give you antiplatelet medicine that helps stop platelets from clumping together to form blood clots or anticoagulant medicine (blood thinner) that keeps existing blood clots from getting larger. Two common medicines are aspirin and clopidogrel.

Medical Procedures

If you have carotid artery disease, your doctor may recommend a carotid endarterectomy or carotid artery angioplasty. Both procedures open blocked carotid arteries. Researchers are testing other treatments for ischemic stroke, such as intra-arterial thrombolysis and mechanical clot removal in cerebral ischemia (MERCI). In intra-arterial thrombolysis, a long flexible tube called a catheter is put into your groin (upper thigh) and threaded to the tiny arteries of the brain. Your doctor can deliver medicine through this catheter to break up a blood clot in the brain. MERCI is a device that can remove blood clots from an artery. During the procedure, a catheter is threaded through a carotid artery to the affected artery in the brain. The device is then used to pull the blood clot out through the catheter.

Treating a Hemorrhagic Stroke

A hemorrhagic stroke occurs if an artery in the brain leaks blood or ruptures. The first steps in treating a hemorrhagic stroke are to find the cause of bleeding in the brain and then control it. Unlike ischemic strokes, hemorrhagic strokes aren't treated with antiplatelet medicines and blood thinners because these medicines can make bleeding worse.

If you're taking antiplatelet medicines or blood thinners and have a hemorrhagic stroke, you'll be taken off the medicine. If high blood pressure is the cause of bleeding in the brain, your doctor may prescribe medicines to lower your blood pressure. This can help prevent further bleeding.

Surgery also may be needed to treat a hemorrhagic stroke. The types of surgery used include aneurysm clipping, coil embolization, and arteriovenous malformation (AVM) repair.

Aneurysm Clipping and Coil Embolization

If an aneurysm (a balloon-like bulge in an artery) is the cause of a stroke, your doctor may recommend aneurysm clipping or coil embolization.

Aneurysm clipping is done to block off the aneurysm from the blood vessels in the brain. This surgery helps prevent further leaking of blood from the aneurysm. It also can help prevent the aneurysm from bursting again. During the procedure, a surgeon will make an incision (cut) in the brain and place a tiny clamp at the base of the aneurysm. You'll be given medicine to make you sleep during the surgery. After the surgery, you'll need to stay in the hospital's intensive care unit for a few days.

Coil embolization is a less complex procedure for treating an aneurysm. The surgeon will insert a tube called a catheter into an artery in the groin. He or she will thread the tube to the site of the aneurysm. Then, a tiny coil will be pushed through the tube and into the aneurysm. The coil will cause a blood clot to form, which will block blood flow through the aneurysm and prevent it from bursting again. Coil embolization is done in a hospital. You'll be given medicine to make you sleep during the surgery.

Arteriovenous Malformation Repair

If an AVM is the cause of a stroke, your doctor may recommend an AVM repair. (An AVM is a tangle of faulty arteries and veins that can rupture within the brain.) AVM repair helps prevent further bleeding in the brain.

Doctors use several methods to repair AVMs. These methods include:

- Injecting a substance into the blood vessels of the AVM to block blood flow

- Surgery to remove the AVM

- Using radiation to shrink the blood vessels of the AVM

How Can a Stroke Be Prevented?

Taking action to control your risk factors can help prevent or delay a stroke. If you've already had a stroke. Talk to your doctor about whether you may benefit from aspirin primary prevention, or using aspirin to help prevent your first stroke. The following heart-healthy lifestyle changes can help prevent your first stroke and help prevent you from having another one.

- Be physically active

- Don't smoke

- Aim for a healthy weight

- Make heart-healthy eating choices

- Manage stress

If you or someone in your family has had a stroke, be sure to tell your doctor. By knowing your family history of stroke, you may be able to lower your risk factors and prevent or delay a stroke. If you've had a TIA, don't ignore it. TIAs are warnings, and it's important for your doctor to find the cause of the TIA so you can take steps to prevent a stroke.

What to Expect after a Stroke

If you have had a stroke, you can make great progress in regaining your independence. However, some problems may continue:

- Paralysis (inability to move some parts of the body), weakness, or both on one side of the body
- Trouble with thinking, awareness, attention, learning, judgment, and memory
- Problems understanding or forming speech
- Trouble controlling or expressing emotions
- Numbness or strange sensations
- Pain in the hands and feet that worsens with movement and temperature changes
- Trouble with chewing and swallowing
- Problems with bladder and bowel control
- Depression

Stroke Rehabilitation

Rehab can include working with speech, physical, and occupational therapists.

- **Speech therapy** helps people who have problems producing or understanding speech.
- **Physical therapy** uses exercises to help you relearn movement and coordination skills you may have lost because of the stroke.
- **Occupational therapy** focuses on improving daily activities, such as eating, drinking, dressing, bathing, reading, and writing.

Therapy and medicine may help with depression or other mental health conditions following a stroke. Joining a patient support group may help you adjust to life after a stroke. Talk with your health-care team about local support groups, or check with an area medical center.

Support from family and friends can also help relieve fear and anxiety following a stroke. Let your loved ones know how you feel and what they can do to help you.

Preventing Another Stroke

If you have had a stroke, you are at high risk for another stroke:

• One in four strokes each year are recurrent.

• The chance of stroke within 90 days of a TIA may be as high as 17 percent, with the greatest risk during the first week.

That's why it's important to treat the causes of stroke, including heart disease, high blood pressure, atrial fibrillation (fast, irregular heartbeat), high cholesterol, and diabetes. Your doctor may prescribe you medicine or tell you to change your diet, exercise, or adopt other healthy lifestyle habits. Surgery may also be helpful in some cases.

Chapter 17

Eye Disorders

Chapter Contents

Section 17.1

Cataracts

This section includes text excerpted from "Facts about Cataract,"
National Eye Institute (NEI), September 2015.

What Is a Cataract?

A cataract is a clouding of the lens in the eye that affects vision.
Most cataracts are related to aging. Cataracts are very common in
older people. By age 80, more than half of all Americans either have a
cataract or have had cataract surgery. A cataract can occur in either
or both eyes. It cannot spread from one eye to the other.

What Is the Lens?

The lens is a clear part of the eye that helps to focus light, or an
image, on the retina. The retina is the light-sensitive tissue at the back
of the eye. In a normal eye, light passes through the transparent lens
to the retina. Once it reaches the retina, light is changed into nerve

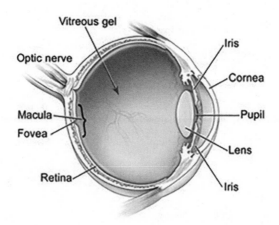

Figure 17.1. *Eye*

signals that are sent to the brain. The lens must be clear for the retina to receive a sharp image. If the lens is cloudy from a cataract, the image you see will be blurred.

What Causes Cataracts?

The lens lies behind the iris and the pupil. It works much like a camera lens. It focuses light onto the retina at the back of the eye, where an image is recorded. The lens also adjusts the eye's focus, letting us see things clearly both up close and far away. The lens is made of mostly water and protein. The protein is arranged in a precise way that keeps the lens clear and lets light pass through it.

But as we age, some of the protein may clump together and start to cloud a small area of the lens. This is a cataract. Over time, the cataract may grow larger and cloud more of the lens, making it harder to see. Researchers suspect that there are several causes of cataract, such as smoking and diabetes. Or, it may be that the protein in the lens just changes from the wear and tear it takes over the years.

How Do Cataracts Affect Vision?

Age-related cataracts can affect your vision in two ways:

1. Clumps of protein reduce the sharpness of the image reaching the retina. The lens consists mostly of water and protein. When the protein clumps up, it clouds the lens and reduces the light that reaches the retina. The clouding may become severe enough to cause blurred vision. Most age-related cataracts develop from protein clumpings. When a cataract is small, the cloudiness affects only a small part of the lens. You may not notice any changes in your vision. Cataracts tend to "grow" slowly, so vision gets worse gradually. Over time, the cloudy area in the lens may get larger, and the cataract may increase in size. Seeing may become more difficult. Your vision may get duller or blurrier.

2. The clear lens slowly changes to a yellowish/brownish color, adding a brownish tint to vision. As the clear lens slowly colors with age, your vision gradually may acquire a brownish shade. At first, the amount of tinting may be small and may not cause a vision problem. Over time, increased tinting may make it more difficult to read and perform other routine activities. This gradual change in the amount of tinting does not affect the sharpness of the image transmitted to the retina. If you have advanced lens discoloration, you may not be able

to identify blues and purples. You may be wearing what you believe to be a pair of black socks, only to find out from friends that you are wearing purple socks.

Who Is at Risk for Cataract?

The risk of cataract increases as you get older. Other risk factors for cataract include:

- Certain diseases (for example, diabetes).

- Personal behavior (smoking, alcohol use).

- The environment (prolonged exposure to ultraviolet sunlight).

What Are the Symptoms of a Cataract?

The most common symptoms of a cataract are:

- Cloudy or blurry vision.

- Colors seem faded.

- Glare. Headlights, lamps, or sunlight may appear too bright. A halo may appear around lights.

- Poor night vision.

- Double vision or multiple images in one eye. (This symptom may clear as the cataract gets larger.)

- Frequent prescription changes in your eyeglasses or contact lenses.

These symptoms also can be a sign of other eye problems. If you have any of these symptoms, check with your eye care professional.

How Is a Cataract Treated?

The symptoms of early cataract may be improved with new eyeglasses, brighter lighting, antiglare sunglasses, or magnifying lenses. If these measures do not help, surgery is the only effective treatment. Surgery involves removing the cloudy lens and replacing it with an artificial lens.

A cataract needs to be removed only when vision loss interferes with your everyday activities, such as driving, reading, or watching TV. You and your eye care professional can make this decision together. Once you understand the benefits and risks of surgery, you can make an informed decision about whether cataract surgery is right for you. In most cases, delaying cataract surgery will not cause long-term damage to your eye or make the surgery more difficult. You do not have to rush into surgery.

Sometimes a cataract should be removed even if it does not cause problems with your vision. For example, a cataract should be removed if it prevents examination or treatment of another eye problem, such as age-related macular degeneration (AMD) or diabetic retinopathy.

If you choose surgery, your eye care professional may refer you to a specialist to remove the cataract. If you have cataracts in both eyes that require surgery, the surgery will be performed on each eye at separate times, usually four weeks apart.

Is Cataract Surgery Effective?

Cataract removal is one of the most common operations performed in the United States. It also is one of the safest and most effective types of surgery. In about 90 percent of cases, people who have cataract surgery have better vision afterward.

What Are the Risks of Cataract Surgery?

As with any surgery, cataract surgery poses risks, such as infection and bleeding. Before cataract surgery, your doctor may ask you to temporarily stop taking certain medications that increase the risk of bleeding during surgery. After surgery, you must keep your eye clean, wash your hands before touching your eye, and use the prescribed medications to help minimize the risk of infection. Serious infection can result in loss of vision.

Cataract surgery slightly increases your risk of retinal detachment. Other eye disorders, such as high myopia (near-sightedness), can further increase your risk of retinal detachment after cataract surgery. One sign of a retinal detachment is a sudden increase in flashes or floaters. Floaters are little "cobwebs" or specks that seem to float about in your field of vision. If you notice a sudden increase in floaters or flashes, see an eye care professional immediately. A retinal detachment is a medical emergency. If necessary, go to an emergency service or hospital. Your eye must be examined by an eye surgeon as soon as possible. A retinal detachment causes no pain. Early treatment for retinal detachment often can prevent permanent loss of vision. The sooner you get treatment, the more likely you will regain good vision.

Even if you are treated promptly, some vision may be lost. Talk to your eye care professional about these risks. Make sure cataract surgery is right for you.

What If I Have Other Eye Conditions and Need Cataract Surgery?

Many people who need cataract surgery also have other eye conditions, such as age-related macular degeneration or glaucoma. If you have other eye conditions in addition to cataract, talk with your doctor. Learn about the risks, benefits, alternatives, and expected results of cataract surgery.

When Will My Vision Be Normal Again?

You can return quickly to many everyday activities, but your vision may be blurry. The healing eye needs time to adjust so that it can focus properly with the other eye, especially if the other eye has a cataract. Ask your doctor when you can resume driving. If you received an IOL (intraocular lens), you may notice that colors are very bright. The IOL is clear, unlike your natural lens that may have had a yellowish/brownish tint. Within a few months after receiving an IOL, you will become used to improved color vision. Also, when your eye heals, you may need new glasses or contact lenses.

What Can I Do If I Already Have Lost Some Vision from Cataract?

If you have lost some vision, speak with your surgeon about options that may help you make the most of your remaining vision.

What Can I Do to Protect My Vision?

Wearing sunglasses and a hat with a brim to block ultraviolet sunlight may help to delay cataract. If you smoke, stop. Researchers also believe good nutrition can help reduce the risk of age-related cataract. They recommend eating green leafy vegetables, fruit, and other foods with antioxidants. If you are age 60 or older, you should have a comprehensive dilated eye exam at least once every two years. In addition to cataract, your eye care professional can check for signs of age-related macular degeneration, glaucoma, and other vision disorders. Early treatment for many eye diseases may save your sight.

Section 17.2

Corneal Diseases and Conditions

This section includes text excerpted from "Facts about the Cornea and Corneal Disease," National Eye Institute (NEI), May 2016.

What Is the Cornea?

The cornea is the eye's outermost layer. It is the clear, dome-shaped surface that covers the front of the eye. It plays an important role in focusing your vision.

Why Are Tears Important to the Cornea?

Every time we blink, tears are distributed across the cornea to keep the eye moist, help wounds heal, and protect against infection. Tears form in three layers:

- An outer, oily (lipid) layer that keeps tears from evaporating too quickly and helps tears remain on the eye;

- A middle (aqueous) layer that nourishes the cornea and the conjunctiva—the mucous membrane that covers the front of the eye and the inside of the eyelids;

- A bottom (mucin) layer that helps spread the aqueous layer across the eye to ensure that the eye remains wet.

What Are Some Common Conditions That Affect the Cornea?

Injuries

After minor injuries or scratches, the cornea usually heals on its own. Deeper injuries can cause corneal scarring, resulting in a haze on the cornea that impairs vision. If you have a deep injury, or a corneal disease or disorder, you could experience:

- Pain in the eye

- Sensitivity to light

- Reduced vision or blurry vision

- Redness or inflammation in the eye

- Headache, nausea, fatigue

If you experience any of these symptoms, seek help from an eye care professional.

Allergies

The most common allergies that affect the eye are those related to pollen, particularly when the weather is warm and dry. Symptoms in the eye include redness, itching, tearing, burning, stinging, and watery discharge, although usually not severe enough to require medical attention. Antihistamine decongestant eye drops effectively reduce these symptoms. Rain and cooler weather, which decreases the amount of pollen in the air, can also provide relief.

Keratitis

Keratitis is an inflammation of the cornea. Noninfectious keratitis can be caused by a minor injury, or from wearing contact lenses too long. Infection is the most common cause of keratitis. Infectious keratitis can be caused by bacteria, viruses, fungi or parasites. Often, these infections are also related to contact lens wear, especially improper cleaning of contact lenses or overuse of old contact lenses that should be discarded. Minor corneal infections are usually treated with antibacterial eye drops. If the problem is severe, it may require more intensive antibiotic or antifungal treatment to eliminate the infection, as well as steroid eye drops to reduce inflammation.

What Are Corneal Dystrophies?

A corneal dystrophy is a condition in which one or more parts of the cornea lose their normal clarity due to a build-up of material that clouds the cornea. These diseases:

- Are usually inherited

- Affect both eyes

- Progress gradually

- Don't affect other parts of the body, and aren't related to diseases affecting other parts of the eye or body

- Happen in otherwise healthy people.

Corneal dystrophies affect vision in different ways. Some cause severe visual impairment, while a few cause no vision problems and are only discovered during a routine eye exam. Other dystrophies may cause repeated episodes of pain without leading to permanent vision loss. Some of the most common corneal dystrophies include keratoconus, Fuchs dystrophy, lattice dystrophy, and map—dot—fingerprint dystrophy.

Fuchs Dystrophy

Fuchs dystrophy is a slowly progressing disease that usually affects both eyes and is slightly more common in women than in men. It can cause your vision to gradually worsen over many years, but most people with Fuchs dystrophy won't notice vision problems until they reach their 50s or 60s.

Fuchs dystrophy is caused by the gradual deterioration of cells in the corneal endothelium; the causes aren't well understood. Normally, these endothelial cells maintain a healthy balance of fluids within the cornea. Healthy endothelial cells prevent the cornea from swelling and keep the cornea clear. In Fuchs dystrophy, the endothelial cells slowly die off and cause fluid buildup and swelling within the cornea. The cornea thickens and vision becomes blurred.

As the disease progresses, Fuchs dystrophy symptoms usually affect both eyes and include:

- Glare, which affects vision in low light

- Blurred vision that occurs in the morning after waking and gradually improves during the day

- Distorted vision, sensitivity to light, difficulty seeing at night, and seeing halos around light at night

- Painful, tiny blisters on the surface of the cornea

- A cloudy or hazy looking cornea

The first step in treating Fuchs dystrophy is to reduce the swelling with drops, ointments, or soft contact lenses. If you have severe disease, your eye care professional may suggest a corneal transplant.

Map—Dot—Fingerprint Dystrophy

Map-Dot-Fingerprint dystrophy, also known as epithelial basement membrane dystrophy, occurs when the basement membrane develops abnormally and forms folds in the tissue. The folds create gray shapes that look like continents on a map. There also may be clusters of opaque dots underneath or close to the maplike patches. Less frequently, the folds form concentric lines in the central cornea that resemble small fingerprints.

Symptoms include blurred vision, pain in the morning that lessens during the day, sensitivity to light, excessive tearing, and a feeling that there's something in the eye.

Map—dot—fingerprint dystrophy usually occurs in both eyes and affects adults between the ages of 40 and 70, although it can develop earlier in life. Typically, map—dot—fingerprint dystrophy will flare up now and then over the course of several years and then go away, without vision loss. Some people can have map-dot-fingerprint dystrophy but not experience any symptoms.

Others with the disease will develop recurring epithelial erosions, in which the epithelium's outermost layer rises slightly, exposing a small gap between the outermost layer and the rest of the cornea. These erosions alter the cornea's normal curvature and cause blurred vision. They may also expose the nerve endings that line the tissue, resulting in moderate to severe pain over several days.

The discomfort of epithelial erosions can be managed with topical lubricating eye drops and ointments. If drops or ointments don't relieve the pain and discomfort, there are outpatient surgeries including:

- Anterior corneal puncture, which help the cells adhere better to the tissue

- Corneal scraping to remove eroded areas of the cornea and allow healthy tissue to regrow

- Laser surgery to remove surface irregularities on the cornea

What Other Diseases Can Affect the Cornea?

Herpes Zoster (Shingles)

Shingles is a reactivation of the varicel-lazoster virus (VZV), the same virus that causes chickenpox. If you have had chickenpox, the virus can live on within your nerve cells for years after the sores have gone away. In some people, the varicel-lazoster virus (VZV) reactivates later in life, travels through the nerve fibers, and emerges in the cornea. If this happens, your eye care professional may prescribe oral antiviral treatment to reduce the risk of inflammation and scarring in the cornea. Shingles can also cause decreased sensitivity in the cornea.

Corneal problems may arise months after the shingles are gone from the rest of the body. If you experience shingles in your eye, or nose, or on your face, it's important to have your eyes examined several months after the shingles have cleared.

Ocular Herpes

Herpes of the eye, or ocular herpes, is a recurrent viral infection that is caused by the herpes simplex virus (HSV-1). This is the same virus that causes cold sores. Ocular herpes can also be caused by the sexually transmitted herpes simplex virus (HSV-2) that causes genital herpes.

Ocular herpes can produce sores on the eyelid or surface of the cornea and over time the inflammation may spread deeper into the cornea and eye, and develop into a more severe infection called stromal keratitis. There is no cure for ocular herpes, but it can be controlled with antiviral drugs.

Glaucoma

ICE is usually present in only one eye. It is caused by the movement of endothelial cells from the cornea to the iris. This loss of cells from the cornea leads to corneal swelling and distortion of the iris and pupil. This cell movement also blocks the fluid outflow channels of the eye, which causes glaucoma.

There is no treatment to stop the progression of ICE, but the glaucoma is treatable. If the cornea becomes so swollen that vision is significantly impaired, a corneal transplant may be necessary.

Pterygium

A pterygium is a pinkish, triangular tissue growth on the cornea. Some pterygia (plural for pyterygium) grow slowly throughout a lifetime, while others stop growing. A pterygium rarely grows so large that it covers the pupil of the eye.

Pterygia are more common in sunny climates and in adults 20–40 years of age. It's unclear what causes pterygia. However, since people who develop pterygia usually have spent significant time outdoors, researchers believe chronic exposure to UV light from the sun may be a factor.

To protect yourself from developing pterygia, wear sunglasses, or a wide-brimmed hat in places where the sunlight is strong. If you have one or more pterygia, lubricating eye drops may be recommended to reduce redness and soothe irritation.

Because a pterygium is visible, some people might want to have it removed for cosmetic reasons. However, unless it affects vision, surgery to remove a pterygium is not recommended. Even if it is surgically removed, a pterygium may grow back, particularly if removed before age 40.

What Treatments Are There for Advanced Corneal Disease?

Laser Surgery

Phototherapeutic keratectomy (PTK) is a surgical technique that uses UV light and laser technology to reshape and restore the cornea. PTK has been used to treat recurrent erosions and corneal dystrophies, such as map-dot-fingerprint dystrophy and basal membrane dystrophy. PTK helps delay or postpone corneal grafting or replacement.

Section 17.3

Dry Eye

This section includes text excerpted from "Facts about Dry Eye," National Eye Institute (NEI), July 2017.

What Is Dry Eye?

Dry eye occurs when the quantity and/or quality of tears fails to keep the surface of the eye adequately lubricated. Experts estimate that dry eye affects millions of adults in the United States. The risk of developing dry eye increases with advancing age. Women have a higher prevalence of dry eye compared with men.

What Are the Symptoms of Dry Eye?

Dry eye causes a scratchy sensation or the feeling that something is in the eye. Other symptoms include stinging or burning, episodes of excess tearing that follow periods of dryness, discharge, pain, and redness in the eye. People with dry eye may also feel as if their eyelids are heavy and may experience blurred vision.

What Are Tears and How Do They Relate to Dry Eye?

In a healthy eye, lubricating tears called basal tears continuously bathe the cornea, the clear, dome-shaped outer surface of the eye. With every blink of the eye, basal tears flow across the cornea, nourishing its cells and providing a layer of liquid protection from the environment. When the glands nearby each eye fail to produce enough basal tears, or when the composition of the tears changes, the health of the eye and vision are compromised. Vision may be affected because tears on the surface of the eye play an important role in focusing light.

Tears are a complex mixture of fatty oils, water, mucus, and more than 1500 different proteins that keep the surface of the eye smooth and protected from the environment, irritants, and infectious pathogens. Tears form in three layers:

- An outer, oily (lipid) layer, produced by the Meibomian glands, keeps tears from evaporating too quickly and helps tears remain on the eye.

- A middle (aqueous) layer contains the watery portion of tears as well as water-soluble proteins. This layer is produced by the main lacrimal gland and accessory lacrimal glands. It nourishes the cornea and the conjunctiva, the mucous membrane that covers the entire front of the eye and the inside of the eyelids.

- An inner (mucin) layer, produced by goblet cells, binds water from the aqueous layer to ensure that the eye remains wet.

What Causes Dry Eye?

Dry eye can occur when basal tear production decreases, tear evaporation increases, or tear composition is imbalanced. Factors that can contribute to dry eye include the following:

- Medications including antihistamines, decongestants, antidepressants, birth control pills, hormone replacement therapy to relieve symptoms of menopause, and medications for anxiety, Parkinson disease, and high blood pressure have been associated with dry eye.

- Advancing age is a risk factor for declines in tear production. Dry eye is more common in people age 50 years or older.

- Rosacea (an inflammatory skin disease) and blepharitis (an inflammatory eyelid disease) can disrupt the function of the Meibomian glands.

- Autoimmune disorders such as Sjögren syndrome, lupus, scleroderma, and rheumatoid arthritis and other disorders such as diabetes, thyroid disorders, and Vitamin A deficiency are associated with dry eye.

- Women are more likely to develop dry eye. Hormonal changes during pregnancy and after menopause have been linked with dry eye. Women also have an increased risk for autoimmune disorders.

- Windy, smoky, or dry environments increase tear evaporation.

- Seasonal allergies can contribute to dry eye.

- Prolonged periods of screen time encourage insufficient blinking.

- Laser eye surgery may cause temporary dry eye symptoms.

How Is Dry Eye Diagnosed and Treated?

People experiencing dry eye symptoms should consult an eye care professional to determine the cause, which guides treatment strategy.

Change medications. Consult a physician about switching medications to alternative ones that are not associated with dry eye. This may alleviate dry eye symptoms.

Over-the-counter (OTC) topical medications. Mild dry eye symptoms may be treated with over-the-counter medications such as artificial tears, gels, and ointments.

Environmental and lifestyle changes. Cutting back on-screen time and taking periodic eye breaks may help. Closing the eyes for a few minutes, or blinking repeatedly for a few seconds, may replenish basal tears and spread them more evenly across the eye. Sunglasses that wrap around the face and have side shields that block wind and dry air can reduce symptoms in windy or dry conditions. In cases of Meibomian gland dysfunction, warm lid compresses and scrubs may be helpful. Smoking cessation and limiting exposure to second-hand smoke also may help.

Prescription dry eye medications. Cyclosporine and lifitegrast are the only prescription medications approved by the U.S.

Food and Drug Administration (FDA) for treating dry eye. Corticosteroid eye drops also may be prescribed short term to reduce eye inflammation.

Devices. FDA-approved devices provide temporary relief from dry eye by stimulating glands and nerves associated with tear production.

Surgical options. Punctal plugs made of silicone or collagen may be inserted by an eye care professional to partially or completely plug the tear ducts at the inner corners of the eye to keep tears from draining from the eye. In severe cases, surgical closure of the drainage ducts by thermal punctal cautery may be recommended to close the tear ducts permanently.

Section 17.4

Glaucoma

This section includes text excerpted from "Healthy Living—Don't Let Glaucoma Steal Your Sight!" Centers for Disease Control and Prevention (CDC), January 11, 2017.

Know the Facts

- Glaucoma is a group of diseases that damage the eye's optic nerve and can result in vision loss and even blindness.

- About 3 million Americans have glaucoma. It is the 2nd leading cause of blindness worldwide.

- Open-angle glaucoma, the most common form, results in increased eye pressure. There are often no early symptoms, which is why 50 percent of people with glaucoma don't know they have the disease.

- There is no cure (yet) for glaucoma, but if it's caught early, you can preserve your vision and prevent vision loss. Taking action to preserve your vision health is key.

Know Your Risk

Anyone can get glaucoma, but certain groups are at higher risk. These groups include African Americans over age 40, all people over age 60, people with a family history of glaucoma, and people who have diabetes. African Americans are 6 to 8 times more likely to get glaucoma than whites. People with diabetes are 2 times more likely to get glaucoma than people without diabetes.

Take Action

There are many steps you can take to help protect your eyes and lower your risk of vision loss from glaucoma.

• If you are in a high-risk group, get a comprehensive dilated eye exam to catch glaucoma early and start treatment. Prescription eye drops can stop glaucoma from progressing. Your eye care specialist will recommend how often to return for follow-up exams. Medicare covers a glaucoma test once a year for people in high-risk groups.

• Even if you are not in a high-risk group, getting a comprehensive dilated eye exam by the age of 40 can help catch glaucoma and other eye diseases early.

• Open-angle glaucoma does not have symptoms and is hereditary, so talk to your family members about their vision health to help protect your eyes—and theirs.

• Maintaining a healthy weight, controlling your blood pressure, being physically active, and avoiding smoking will help you avoid vision loss from glaucoma. These healthy behaviors will also help prevent type 2 diabetes and other chronic conditions.

Manage and Treat

Vision loss from glaucoma usually affects peripheral vision (what you can see on the side of your head when looking ahead) first. Later, it will affect your central vision, which is needed for seeing objects clearly and for common daily tasks like reading and driving.

Glaucoma is treated with eye drops, oral medicine, or surgery (or a combination of treatments) to reduce pressure in the eye and prevent permanent vision loss. Take medicine as prescribed, and tell your eye care specialist about any side effects. You and your doctor are a team. If laser or surgical procedures are recommended to reduce the pressure in your eye, make sure to schedule regular follow-up visits to continue to monitor eye pressure. Some people with glaucoma have low vision, which means they have a hard time doing routine activities even with the help of glasses or contacts.

Section 17.5

Low Vision

This section includes text excerpted from "Low Vision—What You Should Know," National Eye Institute (NEI), January 24, 2013. Reviewed September 2017.

What Is Low Vision?

When you have low vision, eyeglasses, contact lenses, medicine, or surgery may not help. Activities like reading, shopping, cooking, writing, and watching TV may be hard to do.

In fact, millions of Americans lose some of their sight every year. While vision loss can affect anyone at any age, low vision is most common for those over age 65.

Low vision is usually caused by eye diseases or health conditions. Some of these include age-related macular degeneration (AMD), cataract, diabetes, and glaucoma. Eye injuries and birth defects are some other causes. Whatever the cause, lost vision cannot be restored. It can, however, be managed with proper treatment and vision rehabilitation.

You should visit an eye care professional if you experience any changes to your eyesight.

How Do I Know If I Have Low Vision?

Below are some signs of low vision. Even when wearing your glasses or contact lenses, do you still have difficulty with—

- Recognizing the faces of family and friends?

- Reading, cooking, sewing, or fixing things around the house?

- Selecting and matching the color of your clothes?

- Seeing clearly with the lights on or feeling like they are dimmer than normal?

- Reading traffic signs or the names of stores?

These could all be early warning signs of vision loss or eye disease. The sooner vision loss or eye disease is detected by an eye care professional, the greater your chances of keeping your remaining vision.

How Do I Know When to Get an Eye Exam?

Visit your eye care professional regularly for a comprehensive dilated eye exam. However, if you notice changes to your eyes or eyesight, visit your eye care professional right away!

What Can I Do If I Have Low Vision?

To cope with vision loss, you must first **have an excellent support team**. This team should include you, your primary eye care professional, and an optometrist or ophthalmologist specializing in low vision.

Occupational therapists, orientation and mobility specialists, certified low vision therapists, counselors, and social workers are also available to help.

Together, the low vision team can help you make the most of your remaining vision and maintain your independence.

Second, **talk with your eye care professional** about your vision problems. Even though it may be difficult, ask for help. Find out where you can get more information about support services and adaptive devices. Also, find out which services and devices are best for you and which will give you the most independence.

Third, **ask about vision rehabilitation**, even if your eye care professional says that "nothing more can be done for your vision."

Vision rehabilitation programs offer a wide range of services, including training for magnifying and adaptive devices, ways to complete daily living skills safely and independently, guidance on modifying your home, and information on where to locate resources and support to help you cope with your vision loss.

Medicare may cover part or all of a patient's occupational therapy, but the therapy must be ordered by a doctor and provided by a Medicare-approved healthcare provider. To see if you are eligible for Medicare-funded occupational therapy, call 800-633-4227 (800-MEDICARE).

Finally, **be persistent**. Remember that you are your best health-care advocate. Explore your options, learn as much as you can, and keep asking questions about vision rehabilitation. In fact, write down questions to ask your doctor before your exam, and bring along a notepad to jot down answers.

There are many resources to help people with low vision, and many of these programs, devices, and technologies can help you maintain your normal, everyday way of life.

What Questions Should I Ask My Eye Care Team?

An important part of any doctor patient relationship is effective communication. Here are some questions to ask your eye care professional or specialist in low vision to jumpstart the discussion about vision loss.

Questions to Ask Your Eye Care Professional

* What changes can I expect in my vision?

* Will my vision loss get worse? How much of my vision will I lose?

* Will regular eyeglasses improve my vision?

* What medical or surgical treatments are available for my condition?

* What can I do to protect or prolong my vision?

* Will diet, exercise, or other lifestyle changes help?

* If my vision can't be corrected, can you refer me to a specialist in low vision?

* Where can I get vision rehabilitation services?

Questions to Ask Your Specialist in Low Vision

* How can I continue my normal, routine activities?

* Are there resources to help me in my job?

* Will any special devices help me with daily activities like reading, sewing, cooking, or fixing things around the house?

* What training and services are available to help me live better and more safely with low vision?

• Where can I find individual or group support to cope with my vision loss?

Section 17.6

Macular Degeneration

This section includes text excerpted from "Facts about Age-Related Macular Degeneration," National Eye Institute (NEI), September 2015.

What Is Age-Related Macular Degeneration (AMD)?

AMD is a common eye condition and a leading cause of vision loss among people age 50 and older. It causes damage to the macula, a small spot near the center of the retina and the part of the eye needed for sharp, central vision, which lets us see objects that are straight ahead.

In some people, AMD advances so slowly that vision loss does not occur for a long time. In others, the disease progresses faster and may lead to a loss of vision in one or both eyes. As AMD progresses, a blurred area near the center of vision is a common symptom. Over time, the blurred area may grow larger or you may develop blank spots in your central vision. Objects also may not appear to be as bright as they used to be.

AMD by itself does not lead to complete blindness, with no ability to see. However, the loss of central vision in AMD can interfere with simple everyday activities, such as the ability to see faces, drive, read, write, or do close work, such as cooking or fixing things around the house.

The Macula

The macula is made up of millions of light-sensing cells that provide sharp, central vision. It is the most sensitive part of the retina, which is located at the back of the eye. The retina turns light into electrical signals and then sends these electrical signals through the optic nerve to the brain, where they are translated into the images we see. When the macula is damaged, the center of your field of view may appear blurry, distorted, or dark.

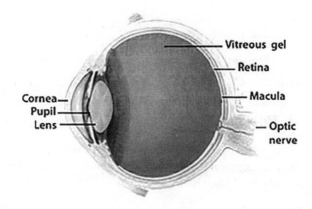

Figure 17.2. *Parts of the Eye*

Who Is at Risk?

Age is a major risk factor for AMD. The disease is most likely to occur after age 60, but it can occur earlier. Other risk factors for AMD include:

- **Smoking.** Research shows that smoking doubles the risk of AMD.

- **Race.** AMD is more common among Caucasians than among African-Americans or Hispanics/Latinos.

- **Family history and Genetics.** People with a family history of AMD are at higher risk. At last count, researchers had identified nearly 20 genes that can affect the risk of developing AMD. Many more genetic risk factors are suspected. You may see offers for genetic testing for AMD. Because AMD is influenced by so many genes plus environmental factors such as smoking and nutrition, there are currently no genetic tests that can diagnose AMD, or predict with certainty who will develop it. The American Academy of Ophthalmology (AAO) currently recommends against routine genetic testing for AMD, and insurance generally does not cover such testing.

Does Lifestyle Make a Difference?

Researchers have found links between AMD and some lifestyle choices, such as smoking. You might be able to reduce your risk of AMD or slow its progression by making these healthy choices:

- Avoid smoking

- Exercise regularly

- Maintain normal blood pressure and cholesterol levels

- Eat a healthy diet rich in green, leafy vegetables and fish

How Is AMD Detected?

The early and intermediate stages of AMD usually start without symptoms. Only a comprehensive dilated eye exam can detect AMD. The eye exam may include the following:

- **Visual acuity test.** This eye chart measures how well you see at distances.

- **Dilated eye exam.** Your eye care professional place drops in your eyes to widen or dilate the pupils. This provides a better view of the back of your eye. Using a special magnifying lens, he or she then looks at your retina and optic nerve for signs of AMD and other eye problems.

- **Amsler grid.** Your eye care professional also may ask you to look at an Amsler grid. Changes in your central vision may cause the lines in the grid to disappear or appear wavy, a sign of AMD.

- **Fluorescein angiogram.** In this test, which is performed by an ophthalmologist, a fluorescent dye is injected into your arm. Pictures are taken as the dye passes through the blood vessels in your eye. This makes it possible to see leaking blood vessels, which occur in a severe, rapidly progressive type of AMD. In rare cases, complications to the injection can arise, from nausea to more severe allergic reactions.

- **Optical coherence tomography (OCT).** You have probably heard of ultrasound, which uses sound waves to capture images of living tissues. OCT is similar except that it uses light waves, and can achieve very high-resolution images of any tissues that can be penetrated by light—such as the eyes. After your eyes are dilated, you'll be asked to place your head on a chin rest and hold still for several seconds while the images are obtained. The light beam is painless.

During the exam, your eye care professional will look for drusen, which are yellow deposits beneath the retina. Most people develop some very small drusen as a normal part of aging. The presence of medium-to-large drusen may indicate that you have AMD. Another sign of AMD is the appearance of pigmentary changes under the retina. In addition to the pigmented cells in the iris (the colored part of the eye), there are pigmented cells beneath the retina. As these cells break down and release their pigment, your eye care professional may see dark clumps of released pigment and later, areas that are less pigmented. These changes will not affect your eye color.

What Are the Stages of AMD?

There are three stages of AMD defined in part by the size and number of drusen under the retina. It is possible to have AMD in one eye only, or to have one eye with a later stage of AMD than the other.

- **Early AMD.** Early AMD is diagnosed by the presence of medium-sized drusen, which are about the width of an average human hair. People with early AMD typically do not have vision loss.

- **Intermediate AMD.** People with intermediate AMD typically have large drusen, pigment changes in the retina, or both. Again, these changes can only be detected during an eye exam. Intermediate AMD may cause some vision loss, but most people will not experience any symptoms.

- **Late AMD.** In addition to drusen, people with late AMD have vision loss from damage to the macula. There are two types of late AMD:

- In geographic atrophy (also called dry AMD), there is a gradual breakdown of the light-sensitive cells in the macula that convey visual information to the brain, and of the supporting tissue beneath the macula. These changes cause vision loss.

- In neovascular AMD (also called wet AMD), abnormal blood vessels grow underneath the retina. ("Neovascular" literally means "new vessels.") These vessels can leak fluid and blood, which may lead to swelling and damage of the macula. The damage may be rapid and severe, unlike the more gradual course of geographic atrophy. It is possible to have both geographic atrophy and neovascular AMD in the same eye, and either condition can appear first.

AMD has few symptoms in the early stages, so it is important to have your eyes examined regularly. If you are at risk for AMD because of age, family history, lifestyle, or some combination of these factors, you should not wait to experience changes in vision before getting checked for AMD.

Not everyone with early AMD will develop late AMD. For people who have early AMD in one eye and no signs of AMD in the other eye, about five percent will develop advanced AMD after 10 years. For people who have early AMD in both eyes, about 14 percent will develop late AMD in at least one eye after 10 years. With prompt detection of AMD, there are steps you can take to further reduce your risk of vision loss from late AMD.

If you have late AMD in one eye only, you may not notice any changes in your overall vision. With the other eye seeing clearly, you may still be able to drive, read, and see fine details. However, having late AMD in one eye means you are at increased risk for late AMD in your other eye. If you notice distortion or blurred vision, even if it doesn't have much effect on your daily life, consult an eye care professional.

How Is AMD Treated?

Early AMD

Currently, no treatment exists for early AMD, which in many people shows no symptoms or loss of vision. Your eye care professional may recommend that you get a comprehensive dilated eye exam at least once a year. The exam will help determine if your condition is advancing.

As for prevention, AMD occurs less often in people who exercise, avoid smoking, and eat nutritious foods including green leafy vegetables and fish. If you already have AMD, adopting some of these habits may help you keep your vision longer.

Intermediate and Late AMD

Researchers at the National Eye Institute (NEI) tested whether taking nutritional supplements could protect against AMD in the

Age-Related Eye Disease Studies (AREDS and AREDS2). They found that daily intake of certain high-dose vitamins and minerals can slow progression of the disease in people who have intermediate AMD, and those who have late AMD in one eye.

If you have intermediate or late AMD, you might benefit from taking supplements containing these ingredients. But first, be sure to review and compare the labels. Many supplements have different ingredients, or different doses, from those tested in the AREDS trials. Also, consult your doctor or eye care professional about which supplement, if any, is right for you. For example, if you smoke regularly, or used to, your doctor may recommend that you avoid supplements containing beta-carotene.

Even if you take a daily multivitamin, you should consider taking an AREDS supplement if you are at risk for late AMD. The formulations tested in the AREDS trials contain much higher doses of vitamins and minerals than what is found in multivitamins. Tell your doctor or eye care professional about any multivitamins you are taking when you are discussing possible AREDS formulations.

Finally, remember that the AREDS formulation is not a cure. It does not help people with early AMD, and will not restore vision already lost from AMD. But it may delay the onset of late AMD. It also may help slow vision loss in people who already have late AMD.

Advanced Neovascular AMD

Neovascular AMD typically results in severe vision loss. However, eye care professionals can try different therapies to stop further vision loss. You should remember that the therapies described below are not a cure. The condition may progress even with treatment.

- Injections
- Photodynamic therapy
- Laser surgery

Coping with AMD

AMD and vision loss can profoundly affect your life. This is especially true if you lose your vision rapidly.

Even if you experience gradual vision loss, you may not be able to live your life the way you used to. You may need to cut back on working, volunteering, and recreational activities. Your relationships may change, and you may need more help from family and friends than you are used to. These changes can lead to feelings of loss, lowered self-esteem, isolation, and depression.

In addition to getting medical treatment for AMD, there are things you can do to cope:

- Learn more about your vision loss.

- Visit a specialist in low vision and get devices and learning skills to help you with the tasks of everyday living.

- Try to stay positive. People who remain hopeful say they are better able to cope with AMD and vision loss.

- Stay engaged with family and friends.

- Seek a professional counsellor or support group. Your doctor or eye care professional may be able to refer you to one.

Chapter 18

Gastrointestinal (GI) Disorders

Chapter Contents

Section 18.1

Constipation

This section includes text excerpted from "Constipation," National Institute of Diabetes and Digestive and Kidney Diseases (NIDDK), November 2014. Reviewed September 2017.

Definition and Facts

What Is Constipation?

Constipation is a condition in which you typically have:

- fewer than three bowel movements a week

- bowel movements with stools that are hard, dry, and small, making them painful or difficult to pass

Some people think they are constipated if they don't have a bowel movement every day. However, people can have different bowel movement patterns. Some people may have three bowel movements a day. Other people may only have three bowel movements a week.

Constipation most often lasts for only a short time and is not dangerous. You can take steps to prevent or relieve constipation.

How Common Is Constipation?

Constipation is one of the most common gastrointestinal (GI) problems, affecting about 42 million people in the United States.

Who Is More Likely to Become Constipated?

Constipation is common among all ages and populations in the United States, yet certain people are more likely to become constipated, including:

- older adults

- women, especially during pregnancy or after giving birth

246

- non-Caucasians
- people with lower incomes
- people who just had surgery
- people taking medicines to treat depression or to relieve pain from things such as a broken bone, a pulled tooth, or back pain

What Are the Complications of Constipation?

Chronic, or long-lasting, constipation can lead to health problems such as hemorrhoids, anal fissures, rectal prolapse, or fecal impaction.

Hemorrhoids

Hemorrhoids are swollen and inflamed veins around your anus or in your lower rectum. You can develop hemorrhoids if you strain to have a bowel movement. If you have hemorrhoids, you may have bleeding in your rectum. You have bleeding in the rectum when you see bright red blood in your stool, on toilet paper, or in the toilet after a bowel movement.

Anal Fissures

Anal fissures are small tears in your anus that may cause itching, pain, or bleeding.

Rectal Prolapse

Rectal prolapse happens when your rectum slips so that it sticks out of your anus. Rectal prolapse can happen if you strain during bowel movements, among other reasons. Rectal prolapse may cause mucus to leak from your anus. Rectal prolapse is most common in older adults with a history of constipation, and is also more common in women than men, especially postmenopausal women.

Fecal impaction

Fecal impaction happens when hard stool packs your intestine and rectum so tightly that the normal pushing action of your colon is not enough to push the stool out. Fecal impaction occurs most often in children and older adults.

Symptoms and Causes

What Are the Symptoms of Constipation?

The most common symptoms of constipation are:

- fewer-than-normal bowel movements
- stool that is difficult or painful to pass
- pain or bloating in your abdomen

What Causes Constipation?

Constipation can happen for many reasons, and constipation may have more than one cause at a time. Among the most common causes of constipation are:

- slow movement of stool through the colon
- delayed emptying of the colon from pelvic disorders, especially in women
- a form of irritable bowel syndrome (IBS) that has symptoms of both IBS and constipation, also called IBS with constipation, or IBS-C

Constipation may become worse because of the following factors:

Diets Low in Fiber

Fiber helps stool stay soft. Drink liquids to help fiber keep stool soft. Older adults commonly have constipation because of limited dietary fiber, lack of physical activity, and medications.

Lack of Physical Activity

If you don't exercise or move around regularly you may get constipated. For example, people may be less active because they:

- have other health problems
- sit all day and don't exercise regularly
- have to stay in bed most of the time because of an illness or accident

Medicines

Some medicines that doctors prescribe to treat other health problems can cause constipation. Medicines that can cause constipation include:

- antacids—used to neutralize stomach acid—that contain aluminum and calcium

- anticholinergics—used to treat muscle spasms in the intestines

- anticonvulsants—used to decrease abnormal electrical activity in the brain to prevent seizures

- antispasmodics—used to reduce muscle spasms in the intestines

- calcium channel blockers—used to treat high blood pressure and heart disease

- diuretics—used to help the kidneys remove fluid from the blood

- iron supplements—used to build up higher iron levels in the blood

- medicines used to treat Parkinson disease

- narcotics—used to treat severe pain

- some medicines used to treat depression

Life Changes or Daily Routine Changes

Constipation can happen when your life or daily routine changes. For example, your bowel movements can change:

- when you travel

- if you become pregnant

- as you get older

Ignoring the Urge to Have a Bowel Movement

If you ignore the urge to have a bowel movement, over time, you may stop feeling the need to have one. You may delay having a bowel movement because you do not want to use toilets outside of your home, do not have access to a toilet, or may feel you are too busy. This habit can lead to constipation.

Certain Health Problems

Some health problems can make stool move more slowly through your colon, rectum, or anus, causing constipation. These health problems include:

- disorders that affect your brain and spine, such as Parkinson disease
- spinal cord or brain injuries
- diabetes
- hypothyroidism

Gastrointestinal (GI) Tract Problems

Problems in your GI tract that compress or narrow your colon and rectum can cause constipation. These problems include:

- tumors
- inflammation, or swelling, such as diverticulitis or inflammatory bowel disease

Functional GI Disorders

Functional GI disorders happen when your GI tract behaves in an abnormal way, yet without evidence of damage due to a disease. For example, IBS is a common functional GI disorder, and many people with IBS can have IBS with constipation.

Diagnosis

How Do Doctors Diagnose Constipation?

Doctors diagnose constipation by:

- taking a medical history
- performing a physical exam
- performing diagnostic tests, such as a blood test

Medical History

The medical history will include questions about your constipation, such as:

- how often you have a bowel movement
- how long you've had symptoms
- what your stools look like and whether you have blood in your stool

- your eating habits
- your level of physical activity
- the medicines you take

Physical Exam

The physical exam may include a digital rectal exam. During a digital rectal exam, your doctor will have you bend over a table or lie on your side while holding your knees close to your chest. After putting on a glove, the doctor slides a lubricated finger into your anus to check for tenderness, blockage, or blood, and will ask you to squeeze your anal muscles.

Diagnostic Tests

The tests your doctor may order for constipation depend on:

- how long you've been constipated
- how severe your constipation is
- your age
- whether you've had blood in your stool, recent changes in your bowel movement pattern, or weight loss

What Tests Do Doctors Use to Diagnose Constipation?

A doctor may use one or more of the following tests to diagnose constipation.

- Blood test
- Flexible sigmoidoscopy or colonoscopy
- Colorectal transit studies
  - Radiopaque markers
  - Scintigraphy
- Anorectal function tests
- Lower GI series
- Defecography
- Magnetic resonance imaging (MRI)
- Computerized tomography (CT) scan

Treatment

How Do Doctors Treat Constipation?

Treatment for constipation depends on:

- what's causing your constipation
- how bad your constipation is
- how long you've been constipated

Treatment for constipation may include the following:

- Changes in eating, diet, and nutrition
- Changes in your eating, diet, and nutrition can treat constipation. These changes include:

  - Drinking liquids throughout the day. A healthcare professional can recommend how much and what kind of liquids you should drink.
  - Eating more fruits and vegetables.
  - Eating more fiber.

Exercise and Lifestyle Changes

Exercising every day may help prevent and relieve constipation. You can also try to have a bowel movement at the same time each day. Picking a specific time of day may help you have a bowel movement regularly. For example, some people find that trying to have a bowel movement 15 to 45 minutes after breakfast helps them have a bowel movement. Eating helps your colon move stool. Make sure you give yourself enough time to have a bowel movement. You should also use the bathroom as soon as you feel the urge to have a bowel movement.

Over-the-Counter Medicines

Your doctor may suggest using a laxative for a short time if you're doing all the right things and are still constipated. Your doctor will tell you what type of laxative is best for you. Over-the-counter laxatives come in many forms, including liquid, tablet, capsule, powder, and granules.

If you're taking an over-the-counter or prescription medicine or supplement that can cause constipation, your doctor may suggest you stop taking it or switch to a different one.

Bulk-forming agents. Bulk-forming agents absorb fluid in your intestines, making your stool bulkier. Bulkier stool helps trigger the bowel to contract and push stool out. Be sure to take bulk-forming agents with water or they can cause an obstruction or a blockage in your bowel. They can also cause bloating and pain in your abdomen.

Osmotic agents. Osmotic agents help stool retain fluid. Stools with more fluid increase your number of bowel movements and soften stool. Older adults and people with heart or kidney failure should be careful when taking osmotic agents. They can cause dehydration or a mineral imbalance.

Stool softeners. Stool softeners help mix fluid into stools to soften them. Doctors recommend stool softeners for people who should avoid straining while having a bowel movement. Doctors often recommend stool softeners after surgery or for women after childbirth.

Lubricants. Lubricants work by coating the surface of stool, which helps the stool hold in fluid and pass more easily. Lubricants are simple, inexpensive laxatives. Doctors may recommend lubricants for people with anorectal blockage.

If these laxatives don't work for you, your doctor may recommend other types of laxatives, including:

Stimulants. Stimulant laxatives cause the intestines to contract, which moves stool. You should only use stimulants if your constipation is severe or other treatments have not worked.

People should not use stimulant laxatives containing phenolphthalein. Phenolphthalein may increase your chances of cancer. Most laxatives sold in the United States do not contain phenolphthalein. Make sure to check the ingredients on the medicine's package or bottle.

If you've been taking laxatives for a long time and can't have a bowel movement without taking a laxative, talk with your doctor about how you can slowly stop using them. If you stop taking laxatives, over time, your colon should start moving stool normally.

Prescription Medicines

If over-the-counter medicines do not relieve your symptoms, your doctor may prescribe one of the following medicines:

Chloride channel activator. If you have irritable bowel syndrome (IBS) with long-lasting or idiopathic—meaning the cause is not known—constipation, your doctor may prescribe lubiprostone (Amitiza). Lubiprostone is a chloride channel activator available with a prescription. Research has shown lubiprostone to be safe when used for 6 to 12 months. This type of medicine increases fluid in your GI tract, which helps to:

- reduce pain or discomfort in your abdomen
- make your stool softer
- reduce your need to strain when having a bowel movement
- increase how often you have bowel movements

Guanylate cyclase-C agonist. If you have IBS with long-lasting or idiopathic constipation, your doctor may prescribe linaclotide (Linzess) to help make your bowel movements regular. Linaclotide is a guanylate cyclase-C agonist that eases pain in your abdomen and speeds up how often you have bowel movements.

Biofeedback

If you have problems with the muscles that control bowel movements, your doctor may recommend biofeedback to retrain your muscles. Biofeedback uses special sensors to measure bodily functions. A video monitor shows the measurements as line graphs, and sounds from the equipment tell you when you're using the correct muscles. By watching the monitor and listening to the sounds, you learn how to change the muscle function. Practicing at home can improve muscle function. You may have to practice for 3 months before you get all the benefit from the training.

Surgery

You may need surgery to treat an anorectal blockage caused by rectal prolapse if other treatments don't work. You may need surgery to remove your colon if your colon muscles don't work correctly. Your doctor can tell you about the benefits and risks of surgery.

How Do Doctors Treat Complications of Constipation?

Doctors can treat or tell you how to treat complications of constipation. Hemorrhoids, anal fissures, rectal prolapse, and fecal impaction all have different treatments.

Hemorrhoids

You can treat hemorrhoids at home by:

- making dietary changes to prevent constipation
- taking warm tub baths
- applying over-the-counter hemorrhoid cream to the area or using suppositories—a medicine you insert into your rectum—before bedtime

Talk with your doctor about hemorrhoids that do not respond to at-home treatments.

Anal Fissures

You can treat anal fissures at home by:

- making changes in your diet to prevent constipation
- applying over-the-counter hemorrhoid cream to numb the area or relax your muscles
- using stool softeners
- taking warm tub baths

Your doctor may recommend surgery to treat anal fissures that don't heal with at-home treatments.

Rectal Prolapse

Your doctor may be able to treat your rectal prolapse in his or her office by manually pushing the rectum back through your anus. If you have a severe or chronic—long-lasting—rectal prolapse, you may need surgery. The surgery will strengthen and tighten your anal sphincter muscle and repair the prolapsed lining. You can help prevent rectal prolapse caused by constipation by not straining during a bowel movement.

Fecal Impaction

You can soften a fecal impaction with mineral oil that you take by mouth or through an enema. After softening the impaction, a health-care professional may break up and remove part of the hardened stool by inserting one or two gloved, lubricated fingers into your anus.

Eating, Diet, and Nutrition

How Can My Diet Help Prevent and Relieve Constipation?

You can drink water and other fluids, such as fruit and vegetable juices and clear soups, to help the fiber in your diet work better. This change should make your stools more normal and regular. Ask your doctor about how much you should drink each day based on your health and activity level and where you live.

Depending on their age and sex, adults should get 22 to 34 grams of fiber a day. Older adults sometimes don't get enough fiber in their diets, because they may lose interest in food. If you are older and have lost interest in food, talk with your doctor if:

- food doesn't taste the same as it once did
- you don't feel hungry as often
- you don't want to cook
- you have problems chewing or swallowing

Talk with your doctor to plan a diet with the right amount of fiber for you. Be sure to add fiber to your diet a little at a time so that your body gets used to the change.

Use the following table as a tool to help replace less healthy foods with foods that have fiber.

Table 18.1. Fiber-Rich Food

Examples of Foods That Have Fiber	
Beans, Cereals, and Breads	**Fiber**
½ cup of beans (navy, pinto, kidney, etc.), cooked	6.2–9.6 grams
½ cup of shredded wheat, ready-to-eat cereal	2.7–3.8 grams
? cup of 100 percent bran, ready-to-eat cereal	9.1 grams
1 small oat bran muffin	3.0 grams
1 whole-wheat English muffin	4.4 grams
Fruits	
1 small apple, with skin	3.6 grams
1 medium pear, with skin	5.5 grams
½ cup of raspberries	4.0 grams
½ cup of stewed prunes	3.8 grams

Table 18.1. Continued

Examples of Foods That Have Fiber	
Beans, Cereals, and Breads	**Fiber**
Vegetables	
½ cup of winter squash, cooked	2.9 grams
1 medium sweet potato, baked in skin	3.8 grams
½ cup of green peas, cooked	3.5–4.4 grams
1 small potato, baked, with skin	3.0 grams
½ cup of mixed vegetables, cooked	4.0 grams
½ cup of broccoli, cooked	2.6–2.8 grams
½ cup of greens (spinach, collards, turnip greens), cooked	2.5–3.5 grams

What Should I Avoid Eating If I'm Constipated?

If you're constipated, try not to eat too many foods with little or no fiber, such as:

- cheese

- chips

- fast food

- ice cream

- meat

- prepared foods, such as some frozen meals and snack foods

- processed foods, such as hot dogs or some microwavable dinners

Section 18.2

Diverticulosis

This section includes text excerpted from "Diverticular Disease," National Institute of Diabetes and Digestive and Kidney Diseases (NIDDK), May 2016.

Definition and Facts

What Is Diverticulosis?

Diverticulosis is a condition that occurs when small pouches, or sacs, form and push outward through weak spots in the wall of your colon. These pouches are most common in the lower part of your colon, called the sigmoid colon. One pouch is called a diverticulum. Multiple pouches are called diverticula. Most people with diverticulosis do not have symptoms or problems.

When diverticulosis does cause symptoms or problems, doctors call this diverticular disease. For some people, diverticulosis causes symptoms such as changes in bowel movement patterns or pain in the abdomen. Diverticulosis may also cause problems such as diverticular bleeding and diverticulitis.

Diverticular Bleeding

Diverticular bleeding occurs when a small blood vessel within the wall of a pouch, or diverticulum, bursts.

Diverticulitis

Diverticulitis occurs when you have diverticulosis and one or a few of the pouches in the wall of your colon become inflamed. Diverticulitis can lead to serious complications.

What Are the Complications of Diverticulitis?

Diverticulitis can come on suddenly and cause other problems, such as the following:

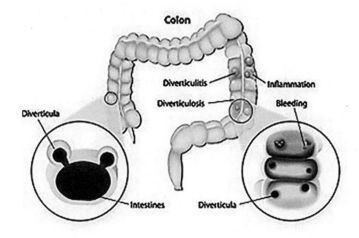

Figure 18.1. *Diverticulosis and Diverticulitis*

Abscess. An abscess is a painful, swollen, infected, and pus-filled area just outside your colon wall that may make you ill with nausea, vomiting, fever, and severe tenderness in your abdomen.

Perforation. A perforation is a small tear or hole in a pouch in your colon.

Peritonitis. Peritonitis is inflammation or infection of the lining of your abdomen. Pus and stool that leak through a perforation can cause peritonitis.

Fistula. A fistula is an abnormal passage, or tunnel, between two organs or between an organ and the outside of your body. The most common types of fistula with diverticulitis occur between the colon and the bladder or between the colon and the vagina in women.

Intestinal obstruction. An intestinal obstruction is a partial or total blockage of the movement of food or stool through your intestines.

How Common Are Diverticulosis and Diverticulitis?

Diverticulosis is quite common, especially as people age. Research suggests that about 35 percent of U.S. adults age 50 years or younger have diverticulosis, while about 58 percent of those older than age 60 have diverticulosis. Most people with diverticulosis will never develop symptoms or problems.

Experts used to think that 10 to 25 percent of people with diverticulosis would develop diverticulitis. However, newer research suggests that the percentage who develop diverticulitis may be much lower—less than 5 percent.

In the United States, about 200,000 people are hospitalized for diverticulitis each year. About 70,000 people are hospitalized for diverticular bleeding each year.

Who Is More Likely to Have Diverticulosis and Diverticulitis?

People are more likely to develop diverticulosis and diverticulitis as they age.

Among people ages 50 and older, women are more likely than men to develop diverticulitis. However, among people younger than age 50, men are more likely to develop diverticulitis.

Symptoms and Causes

What Are the Symptoms of Diverticulosis?

Most people with diverticulosis do not have symptoms. If your diverticulosis causes symptoms, they may include:

- bloating

- constipation or diarrhea

- cramping or pain in your lower abdomen

Other conditions, such as irritable bowel syndrome and peptic ulcers, cause similar symptoms, so these symptoms may not mean you have diverticulosis. If you have these symptoms, see your doctor.

If you have diverticulosis and develop diverticular bleeding or diverticulitis, these conditions also cause symptoms.

What Are the Symptoms of Diverticular Bleeding?

In most cases, when you have diverticular bleeding, you will suddenly have a large amount of red or maroon-colored blood in your stool.

Diverticular bleeding may also cause dizziness or light-headedness, or weakness. See your doctor right away if you have any of these symptoms.

What Are the Symptoms of Diverticulitis?

When you have diverticulitis, the inflamed pouches most often cause pain in the lower left side of your abdomen. The pain is usually severe and comes on suddenly, though it can also be mild and get worse over several days. The intensity of the pain can change over time.
Diverticulitis may also cause:

- constipation or diarrhea

- fevers and chills

- nausea or vomiting

What Causes Diverticulosis and Diverticulitis?

Experts are not sure what causes diverticulosis and diverticulitis. Researchers are studying several factors that may play a role in causing these conditions.

Fiber

For more than 50 years, experts thought that following a low-fiber diet led to diverticulosis. However, research has found that a low-fiber diet may not play a role. This study also found that a high-fiber diet with more frequent bowel movements may be linked with a greater chance of having diverticulosis. Talk with your doctor about how much fiber you should include in your diet.

Genes

Some studies suggest that genes may make some people more likely to develop diverticulosis and diverticulitis. Experts are still studying the role genes play in causing these conditions.

Other factors

Studies have found links between diverticular disease—diverticulosis that causes symptoms or problems such as diverticular bleeding or diverticulitis—and the following factors:

- certain medicines—including nonsteroidal anti-inflammatory drugs (NSAIDs), such as aspirin, and steroids

- lack of exercise

- obesity

- smoking

Diverticulitis may begin when bacteria or stool get caught in a pouch in your colon. A decrease in healthy bacteria and an increase in disease-causing bacteria in your colon may also lead to diverticulitis.

Diagnosis

How Do Doctors Diagnose Diverticulosis and Diverticulitis?

If your doctor suspects you may have diverticulosis or diverticulitis, your doctor may use your medical history, a physical exam, and tests to diagnose these conditions.

Doctors may also diagnose diverticulosis if they notice pouches in the colon wall while performing tests, such as routine X-rays or colonoscopy, for other reasons.

Medical History

Your doctor will ask about your medical history, including your:

- bowel movement patterns
- diet
- health
- medicines
- symptoms

Physical Exam

Your doctor will perform a physical exam, which may include a digital rectal exam. During a digital rectal exam, your doctor will have you bend over a table or lie on your side while holding your knees close to your chest. After putting on a glove, the doctor will slide a lubricated finger into your anus to check for pain, bleeding, hemorrhoids, or other problems.

What Tests Do Doctors Use to Diagnose Diverticulosis and Diverticulitis?

Your doctor may use the following tests to help diagnose diverticulosis and diverticulitis:

- Blood test
- Computerized tomography (CT) scan

- Lower GI series
- Colonoscopy

Treatment

How Do Doctors Treat Diverticulosis?

The goal of treating diverticulosis is to prevent the pouches from causing symptoms or problems. Your doctor may recommend the following treatments:

High-fiber diet. Although a high-fiber diet may not prevent diverticulosis, it may help prevent symptoms or problems in people who already have diverticulosis. A doctor may suggest that you increase fiber in your diet slowly to reduce your chances of having gas and pain in your abdomen. Learn more about foods that are high in fiber.

Fiber supplements. Your doctor may suggest you take a fiber product such as methylcellulose (Citrucel) or psyllium (Metamucil) one to three times a day. These products are available as powders, pills, or wafers and provide 0.5 to 3.5 grams of fiber per dose. You should take fiber products with at least 8 ounces of water.

Medicines. Some studies suggest that mesalazine (Asacol) taken every day or in cycles may help reduce symptoms that may occur with diverticulosis, such as pain in your abdomen or bloating. Studies suggest that the antibiotic rifaximin (Xifaxan) may also help with diverticulosis symptoms.

Probiotics. Some studies show that probiotics may help with diverticulosis symptoms and may help prevent diverticulitis. However, researchers are still studying this subject. Probiotics are live bacteria like those that occur normally in your stomach and intestines. You can find probiotics in dietary supplements—in capsule, tablet, and powder form—and in some foods, such as yogurt.

For safety reasons, talk with your doctor before using probiotics or any complementary or alternative medicines or medical practices.

How Do Doctors Treat Diverticular Bleeding?

Diverticular bleeding is rare. If you have bleeding, it can be severe. In some people, the bleeding may stop by itself and may not require treatment. However, if you have bleeding from your rectum—even a small amount—you should see a doctor right away.

To find the site of the bleeding and stop it, a doctor may perform a colonoscopy. Your doctor may also use a CT scan or an angiogram to find the bleeding site. An angiogram is a special kind of X-ray in which your doctor threads a thin, flexible tube through a large artery, often from your groin, to the bleeding area.

Colon Resection

If your bleeding does not stop, a surgeon may perform abdominal surgery with a colon resection. In a colon resection, the surgeon removes the affected part of your colon and joins the remaining ends of your colon together. You will receive general anesthesia for this procedure.

In some cases, during a colon resection, it may not be safe for the surgeon to rejoin the ends of your colon right away. In this case, the surgeon performs a temporary colostomy. Several months later, in a second surgery, the surgeon rejoins the ends of your colon and closes the opening in your abdomen.

How Do Doctors Treat Diverticulitis?

If you have diverticulitis with mild symptoms and no other problems, a doctor may recommend that you rest, take oral antibiotics, and follow a liquid diet for a period of time. If your symptoms ease after a few days, the doctor will recommend gradually adding solid foods back into your diet.

Severe cases of diverticulitis that come on quickly and cause complications, will likely require a hospital stay and involve intravenous (IV) antibiotics. A few days without food or drink will help your colon rest.

If the period without food or drink is longer than a few days, your doctor may give you an IV liquid food mixture. The mixture contains:

- carbohydrates
- proteins
- fats
- vitamins
- minerals

Eating, Diet, and Nutrition

What Should I Eat If I Have Diverticulosis or Diverticulitis?

If you have diverticulosis or if you have had diverticulitis in the past, your doctor may recommend eating more foods that are high in fiber.

The *Dietary Guidelines for Americans,* 2015–2020, recommends a dietary fiber intake of 14 grams per 1,000 calories consumed. For example, for a 2,000-calorie diet, the fiber recommendation is 28 grams per day.

The amount of fiber in a food is listed on the food's nutrition facts label. Some fiber-rich foods are listed in the table below.

Table 18.2. Fiber Rich Foods

Grains	
Food and Portion Size	**Amount of Fiber**
1/3–3/4 cup high-fiber bran ready-to-eat cereal	9.1–14.3 grams
1–1 1/4 cup of shredded wheat ready-to-eat cereal	5.0–9.0 grams
1 1/2 cup whole wheat spaghetti, cooked	3.2 grams
1 small oat bran muffin	3.0 grams
Fruits	
Food and Portion Size	Amount of Fiber
1 medium pear, with skin	5.5 grams
1 medium apple, with skin	4.4 grams
1/2 cup of raspberries	4.0 grams
1/2 cup of stewed prunes	3.8 grams
Vegetables	
Food and Portion Size	Amount of Fiber
1/2 cup of green peas, cooked	3.5–4.4 grams
1/2 cup of mixed vegetables, cooked from frozen	4.0 grams
1/2 cup of collards, cooked	3.8 grams
1 medium sweet potato, baked in skin	3.8 grams
1 medium potato, baked, with skin	3.6 grams
1/2 cup of winter squash, cooked	2.9 grams
Beans	
Food and Portion Size	Amount of Fiber
1/2 cup navy beans, cooked	9.6 grams
1/2 cup pinto beans, cooked	7.7 grams
1/2 kidney beans, cooked	5.7 grams

(Source: U.S. Department of Agriculture (USDA) and U.S. Department of Health and Human Services (HHS). 2015–2020 Dietary Guidelines for Americans. 8th Edition. December 2015.)

A doctor or dietitian can help you learn how to add more high-fiber foods to your diet.

Should I Avoid Certain Foods If I Have Diverticulosis or Diverticulitis?

Experts now believe you do not need to avoid certain foods if you have diverticulosis or diverticulitis.

In the past, doctors might have asked you to avoid nuts; popcorn; and seeds such as sunflower, pumpkin, caraway, and sesame. Research suggests that these foods are not harmful to people with diverticulosis or diverticulitis. The seeds in tomatoes, zucchini, cucumbers, straw-berries, and raspberries, as well as poppy seeds, are also fine to eat.

Even so, each person is different. You may find that certain types or amounts of foods worsen your symptoms.

Section 18.3

Peptic Ulcers

This section contains text excerpted from the following sources: Text beginning with the heading "Definition and Facts" is excerpted from "Peptic Ulcer," MedlinePlus, National Institutes of Health (NIH), May 20, 2016; Text under the heading "Symptoms and Causes" is excerpted from "Peptic Ulcers (Stomach Ulcers)," National Institute of Diabetes and Digestive and Kidney Diseases (NIDDK), November 2014. Reviewed September 2017.

Definition and Facts

A peptic ulcer is a sore in the lining of your stomach or your duo-denum, the first part of your small intestine. A burning stomach pain is the most common symptom. The pain:

- starts between meals or during the night

- briefly stops if you eat or take antacids

- lasts for minutes to hours

- comes and goes for several days or weeks

Peptic ulcers happen when the acids that help you digest food dam-age the walls of the stomach or duodenum. The most common cause is infection with a bacterium called *Helicobacter pylori.* Another cause is the long-term use of nonsteroidal anti-inflammatory medicines (NSAIDs) such as aspirin and ibuprofen. Stress and spicy foods do not cause ulcers, but can make them worse.

To see if you have an *H. pylori infection,* your doctor will test your blood, breath, or stool. Your doctor also may look inside your stomach and duodenum by doing an endoscopy or X-ray.

Peptic ulcers will get worse if not treated. Treatment may include medicines to reduce stomach acids or antibiotics to kill *H. pylori.* Antacids and milk can't heal peptic ulcers. Not smoking and avoiding alcohol can help. You may need surgery if your ulcers don't heal.

Symptoms and Causes

What Are the Symptoms of a Peptic Ulcer?

A dull or burning pain in your stomach is the most common symptom of a peptic ulcer. You may feel the pain anywhere between your belly button and breastbone. The pain most often:

- happens when your stomach is empty—such as between meals or during the night

- stops briefly if you eat or if you take antacids

- lasts for minutes to hours

- comes and goes for several days, weeks, or months

Less common symptoms may include:

- bloating

- burping

- feeling sick to your stomach

- poor appetite

- vomiting

- weight loss

Even if your symptoms are mild, you may have a peptic ulcer. You should see your doctor to talk about your symptoms. Without treatment, your peptic ulcer can get worse.

What Causes a Peptic Ulcer?

Causes of peptic ulcers include:

- long-term use of nonsteroidal anti-inflammatory drugs (NSAIDs), such as aspirin and ibuprofen

- an infection with the bacteria *Helicobacter pylori (H. pylori)*

- rare cancerous and noncancerous tumors in the stomach, duodenum, or pancreas—known as Zollinger-Ellison syndrome (ZES)

Sometimes peptic ulcers are caused by both NSAIDs and *H. pylori.*

How Do NSAIDs Cause a Peptic Ulcer?

To understand how NSAIDs cause peptic ulcer disease, it is important to understand how NSAIDs work. Nonsteroidal anti-inflammatory drugs reduce pain, fever, and inflammation, or swelling.

Everyone has two enzymes that produce chemicals in your body's cells that promote pain, inflammation, and fever. NSAIDs work by blocking or reducing the amount of these enzymes that your body makes. However, one of the enzymes also produces another type of chemical that protects the stomach lining from stomach acid and helps control bleeding. When NSAIDs block or reduce the amount of this enzyme in your body, they also increase your chance of developing a peptic ulcer.

How Do H. Pylori Cause a Peptic Ulcer and Peptic Ulcer Disease?

H. pylori are spiral-shaped bacteria that can cause peptic ulcer disease by damaging the mucous coating that protects the lining of the stomach and duodenum. Once *H. pylori* have damaged the mucous coating, powerful stomach acid can get through to the sensitive lining. Together, the stomach acid and *H. pylori* irritate the lining of the stomach or duodenum and cause a peptic ulcer.

When Should You Call or See a Doctor?

You should call or see your doctor right away if you:

- feel weak or faint

- have difficulty breathing

- have red blood in your vomit or vomit that looks like coffee grounds

- have red blood in your stool or black stools

- have sudden, sharp stomach pain that doesn't go away

These symptoms could be signs that a peptic ulcer has caused a more serious problem.

Diagnosis

How Do Doctors Diagnose a Peptic Ulcer?

Your doctor will use information from your medical history, a physical exam, and tests to diagnose an ulcer and its cause. The presence of an ulcer can only be determined by looking directly at the stomach with endoscopy or an X-ray test.

Medical History

To help diagnose a peptic ulcer, your doctor will ask you questions about your medical history, your symptoms, and the medicines you take.

Be sure to mention medicines that you take without a prescription, especially NSAIDs, such as:

- aspirin (Bayer Aspirin)

- ibuprofen (Motrin, Advil)

- naproxen (Aleve)

Physical Exam

A physical exam may help a doctor diagnose a peptic ulcer. During a physical exam, a doctor most often:

- checks for bloating in your abdomen

- listens to sounds within your abdomen using a stethoscope

- taps on your abdomen checking for tenderness or pain

Lab Tests

To see if you have *Helicobacter pylori (H. pylori)* infection, your doctor will order these tests:

Blood test. A blood test involves drawing a sample of your blood at your doctor's office or a commercial facility. A healthcare professional tests the blood sample to see if the results fall within the normal range for different disorders or infections.

Urea breath test. For a urea breath test, you will drink a special liquid that contains urea, a waste product that your body makes as it breaks down protein. If *H. pylori* are present, the bacteria will change this waste product into carbon dioxide—a harmless gas. Carbon dioxide normally appears in your breath when you exhale.

A healthcare professional will take a sample of your breath by having you breathe into a bag at your doctor's office or at a lab. He or she then sends your breath sample to a lab for testing. If your breath sample has higher levels of carbon dioxide than normal, you have *H. pylori* in your stomach or small intestine.

Stool test. Doctors use a stool test to study a sample of your stool. A doctor will give you a container for catching and storing your stool at home. You return the sample to the doctor or a commercial facility, who then sends it to a lab for analysis. Stool tests can show the presence of *H. pylori.*

Upper Gastrointestinal (GI) Endoscopy and Biopsy

In an upper GI endoscopy, a gastroenterologist, surgeon, or other trained healthcare professional uses an endoscope to see inside your upper GI tract. This procedure takes place at a hospital or an outpatient center.

An intravenous (IV) needle will be placed in your arm to provide a sedative. Sedatives help you stay relaxed and comfortable during the procedure. In some cases, the procedure can be performed without sedation. You will be given a liquid anesthetic to gargle or spray anesthetic on the back of your throat. The doctor will carefully feed the endoscope down your esophagus and into your stomach and duodenum. A small camera mounted on the endoscope sends a video image to a monitor, allowing close examination of the lining of your upper GI tract. The endoscope pumps air into your stomach and duodenum, making them easier to see.

The doctor may perform a biopsy with the endoscope by taking a small piece of tissue from the lining of your esophagus. You won't feel the biopsy. A pathologist examines the tissue in a lab.

Upper GI Series

An upper GI series looks at the shape of your upper GI tract. An X-ray technician performs this test at a hospital or an outpatient center. A radiologist reads and reports on the X-ray images. You don't need anesthesia. A healthcare professional will tell you how to prepare for the procedure, including when to stop eating and drinking.

During the procedure, you'll stand or sit in front of an X-ray machine and drink barium, a chalky liquid. Barium coats your esophagus, stomach, and small intestine so your doctor can see the shapes of these organs more clearly on X-rays.

You may have bloating and nausea for a short time after the test. For several days afterward, you may have white or light-colored stools from the barium. A healthcare professional will give you instructions about eating and drinking after the test.

Computerized Tomography (CT) Scan

A CT scan uses a combination of X-rays and computer technology to create images. For a CT scan, a healthcare professional may give you a solution to drink and an injection of a special dye, which doctors call contrast medium. You'll lie on a table that slides into a tunnel-shaped device that takes the X-rays. An X-ray technician performs the procedure in an outpatient center or a hospital, and a radiologist interprets the images. You don't need anesthesia.

CT scans can help diagnose a peptic ulcer that has created a hole in the wall of your stomach or small intestine.

Treatment

How Do Doctors Treat Peptic Ulcer Disease?

There are several types of medicines used to treat a peptic ulcer. Your doctor will decide the best treatment based on the cause of your peptic ulcer.

How Do Doctors Treat an NSAID-Induced Peptic Ulcer?

If NSAIDs are causing your peptic ulcer and you don't have an *H. pylori* infection, your doctor may tell you to:

• stop taking the NSAID

• reduce how much of the NSAID you take

• switch to another medicine that won't cause a peptic ulcer

Your doctor may also prescribe medicines to reduce stomach acid and coat and protect your peptic ulcer. Proton pump inhibitors (PPIs), histamine receptor blockers, and protectants can help relieve pain and help your ulcer heal.

PPIs

PPIs reduce stomach acid and protect the lining of your stomach and duodenum. While PPIs can't kill *H. pylori*, they do help fight the *H. pylori* infection.

PPIs include:

- esomeprazole (Nexium)
- dexlansoprazole (Dexilant)
- lansoprazole (Prevacid)
- omeprazole (Prilosec, Zegerid)
- pantoprazole (Protonix)
- rabeprazole (AcipHex)

Histamine Receptor Blockers

Histamine receptor blockers work by blocking histamine, a chemical in your body that signals your stomach to produce acid. Histamine receptor blockers include:

- cimetidine (Tagamet)
- famotidine (Pepcid)
- ranitidine (Zantac)
- nizatidine (Axid) Protectants

Protectants

Protectants coat ulcers and protect them against acid and enzymes so that healing can occur. Doctors only prescribe one protectant—sucralfate (Carafate)—for peptic ulcer disease.

Tell your doctor if the medicines make you feel sick or dizzy or cause diarrhea or headaches. Your doctor can change your medicines.

If you smoke, quit. You also should avoid alcohol. Drinking alcohol and smoking slow the healing of a peptic ulcer and can make it worse.

What If I Still Need to Take NSAIDs?

If you take NSAIDs for other conditions, such as arthritis, you should talk with your doctor about the benefits and risks of using

NSAIDs. Your doctor can help you determine how to continue using an NSAID safely after your peptic ulcer symptoms go away. Your doctor may prescribe a medicine used to prevent NSAID-induced ulcers called Misoprosotol.

Tell your doctor about all the prescription and over-the-counter medicines you take. Your doctor can then decide if you may safely take NSAIDs or if you should switch to a different medicine. In either case, your doctor may prescribe a PPI or histamine receptor blocker to protect the lining of your stomach and duodenum.

If you need NSAIDs, you can reduce the chance of a peptic ulcer returning by:

- taking the NSAID with a meal
- using the lowest effective dose possible
- quitting smoking
- avoiding alcohol

How Do Doctors Treat an NSAID-Induced Peptic Ulcer When You Have an H. Pylori Infection?

If you have an *H. pylori* infection, a doctor will treat your NSAID-induced peptic ulcer with PPIs or histamine receptor blockers and other medicines, such as antibiotics, bismuth subsalicylates, or antacids.

PPIs reduce stomach acid and protect the lining of your stomach and duodenum. While PPIs can't kill *H. pylori,* they do help fight the *H. pylori* infection.

PPIs include:

- esomeprazole (Nexium)
- dexlansoprazole (Dexilant)
- lansoprazole (Prevacid)
- omeprazole (Prilosec, Zegerid)
- pantoprazole (Protonix)
- rabeprazole (AcipHex)

Histamine Receptor Blockers

Histamine receptor blockers work by blocking histamine, a chemical in your body that signals your stomach to produce acid. Histamine receptor blockers include:

- cimetidine (Tagamet)

- famotidine (Pepcid)
- ranitidine (Zantac)
- nizatidine (Axid)

Antibiotics

A doctor will prescribe antibiotics to kill *H. pylori.* How doctors prescribe antibiotics may differ throughout the world. Over time, some types of antibiotics can no longer destroy certain types of *H. pylori.*

Antibiotics can cure most peptic ulcers caused by *H. pylori* or *H. pylori*-induced peptic ulcers. However, getting rid of the bacteria can be difficult. Take all doses of your antibiotics exactly as your doctor prescribes, even if the pain from a peptic ulcer is gone.

Bismuth Subsalicylates

Medicines containing bismuth subsalicylate, such as Pepto-Bismol, coat a peptic ulcer and protect it from stomach acid. Although bismuth subsalicylate can kill *H. pylori,* doctors sometimes prescribe it with antibiotics, not in place of antibiotics.

Antacids

An antacid may make the pain from a peptic ulcer go away temporarily, yet it will not kill *H. pylori.* If you receive treatment for an *H. pylori*-induced peptic ulcer, check with your doctor before taking antacids. Some of the antibiotics may not work as well if you take them with an antacid.

Can a Peptic Ulcer Come Back?

Yes, a peptic ulcer can come back. If you smoke or take NSAIDs, peptic ulcers are more likely to come back. If you need to take an NSAID, your doctor may switch you to a different medicine or add medicines to help prevent a peptic ulcer. Peptic ulcer disease can return, even if you have been careful to reduce your risk.

How Can I Prevent a Peptic Ulcer?

To help prevent a peptic ulcer caused by NSAIDs, ask your doctor if you should:

- stop using NSAIDs

- take NSAIDs with a meal if you still need NSAIDs
- take a lower dose of NSAIDs
- take medicines to protect your stomach and duodenum while taking NSAIDs
- switch to a medicine that won't cause ulcers

To help prevent a peptic ulcer caused by *H. pylori*, your doctor may recommend that you avoid drinking alcohol.

Eating, Diet, and Nutrition

How Can Your Diet Help Prevent or Relieve a Peptic Ulcer?

Researchers have not found that diet and nutrition play an important role in causing or preventing peptic ulcers. Before acid blocking drugs became available, milk was used to treat ulcers. However, milk is not an effective way to prevent or relieve a peptic ulcer.

Alcohol and smoking do contribute to ulcers and should be avoided.

Chapter 19

Hormonal Imbalances

Chapter Contents

Section 19.1

Diabetes

This section includes text excerpted from "Diabetes in Older People," National Institute on Aging (NIA), National Institutes of Health (NIH), July 24, 2017.

Diabetes is a serious disease. People get diabetes when their blood glucose level, sometimes called blood sugar, is too high. The good news is that there are things you can do to take control of diabetes and prevent its problems. And, if you are worried about getting diabetes, there are things you can do to lower your risk.

What Is Diabetes?

Our bodies turn the food we eat into glucose. Insulin helps glucose get into our cells, where it can be used to make energy. If you have diabetes, your body may not make enough insulin, may not use insulin in the right way, or both. That can cause too much glucose in the blood. Your family doctor may refer you to a doctor who specializes in taking care of people with diabetes, called an endocrinologist.

Types of Diabetes

There are two main kinds of diabetes.

- **Type 1 diabetes.** In type 1 diabetes, the body makes little or no insulin. Although adults can develop this type of diabetes, it occurs most often in children and young adults.

- **Type 2 diabetes.** In type 2 diabetes, the body makes insulin but doesn't use it the right way. It is the most common kind of diabetes. It occurs most often in middle-aged and older adults, but it can also affect children. Your chance of getting type 2 diabetes is higher if you are overweight, inactive, or have a family history of diabetes.

Diabetes can affect many parts of your body. It's important to keep diabetes under control. Over time, it can cause serious health problems like heart disease, stroke, kidney disease, blindness, nerve damage, and circulation problems that may lead to amputation. People with type 2 diabetes also have a greater risk for Alzheimer disease.

What Is Prediabetes?

Many people have "prediabetes." This means their glucose levels are higher than normal but not high enough to be called diabetes. Prediabetes is a serious problem because people who have it are at high risk for developing type 2 diabetes.

There are things you can do to prevent or delay getting type 2 diabetes. Losing weight may help. Healthy eating and being physically active can make a big difference. Work with your doctor to set up a plan for good nutrition and regular exercise. Make sure to ask how often you should have your glucose levels checked.

Symptoms of Diabetes

Some people with type 2 diabetes may not know they have it. But, they may feel tired, hungry, or thirsty. They may lose weight without trying, urinate often, or have trouble with blurred vision. They may also get skin infections or heal slowly from cuts and bruises. See your doctor right away if you have one or more of these symptoms.

Tests for Diabetes

Doctors use several blood tests to help diagnose diabetes:

- **Random plasma glucose test**—given at any time during the day

- **A1C test**—given at any time during the day; shows your glucose level for the past 3 months

- **Fasting plasma glucose test**—taken after you have gone without food for at least 8 hours

- **Oral glucose tolerance test**—taken after fasting overnight and then again 2 hours after having a sugary drink

Your doctor may want you to be tested for diabetes twice before making a diagnosis.

Managing Diabetes

Once you've been told you have diabetes, your doctor will choose the best treatment based on the type of diabetes you have, your everyday routine, and any other health problems you have. Many people with type 2 diabetes can control their blood glucose levels with diet and exercise alone. Others need diabetes medicines or insulin injections. Over time, people with diabetes may need both lifestyle changes and medication.

You can keep control of your diabetes by:

- **Tracking your glucose levels.** Very high glucose levels or very low glucose levels (called hypoglycemia) can be risky to your health. Talk to your doctor about how to check your glucose levels at home.

- **Making healthy food choices.** Learn how different foods affect glucose levels. For weight loss, check out foods that are low in fat and sugar. Let your doctor know if you want help with meal planning.

- **Getting exercise.** Daily exercise can help improve glucose levels in older people with diabetes. Ask your doctor to help you plan an exercise program.

- **Taking your diabetes medicines even when you feel good**. Tell your doctor if you have any side effects or cannot afford your medicines.

Your doctor may want you to see other healthcare providers who can help manage some of the extra problems caused by diabetes. He or she can also give you a schedule for other tests that may be needed. Talk to your doctor about how to stay healthy.

Here are some ways to stay healthy with diabetes:

- **Find out your average blood glucose level.** At least twice a year, get the A1C blood test. The result will show your average glucose level for the past 3 months.

- **Watch your blood pressure.** Get your blood pressure checked often.

- **Check your cholesterol.** At least once a year, get a blood test to check your cholesterol and triglyceride levels. High levels may increase your risk for heart problems.

- **Stop smoking.** Smoking raises your risk for many health problems, including heart attack and stroke.

- **Have yearly eye exams.** Finding and treating eye problems early may keep your eyes healthy.

- **Check your kidneys yearly.** Diabetes can affect your kidneys. A urine and blood test will show if your kidneys are okay.

- **Get flu shots every year and the pneumonia vaccine.** A yearly flu shot will help keep you healthy. If you're over 65, make sure you have had the pneumonia vaccine. If you were younger than 65 when you had the pneumonia vaccine, you may need another one. Ask your doctor.

- **Care for your teeth and gums.** Brush your teeth and floss daily. Have your teeth and gums checked twice a year by a dentist to avoid serious problems.

- **Protect your skin.** Keep your skin clean and use skin softeners for dryness. Take care of minor cuts and bruises to prevent infections.

- **Look at your feet.** Take time to look at your feet every day for any red patches. Ask someone else to check your feet if you can't. If you have sores, blisters, breaks in the skin, infections, or build-up of calluses, see a foot doctor, called a podiatrist.

Be Prepared

Make sure you always have at least 3 days' worth of supplies on hand for testing and treating your diabetes in case of an emergency.

Medicare Can Help

Medicare may pay to help you learn how to care for your diabetes. It may also help pay for diabetes tests, supplies, flu and pneumonia shots, special shoes, foot exams, eye tests, and meal planning.

Section 19.2

Hypothyroidism

This section includes text excerpted from
"Hypothyroidism (Underactive Thyroid)," National
Institute of Diabetes and Digestive and Kidney
Diseases (NIDDK), August 2016.

What Is Hypothyroidism?

Hypothyroidism, also called underactive thyroid, is when the thyroid gland doesn't make enough thyroid hormones to meet your body's needs. The thyroid is a small, butterfly-shaped gland in the front of your neck. Thyroid hormones control the way the body uses energy, so they affect nearly every organ in your body, even the way your heart beats. Without enough thyroid hormones, many of your body's functions slow down.

How Common Is Hypothyroidism?

About 4.6 percent of the U.S. population ages 12 and older has hypothyroidism, although most cases are mild. That's almost 5 people out of 100.

Who Is More Likely to Develop Hypothyroidism?

Women are much more likely than men to develop hypothyroidism. The disease is also more common among people older than age 60.
You are more likely to have hypothyroidism if you:

- have had a thyroid problem before, such as a goiter

- have had surgery to correct a thyroid problem

- have received radiation treatment to the thyroid, neck, or chest

- have a family history of thyroid disease

- were pregnant in the past 6 months

- have Turner syndrome, a genetic disorder that affects females

- have other health problems, including:
  - Sjögren syndrome, a disease that causes dry eyes and mouth
  - pernicious anemia, a condition caused by a vitamin B12 deficiency
  - type 1 diabetes
  - rheumatoid arthritis, an autoimmune disease that affects the joints
  - lupus, a chronic inflammatory condition

What Other Health Problems Could I Have Because of Hypothyroidism?

Hypothyroidism can contribute to high cholesterol, so people with high cholesterol should be tested for hypothyroidism. Rarely, severe, untreated hypothyroidism may lead to myxedema coma, an extreme form of hypothyroidism in which the body's functions slow to the point that it becomes life threatening. Myxedema coma requires immediate medical treatment.

What Are the Symptoms of Hypothyroidism?

Hypothyroidism has many symptoms that can vary from person to person. Some common symptoms of hypothyroidism include:

- fatigue
- weight gain
- a puffy face
- trouble tolerating cold
- joint and muscle pain
- constipation
- dry skin
- dry, thinning hair
- decreased sweating
- heavy or irregular menstrual periods
- fertility problems
- depression
- slowed heart rate
- goiter

Because hypothyroidism develops slowly, many people don't notice symptoms of the disease for months or even years. Many of these symptoms, especially fatigue and weight gain, are common and don't always mean that someone has a thyroid problem.

What Causes Hypothyroidism?

Hypothyroidism has several causes, including:

- Hashimoto disease

- thyroiditis, or inflammation of the thyroid

- congenital hypothyroidism, or hypothyroidism that is present at birth

- surgical removal of part or all of the thyroid

- radiation treatment of the thyroid

- Some medicines can interfere with thyroid hormone production and lead to hypothyroidism, including:

  - amiodarone, a heart medicine

  - interferon alpha, a cancer medicine

  - lithium, a bipolar disorder medicine

  - interleukin-2, a kidney cancer medicine

Less often, hypothyroidism is caused by too much or too little iodine in the diet or by pituitary disease.

How Do Doctors Diagnose Hypothyroidism?

Your doctor will take a medical history and do a physical exam, but also will need to do some tests to confirm a diagnosis of hypothyroidism. Many symptoms of hypothyroidism are the same as those of other diseases, so doctors usually can't diagnose hypothyroidism based on symptoms alone. Because hypothyroidism can cause fertility problems, women who have trouble getting pregnant often get tested for thyroid problems. Your doctor may use several blood tests to confirm a diagnosis of hypothyroidism and find its cause.

How Is Hypothyroidism Treated?

Hypothyroidism is treated by replacing the hormone that your own thyroid can no longer make. You will take levothyroxine, a thyroid hormone medicine that is identical to a hormone the thyroid normally makes. Your doctor may recommend taking the medicine in the morning before eating.

Your doctor will give you a blood test about 6 to 8 weeks after you begin taking thyroid hormone and adjust your dose if needed. Each time your dose is adjusted, you'll have another blood test. Once you've reached a dose that's working for you, your healthcare provider will probably repeat the blood test in 6 months and then once a year.

Your hypothyroidism most likely can be completely controlled with thyroid hormone medicine, as long as you take the recommended dose as instructed. Never stop taking your medicine without talking with your healthcare provider first.

What Should I Avoid Eating If I Have Hypothyroidism?

The thyroid uses iodine to make thyroid hormones. However, people with Hashimoto disease or other types of autoimmune thyroid disorders may be sensitive to harmful side effects from iodine. Eating foods that have large amounts of iodine—such as kelp, dulse, or other kinds of seaweed—may cause or worsen hypothyroidism. Taking iodine supplements can have the same effect.

Talk with members of your healthcare team about what foods you should limit or avoid, and let them know if you take iodine supplements. Also, share information about any cough syrups that you take because they may contain iodine.

Women need more iodine when they are pregnant because the baby gets iodine from the mother's diet. If you are pregnant, talk with your healthcare provider about how much iodine you need.

Chapter 20

Falls (Instability)

A simple thing can change your life—like tripping on a rug or slipping on a wet floor. If you fall, you could break a bone, like thousands of older men and women do each year. For older people, a break can be the start of more serious problems, such as a trip to the hospital, injury, or even disability. If you or an older person you know has fallen, you're not alone. More than one in three people age 65 years or older falls each year. The risk of falling—and fall-related problems—rises with age.

Many Older Adults Fear Falling

The fear of falling becomes more common as people age, even among those who haven't fallen. It may lead older people to avoid activities such as walking, shopping, or taking part in social activities.

But don't let a fear of falling keep you from being active. Overcoming this fear can help you stay active, maintain your physical health, and prevent future falls. Doing things like getting together with friends, gardening, walking, or going to the local senior center helps you stay healthy. The good news is, there are simple ways to prevent most falls.

This chapter includes text excerpted from "Prevent Falls and Fractures," National Institute on Aging (NIA), National Institutes of Health (NIH), July 21, 2017.

Causes and Risk Factors for Falls

Many things can cause a fall. Your eyesight, hearing, and reflexes might not be as sharp as they were when you were younger. Diabetes, heart disease, or problems with your thyroid, nerves, feet, or blood vessels can affect your balance. Some medicines can cause you to feel dizzy or sleepy, making you more likely to fall. Other causes include safety hazards in the home or community environment.

Scientists have linked several personal risk factors to falling, including muscle weakness, problems with balance and gait, and blood pressure that drops too much when you get up from lying down or sitting (called postural hypotension). Foot problems that cause pain and unsafe footwear, like backless shoes or high heels, can also increase your risk of falling.

Confusion can sometimes lead to falls. For example, if you wake up in an unfamiliar environment, you might feel unsure of where you are. If you feel confused, wait for your mind to clear or until someone comes to help you before trying to get up and walk around.

Some medications can increase a person's risk of falling because they cause side effects like dizziness or confusion. The more medications you take, the more likely you are to fall.

Take the Right Steps to Prevent Falls

If you take care of your overall health, you may be able to lower your chances of falling. Most of the time, falls and accidents don't "just happen." Here are a few tips to help you avoid falls and broken bones:

- **Stay physically active.** Plan an exercise program that is right for you. Regular exercise improves muscles and makes you stronger. It also helps keep your joints, tendons, and ligaments flexible. Mild weight-bearing activities, such as walking or climbing stairs, may slow bone loss from osteoporosis.

- **Have your eyes and hearing tested.** Even small changes in sight and hearing may cause you to fall. When you get new eyeglasses or contact lenses, take time to get used to them. Always wear your glasses or contacts when you need them If you have a hearing aid, be sure it fits well and wear it.

- **Find out about the side effects of any medicine you take.** If a drug makes you sleepy or dizzy, tell your doctor or pharmacist.

- **Get enough sleep.** If you are sleepy, you are more likely to fall.

- **Limit the amount of alcohol you drink.** Even a small amount of alcohol can affect your balance and reflexes. Studies show that the rate of hip fractures in older adults increases with alcohol use.

- **Stand up slowly.** Getting up too quickly can cause your blood pressure to drop. That can make you feel wobbly. Get your blood pressure checked when lying and standing.

- **Use an assistive device if you need help feeling steady when you walk.** Appropriate use of canes and walkers can prevent falls. If your doctor tells you to use a cane or walker, make sure it is the right size for you and the wheels roll smoothly. This is important when you're walking in areas you don't know well or where the walkways are uneven. A physical or occupational therapist can help you decide which devices might be helpful and teach you how to use them safely.

- **Be very careful when walking on wet or icy surfaces.** They can be very slippery! Try to have sand or salt spread on icy areas by your front or back door.

- **Wear nonskid, rubber-soled, low-heeled shoes, or lace-up shoes with nonskid soles that fully support your feet.** It is important that the soles are not too thin or too thick. Don't walk on stairs or floors in socks or in shoes and slippers with smooth soles.

- **Always tell your doctor if you have fallen since your last checkup, even if you aren't hurt when you fall.** A fall can alert your doctor to a new medical problem or problems with your medications or eyesight that can be corrected. Your doctor may suggest physical therapy, a walking aid, or other steps to help prevent future falls.

What to Do If You Fall

Whether you are at home or somewhere else, a sudden fall can be startling and upsetting. If you do fall, stay as calm as possible. Take several deep breaths to try to relax. Remain still on the floor or ground for a few moments. This will help you get over the shock of falling.

Decide if you are hurt before getting up. Getting up too quickly or in the wrong way could make an injury worse. If you think you can get up safely without help, roll over onto your side. Rest again while your body and blood pressure adjust. Slowly get up on your hands and knees, and crawl to a sturdy chair.

Put your hands on the chair seat and slide one foot forward so that it is flat on the floor. Keep the other leg bent so the knee is on the floor. From this kneeling position, slowly rise and turn your body to sit in the chair. If you are hurt or cannot get up on your own, ask someone for help or call 911. If you are alone, try to get into a comfortable position and wait for help to arrive.

Carrying a mobile or portable phone with you as you move about your house could make it easier to call someone if you need assistance. An emergency response system, which lets you push a button on a special necklace or bracelet to call for help, is another option.

Keep Your Bones Strong to Prevent Falls

Falls are a common reason for trips to the emergency room and for hospital stays among older adults. Many of these hospital visits are for fall-related fractures. You can help prevent fractures by keeping your bones strong.

Having healthy bones won't prevent a fall, but if you fall, it might prevent breaking a hip or other bone, which may lead to a hospital or nursing home stay, disability, or even death. Getting enough calcium and vitamin D can help keep your bones strong. So can physical activity. Try to get at least 150 minutes per week of physical activity.

Other ways to maintain bone health include quitting smoking and limiting alcohol use, which can decrease bone mass and increase the chance of fractures. Also, try to maintain a healthy weight. Being underweight increases the risk of bone loss and broken bones.

Osteoporosis is a disease that makes bones weak and more likely to break. For people with osteoporosis, even a minor fall may be dangerous. Talk to your doctor about osteoporosis.

Chapter 21

Mental Disorders

Chapter Contents

Section 21.1

Delirium

This section contains text excerpted from the following sources:
Text beginning with the heading "What Is Delirium?" is excerpted
from "Delirium," MedlinePlus, National Institutes of Health, May
13, 2016; Text under the heading "Helping People with Delirium" is
excerpted from "Delirium or Sudden Confusion in Elderly Adults,"
U.S. Department of Veterans Affairs (VA), August 9, 2016.

What Is Delirium?

Delirium is a condition that features rapidly changing mental
states. It causes confusion and changes in behavior. Besides falling
in and out of consciousness, there may be problems with:

- Attention and awareness

- Thinking and memory

- Emotion

- Muscle control

- Sleeping and waking

Causes of delirium include medications, poisoning, serious illnesses
or infections, and severe pain. It can also be part of some mental illnesses or dementia.

Delirium and dementia have similar symptoms, so it can be hard
to tell them apart. They can also occur together. Delirium starts suddenly and can cause hallucinations. The symptoms may get better or
worse, and can last for hours or weeks. On the other hand, dementia
develops slowly and does not cause hallucinations. The symptoms are
stable, and may last for months or years.

Delirium tremens is a serious type of alcohol withdrawal syndrome.
It usually happens to people who stop drinking after years of alcohol
abuse.

People with delirium often, though not always, make a full recovery
after their underlying illness is treated.

Helping People with Delirium

Sudden confusion in seniors can be very scary—both for the person who experiences it and the loved ones who witness it. Get medical help as soon as possible, then focus on keeping the older adult safe while they are confused.

People with sudden confusion may focus inward, showing a lack of interest in or attention to the things around them. Or they may become restless and agitated, reacting strongly to things they see, hear, or feel. It is important to remember that feeling confused can be frightening. Do your best to remain calm as you try to figure out the cause of their distress.

Some people with sudden confusion may punch, yell, kick, or act aggressively. That's why it's important to focus on keeping the confused person safe until you find out what's causing their distress. If possible, try to help them walk or change position since this may help ease discomfort.

You may try to gently reorient the person to reality, but remember that their confusion may cause them to see reality in a different way. It will help comfort them to meet them in their world until the confusion is resolved.

Can Delirium be Prevented?

You can take a few simple steps to avoid—or help your loved ones avoid—sudden confusion.

Knowing the risk factors for sudden confusion is the first step. These include:

- Older age
- Dementia
- Sudden confusion in the past
- Multiple medications
- Problems seeing or hearing
- Not getting enough to eat or drink
- Chronic physical illness
- Alcohol or drug use
- Depression
- Problems in the brain or nervous system
- Functional disability

Important steps you can take to counter these risk factors include:

- Making sure the elderly adult gets enough calories and fluids

- Correcting vision or hearing problems with glasses, hearing aids, or other devices

- Helping ensure the elderly adult has good sleep habits and does not become overly tired or nap excessively during the day

- Trying to involve the elderly adult in activities that challenge the brain, like puzzles, reading, talking about current events, or sharing memories of the past

- Reviewing medications and dosages carefully at each doctor visit and asking questions to help make sure they aren't given any longer than necessary

Having one or more risk factors makes an elderly adult more likely to develop sudden confusion. But a sudden event such as a severe illness, infection, or fracture is often what disrupts the brain and causes sudden confusion. This type of confusion is a medical emergency. It's important to identify the cause quickly and to start treatment as soon as possible.

Section 21.2

Depression

This section includes text excerpted from "Depression and Older Adults," National Institute on Aging (NIA), National Institutes of Health (NIH), August 16, 2017.

Depression is more than just feeling sad or blue. It is a common but serious mood disorder that needs treatment. It causes severe symptoms that affect how you feel, think, and handle daily activities, such as sleeping, eating, and working. When you have depression, you have trouble with daily life for weeks at a time. Doctors call this condition "depressive disorder" or "clinical depression." Depression is a real illness. It is not a sign of a person's weakness or a character flaw. You can't "snap out of" clinical depression. Most people who experience depression need treatment to get better.

Depression Is Not a Normal Part of Aging

Depression is a common problem among older adults, but it is NOT a normal part of aging. In fact, studies show that most older adults feel satisfied with their lives, despite having more illnesses or physical problems. However, important life changes that happen as we get older may cause feelings of uneasiness, stress, and sadness. For instance, the death of a loved one, moving from work into retirement, or dealing with a serious illness can leave people feeling sad or anxious. After a period of adjustment, many older adults can regain their emotional balance, but others do not and may develop depression.

Recognizing Symptoms of Depression in Older Adults

Depression in older adults may be difficult to recognize because they may show different symptoms than younger people. For some older adults with depression, sadness is not their main symptom. They may have other, less obvious symptoms of depression, or they may not be willing to talk about their feelings. Therefore, doctors may be less likely to recognize that their patient has depression.

Sometimes older people who are depressed appear to feel tired, have trouble sleeping, or seem grumpy and irritable. Confusion or attention problems caused by depression can sometimes look like Alzheimer disease or other brain disorders. Older adults also may have more medical conditions, such as heart disease, stroke, or cancer, which may cause depressive symptoms. Or they may be taking medications with side effects that contribute to depression.

Types of Depression

There are several types of depressive disorders.

Major depression involves severe symptoms that interfere with the ability to work, sleep, study, eat, and enjoy life. An episode can occur only once in a person's lifetime, but more often, a person has several episodes.

Persistent depressive disorder is a depressed mood that lasts for at least 2 years. A person diagnosed with persistent depressive disorder may have episodes of major depression along with periods of less severe symptoms, but symptoms must last for 2 years to be considered persistent depressive disorder.

Other forms of depression include psychotic depression, postpartum depression, and seasonal affective disorder.

Causes and Risk Factors for Depression

Several factors, or a combination of factors, may contribute to depression.

- **Genes**—People with a family history of depression may be more likely to develop it than those whose families do not have the illness.

- **Personal history**—Older adults who had depression when they were younger are more at risk for developing depression in late life than those who did not have the illness earlier in life.

- **Brain chemistry**—People with depression may have different brain chemistry than those without the illness.

- **Stress**—Loss of a loved one, a difficult relationship, or any stressful situation may trigger depression.

Vascular Depression

For older adults who experience depression for the first time later in life, the depression may be related to changes that occur in the brain and body as a person ages. For example, older adults may suffer from restricted blood flow, a condition called ischemia. Over time, blood vessels may stiffen and prevent blood from flowing normally to the body's organs, including the brain. If this happens, an older adult with no family history of depression may develop what is sometimes called "vascular depression." Those with vascular depression also may be at risk for heart disease, stroke, or other vascular illness.

Depression Can Cooccur with Other Illnesses

Depression, especially in middle-aged or older adults, can cooccur with other serious medical illnesses such as diabetes, cancer, heart disease, and Parkinson disease. Depression can make these conditions worse and vice versa. Sometimes medications taken for these physical illnesses may cause side effects that contribute to depression. A doctor experienced in treating these complicated illnesses can help work out the best treatment strategy. All these factors can cause depression to go undiagnosed or untreated in older people. Yet, treating the depression will help an older adult better manage other conditions he or she may have.

Common Symptoms of Depression

There are many symptoms associated with depression, and some will vary depending on the individual. However, some of the most common symptoms are listed below. If you have several of these symptoms for more than 2 weeks, you may have depression.

- Persistent sad, anxious, or "empty" mood
- Feelings of hopelessness, guilt, worthlessness, or helplessness
- Irritability, restlessness, or having trouble sitting still
- Loss of interest in once pleasurable activities, including sex
- Decreased energy or fatigue
- Moving or talking more slowly
- Difficulty concentrating, remembering, making decisions
- Difficulty sleeping, early-morning awakening, or oversleeping
- Eating more or less than usual, usually with unplanned weight gain or loss
- Thoughts of death or suicide, or suicide attempts
- Aches or pains, headaches, cramps, or digestive problems without a clear physical cause and/or that do not ease with treatment
- Frequent crying

Treatments for Depression

Depression, even severe depression, can be treated. If you think you may have depression, start by making an appointment to see your doctor or healthcare provider. This could be your primary doctor or a provider who specializes in diagnosing and treating mental health conditions (a psychologist or psychiatrist). Certain medications and some medical conditions can cause the same symptoms as depression. A doctor can rule out these possibilities by doing a physical exam, interview, and lab tests. If the doctor can find no medical condition that may be causing the depression, the next step is a psychological evaluation.

Treatment choices differ for each person, and sometimes multiple treatments must be tried to find one that works. It is important to keep trying until you find something that works for you.

The most common forms of treatment for depression are medication and psychotherapy.

Therapy for Depression

Psychotherapy, also called "talk therapy," can help people with depression. Some treatments are short term, lasting 10 to 20 weeks; others are longer, depending on the person's needs. Cognitive behavioral therapy is one type of talk therapy used to treat depression. It focuses on helping people change negative thinking and any behaviors that may be making depression worse. Interpersonal therapy can help an individual understand and work through troubled relationships that may cause the depression or make it worse. Other types of talk therapy, like problem-solving therapy, can be helpful for people with depression.

Medications for Depression

Antidepressants are medicines that treat depression. There are many different types of antidepressants. They may help improve the way your brain uses certain chemicals that control mood or stress. You may need to try several different antidepressant medicines before finding one that improves your symptoms and has manageable side effects.

Antidepressants take time, usually 2 to 4 weeks, to work. Often symptoms such as sleep, appetite, and concentration problems improve before mood lifts, so it is important to give the medication a chance to work before deciding whether it works for you. If you begin taking antidepressants, do not stop taking them without the help of a doctor. Sometimes people taking antidepressants feel better and then stop taking the medication on their own, but then the depression returns. When you and your doctor have decided it is time to stop the medication, usually after 6 to 12 months, the doctor will help you slowly and safely decrease your dose. Stopping antidepressants abruptly can cause withdrawal symptoms.

Most antidepressants are generally safe, but the U.S. Food and Drug Administration (FDA) requires that all antidepressants carry black box warnings, the strictest warnings for prescriptions. The warning says that patients of all ages taking antidepressants should be watched closely, especially during the first few weeks of treatment. Talk to your doctor about any side effects of your medication that you should watch for.

For older adults who are already taking several medications for other conditions, it is important to talk with a doctor about any adverse drug interactions that may occur while taking antidepressants. Do not use herbal medicines such as St. John's Wort before talking with your healthcare provider. It should never be combined with a prescription antidepressant, and you should not use it to replace conventional care or to postpone seeing a healthcare provider.

Preventing Depression

What can be done to lower the risk of depression? How can people cope?

There are a few steps you can take. Try to prepare for major changes in life, such as retirement or moving from your home of many years. Stay in touch with family. Let them know when you feel sad. Regular exercise may also help prevent depression or lift your mood if you are depressed. Pick something you like to do. Being physically fit and eating a balanced diet may help avoid illnesses that can bring on disability or depression.

Section 21.3

Anxiety Disorders

This section includes text excerpted from "Anxiety Disorders: About Anxiety Disorders," NIHSeniorHealth, National Institute on Aging (NIA), January 2016.

Occasional anxiety is a normal part of life. You might feel anxious when faced with a problem at work, before taking a test, or making an important decision.

However, anxiety disorders involve more than temporary worry or fear. For a person with an anxiety disorder, the anxiety does not go away and can get worse over time. These feelings can interfere with daily activities such as job performance, school work, and relationships.

Anxiety Disorders in Older Adults

Studies estimate that anxiety disorders affect up to 15 percent of older adults in a given year. More women than men experience anxiety disorders. They tend to be less common among older adults than younger adults. But developing an anxiety disorder late in life is not a normal part of aging.

Anxiety disorders commonly occur along with other mental or physical illnesses, including alcohol or substance abuse, which may mask anxiety symptoms or make them worse. In older adults, anxiety disorders often occur at the same time as depression, heart disease, diabetes, and other medical problems. In some cases, these other problems need to be treated before a person can respond well to treatment for anxiety.

There are three types of anxiety disorders: generalized anxiety disorder (GAD), social phobia, and panic disorder.

Generalized Anxiety Disorder

All of us worry about things like health, money, or family problems. But people with GAD are extremely worried about these and many other things, even when there is little or no reason to worry about them. They are very anxious about just getting through the day. They think things will always go badly. At times, worrying keeps people with GAD from doing everyday tasks.

Social Phobia

In social phobia, a person fears being judged by others or of being embarrassed. This fear can get in the way of doing everyday things such as going to work, running errands, or meeting with friends. People who have social phobia often know that they shouldn't be so afraid, but they can't control their fear.

Panic Disorder

In panic disorder, a person has sudden, unexplained attacks of terror, and often feels his or her heart pounding. During a panic attack, a person feels a sense of unreality, a fear of impending doom, or a fear of losing control. Panic attacks can occur at any time.

Anxiety Disorders Are Treatable

In general, anxiety disorders are treated with medication, specific types of psychotherapy, or both. Treatment choices depend on the type of disorder, the person's preference, and the expertise of the doctor. If you think you have an anxiety disorder, talk to your doctor.

Chapter 22

Musculoskeletal Disorders

Chapter Contents

Section 22.1

Arthritis

This section includes text excerpted from "Arthritis," Centers for
Disease Control and Prevention (CDC), December 1, 2016.

What is Arthritis?

The word *arthritis* actually means joint inflammation, but the term
has acquired a wider meaning. In public health, arthritis is used as a
shorthand term for arthritis and other rheumatic conditions—a label
for the more than 100 rheumatic diseases and conditions that affect
joints, the tissues which surround joints and other connective tissue.
The pattern, severity, and location of symptoms can vary depending
on the specific form of the disease. Typically, rheumatic conditions are
characterized by pain and stiffness in and around one or more joints.
The symptoms can develop gradually or suddenly. Certain rheumatic
conditions can also involve the immune system and various internal
organs of the body.

Who Is at Risk for Arthritis?

Certain factors are associated with a greater risk of arthritis. Some
of these risk factors are modifiable while others are not.

Nonmodifiable risk factors

- **Age:** The risk of developing most types of arthritis increases
  with age.

- **Gender:** Most types of arthritis are more common in women;
  60 percent of the people with arthritis are women. Gout is more
  common in men.

- **Genetic:** Specific genes are associated with a higher risk of
  certain types of arthritis, such as rheumatoid arthritis (RA)
  and systemic lupus erythematosus (SLE), and ankylosing
  spondylitis.

Modifiable risk factors

- **Overweight and Obesity:** Excess weight can contribute to both the onset and progression of knee osteoarthritis.

- **Joint Injuries:** Damage to a joint can contribute to the development of osteoarthritis in that joint.

- **Infection:** Many microbial agents can infect joints and potentially cause the development of specific forms of arthritis.

- **Occupation:** Certain occupations involving repetitive knee bending and squatting are associated with osteoarthritis of the knee.

What Causes Arthritis?

Elevated uric acid levels cause gout, and specific infections can cause certain forms of arthritis. For many forms of arthritis, the cause is unknown. Scientists are studying the role of factors such as genetics, lifestyle, and environment in the various types of arthritis.

What Are the Most Common Types of Arthritis?

The most common form of arthritis in the Unites States is osteoarthritis followed by gout, fibromyalgia, and rheumatoid arthritis.

What Are the Symptoms of Arthritis?

The pattern and location of symptoms can vary depending on the type of arthritis. Generally, people with arthritis feel pain and stiffness in and around one or more joints. The onset of arthritis symptoms can develop gradually or suddenly. Arthritis is most often a chronic disease, so symptoms may come and go, or persist over time.

What Should I Do If I Think I Have Arthritis?

If you have pain, stiffness, or swelling in or around one or more of your joints, talk to your doctor. It is important to keep in mind that there are many forms of arthritis, and a specific diagnosis of the type you have may help to direct the proper treatment. The earlier you understand your arthritis, the earlier you can start managing your disease and making healthy lifestyle changes to help your arthritis.

Can I Prevent Arthritis?

Depending on the form of arthritis, there are steps that can be taken to reduce your risk of arthritis. Maintaining an appropriate body weight has been shown to decrease the risk of developing osteoarthritis and gout. Protecting your joints from injuries or overuse can reduce the risk of osteoarthritis.

How Is Arthritis Diagnosed?

Diagnosing arthritis often requires a detailed medical history of current and past symptoms, physical examination, X-rays, and blood work. It is possible to have more than one form of arthritis at the same time.

What Are the Treatments for Arthritis?

The focus of treatment for arthritis is to control pain, minimize joint damage, and improve or maintain function and quality of life. In inflammatory types of arthritis, it is also important to control inflammation. According to the American College of Rheumatology (ACR), the treatment of arthritis might involve the following:

- Medications.
- Nonpharmacologic therapies.
- Physical or occupational therapy.
- Splints or joint assistive aids.
- Patient education and support.
- Weight loss.
- Surgery.

How Can I Manage Arthritis Pain?

Both medical treatment and self-management strategies are very important. The Arthritis Self-Management Program (ASMP) and the Chronic Disease Self-Management Program (CDSMP), both developed by Dr. Kate Lorig of Stanford University, are effective self-management education programs. These programs help people learn the techniques needed to manage their arthritis on a day to day basis and gain the confidence to carry it out. Physical activity can also help reduce pain. Programs like Arthritis Foundation Exercise Program (AFEP) and EnhanceFitness® can help can help you safely increase yours physical activity.

Section 22.2

Osteoarthritis

This section includes text excerpted from "Handout on Health: Osteoarthritis," National Institute of Arthritis and Musculoskeletal and Skin Diseases (NIAMS), May 2016.

What Is Osteoarthritis?

Osteoarthritis is the most common type of arthritis and is seen especially among older people. Sometimes it is called degenerative joint disease. Osteoarthritis mostly affects cartilage, the hard but slippery tissue that covers the ends of bones where they meet to form a joint. Healthy cartilage allows bones to glide over one another. It also absorbs energy from the shock of physical movement. In osteoarthritis, the surface layer of cartilage breaks and wears away. This allows bones under the cartilage to rub together, causing pain, swelling, and loss of motion of the joint. Over time, the joint may lose its normal shape. Also, small deposits of bone—called osteophytes or bone spurs—may grow on the edges of the joint. Bits of bone or cartilage can break off and float inside the joint space. This causes more pain and damage.

People with osteoarthritis usually have joint pain and stiffness. Unlike some other forms of arthritis, such as rheumatoid arthritis, osteoarthritis affects only joint function. It does not affect skin tissue, the lungs, the eyes, or the blood vessels.

In rheumatoid arthritis, another common form of arthritis, the immune system attacks the tissues of the joints, leading to pain, inflammation, and eventually joint damage and malformation. It typically begins at a younger age than osteoarthritis, causes swelling and redness in joints, and may make people feel sick, tired, and feverish. Also, the joint involvement of rheumatoid arthritis is symmetrical; that is, if one joint is affected, the same joint on the opposite side of the body is usually similarly affected. Osteoarthritis, on the other hand, can occur in a single joint or can affect a joint on one side of the body much more severely.

Who Has Osteoarthritis?

Osteoarthritis is by far the most common type of arthritis, and the percentage of people who have it grows higher with age. An estimated 27 million Americans age 25 and older have osteoarthritis. Although osteoarthritis becomes more common with age, younger people can develop it, usually as the result of a joint injury, a joint malformation, or a genetic defect in joint cartilage. Both men and women have the disease. Before age 45, more men than women have osteoarthritis; after age 45, it is more common in women. It is also more likely to occur in people who are overweight and in those with jobs that stress particular joints.

How Does Osteoarthritis Affect People?

People with osteoarthritis usually experience joint pain and stiffness. The most commonly affected joints are those at the ends of the fingers (closest to the nail), thumbs, neck, lower back, knees, and hips. Osteoarthritis affects different people differently. It may progress quickly, but for most people, joint damage develops gradually over years. In some people, osteoarthritis is relatively mild and interferes little with day-to-day life; in others, it causes significant pain and disability.

Osteoarthritis Basics: The Joint and Its Parts

A joint is the point where two or more bones are connected. With a few exceptions (in the skull and pelvis, for example), joints are designed to allow movement between the bones and to absorb shock from movements like walking or repetitive motions. These movable joints are made up of the following parts:

- **Cartilage:** A hard but slippery coating on the end of each bone. Cartilage breaks down and wears away in osteoarthritis.

- **Joint capsule:** A tough membrane sac that encloses all the bones and other joint parts.

- **Synovium:** A thin membrane inside the joint capsule that secretes synovial fluid.

- **Synovial fluid:** A fluid that lubricates the joint and keeps the cartilage smooth and healthy.

- **Ligaments, tendons, and muscles:** Tissues that surround the bones and joints, and allow the joints to bend and move. Ligaments are tough, cord-like tissues that connect one bone to another.

- **Tendons:** Tough, fibrous cords that connect muscles to bones. Muscles are bundles of specialized cells that, when stimulated by nerves, either relax or contract to produce movement.

How Do You Know If You Have Osteoarthritis?

Usually, osteoarthritis comes on slowly. Early in the disease, your joints may ache after physical work or exercise. Later on, joint pain may become more persistent. You may also experience joint stiffness, particularly when you first wake up in the morning or have been in one position for a long time.

Although osteoarthritis can occur in any joint, most often it affects the hands, knees, hips, and spine (either at the neck or lower back). Different characteristics of the disease can depend on the specific joint(s) affected. The joints that are most often affected by osteoarthritis includes:

- **Hands:** Osteoarthritis of the hands seems to have some hereditary characteristics; that is, it runs in families. If your mother or grandmother has or had osteoarthritis in their hands, you're at greater-than-average risk of having it too. Women are more likely than men to have osteoarthritis in the hands. For most women, it develops after menopause.

- **Knees:** The knees are among the joints most commonly affected by osteoarthritis. Symptoms of knee osteoarthritis include stiffness, swelling, and pain, which make it hard to walk, climb, and get in and out of chairs and bathtubs. Osteoarthritis in the knees can lead to disability.

- **Hips:** The hips are also common sites of osteoarthritis. As with knee osteoarthritis, symptoms of hip osteoarthritis include pain and stiffness of the joint itself. But sometimes pain is felt in the groin, inner thigh, buttocks, or even the knees. Osteoarthritis of the hip may limit moving and bending, making daily activities such as dressing and putting on shoes a challenge.

- **Spine:** Osteoarthritis of the spine may show up as stiffness and pain in the neck or lower back. In some cases, arthritis-related changes in the spine can cause pressure on the nerves where they exit the spinal column, resulting in weakness, tingling, or numbness of the arms and legs. In severe cases, this can even affect bladder and bowel function.

How Do Doctors Diagnose Osteoarthritis?

No single test can diagnose osteoarthritis; however, sometimes doctors use tests to help confirm a diagnosis or rule out other conditions that could be causing your symptoms. Most doctors use a combination of the following methods:

Clinical History

The doctor begins by asking you to describe the symptoms, when and how the condition started, as well as how the symptoms have changed over time. The doctor will also ask about any other medical problems you and close family members have and about any medications you are taking.

Physical Examination

The doctor will check your reflexes and general health, including muscle strength. The doctor will also examine bothersome joints and observe your ability to walk, bend, and carry out activities of daily living.

X-Rays

X-rays can help doctors determine the form of arthritis a person has and how much joint damage has been done. X-rays of the affected joint can show such things as cartilage loss, bone damage, and bone spurs. But there often is a big difference between the severity of osteoarthritis as shown by the X-ray and the degree of pain and disability you feel. Also, X-rays may not show early osteoarthritis damage until much cartilage loss has taken place.

Magnetic Resonance Imaging (MRI)

Also known as MRI, magnetic resonance imaging provides high-resolution computerized images of internal body tissues. This procedure uses a strong magnet that passes a force through the body to create these images. Doctors often use MRI tests if there is pain, if X-ray findings are minimal, and if the findings suggest damage to other joint tissues such as a ligament or the pad of connective tissue in the knee known as the meniscus.

Other Tests

The doctor may order blood tests to rule out other causes of symptoms. He or she may also order a joint aspiration, which involves drawing fluid from the joint through a needle and examining the fluid under a microscope. Joint fluid samples could reveal bacteria, indicating joint pain is caused by an infection or uric acid crystals, indicating gout. Osteoarthritis is so common, especially in older people, that symptoms seemingly caused by the disease actually may be caused by other medical conditions. The doctor will try to find out what is causing the symptoms by ruling out other disorders and identifying conditions that may make the symptoms worse.

How Is Osteoarthritis Treated?

Most successful treatment programs involve a combination of approaches tailored to the patient's needs, lifestyle, and health. Most programs include ways to manage pain and improve function. These approaches are described below.

Four Goals of Osteoarthritis Treatment

- to control pain
- to improve joint function
- to maintain normal body weight
- to achieve a healthy lifestyle

Treatment Approaches to Osteoarthritis

- exercise
- weight control
- nondrug pain relief techniques and alternative therapies
- medications to control pain
- surgery

Exercise

Research shows that exercise is one of the best treatments for osteoarthritis. Exercise can improve mood and outlook, decrease pain, increase flexibility, strengthen the heart and improve blood flow, maintain weight, and promote general physical fitness. Exercise is also inexpensive and, if done correctly, has few negative side effects. The amount and form of exercise prescribed will depend on which joints are involved, how stable the joints are, and whether a joint replacement has already been done. Walking, swimming, and water aerobics are a few popular types of exercise for people with osteoarthritis. Your doctor and/or physical therapist can recommend specific types of exercise depending on your particular situation. Attention to rest and periods of relief from stress on the joints is also important.

On the Move: Fighting Osteoarthritis with Exercise

You can use exercises to keep strong and limber, improve cardiovascular fitness, extend your joints' range of motion, and reduce your weight. The following types of exercise are part of a well-rounded arthritis treatment plan.

- **Strengthening exercises:** These exercises strengthen muscles that support joints affected by arthritis. They can be performed with weights or with exercise bands, inexpensive devices that add resistance.

- **Aerobic activities:** These are exercises, such as brisk walking or low-impact aerobics, that get your heart pumping and can keep your lungs and circulatory system in shape.

- **Range-of-motion activities:** These keep your joints limber.

- **Balance and agility exercises:** These help you maintain daily living skills.

Ask your doctor or physical therapist what exercises are best for you. Ask for guidelines on exercising.

Weight Control

If you are overweight or obese, you should try to lose weight. Weight loss can reduce stress on weight-bearing joints, limit further injury, increase mobility, and reduce the risk of associated health problems. A dietitian can help you develop healthy eating habits. A healthy diet and regular exercise help reduce weight.

Nondrug Pain Relief and Alternative Therapies

People with osteoarthritis may find many nondrug ways to relieve pain. Below are some examples:

Heat and cold: Heat or cold (or a combination of the two) can be useful for joint pain. Heat can be applied in a number of different ways—with warm towels, hot packs, or a warm bath or shower—to increase blood flow and ease pain and stiffness. In some cases, cold packs (bags of ice or frozen vegetables wrapped in a towel), which reduce inflammation, can relieve pain or numb the sore area. (Check with a doctor or physical therapist to find out if heat or cold is the best treatment.)

Transcutaneous electrical nerve stimulation (TENS): TENS is a technique that uses a small electronic device to direct mild electric pulses to nerve endings that lie beneath the skin in the painful area. TENS may relieve some arthritis pain. It seems to work by blocking pain messages to the brain and by modifying pain perception.

Massage: In this pain-relief approach, a massage therapist will lightly stroke and/or knead the painful muscles. This may increase blood flow and bring warmth to a stressed area. However, arthritis-stressed joints are sensitive, so the therapist must be familiar with the problems of the disease.

Acupuncture: When conventional medical treatment doesn't provide sufficient pain relief, people are more likely to try complementary and alternative therapies to treat osteoarthritis. Some people have found pain relief using acupuncture, a practice in which fine needles are inserted by a licensed acupuncture therapist at specific points on the skin. Scientists think the needles stimulate the release of natural, pain-relieving chemicals produced by the nervous system.

Nutritional supplements: Nutritional supplements such as glucosamine and chondroitin sulfate have been reported to improve symptoms in some people with osteoarthritis, as have certain vitamins. Additional studies have been carried out to further evaluate these claims. It is unknown whether they might change the course of disease.

Medications to Control Pain

Doctors prescribe medicines to eliminate or reduce pain and to improve functioning. Doctors consider a number of factors when choosing medicines for their patients with osteoarthritis. These include the intensity of pain, potential side effects of the medication, your medical history (other health problems you have or are at risk for), and other medications you are taking.

Because some medications can interact with one another and certain health conditions put you at increased risk of drug side effects, it's important to discuss your medication and health history with your doctor before you start taking any new medication, and to see your doctor regularly while you are taking medication. By working together, you and your doctor can find the medication that best relieves your pain with the least risk of side effects.

The following types of medicines are commonly used in treating osteoarthritis:

Over-the-counter pain relievers: Oral pain medications, such as acetaminophen, are often a first-line approach to relieve pain in people with osteoarthritis.

NSAIDs (nonsteroidal anti-inflammatory drugs): A large class of medications useful against both pain and inflammation, (NSAIDs) are a common arthritis treatment. Aspirin and ibuprofen are examples of NSAIDs. Some NSAIDs are available over-the-counter, while more than a dozen others, including a subclass called COX-2 inhibitors, are available only with a prescription.

Narcotic or central acting agents: Prescription pain relievers are sometimes prescribed when over-the-counter medications don't provide sufficient relief or when people have certain medical problems that would make traditional NSAIDs or other first-line therapies unsafe. These medications can carry risks, including the potential for addiction.

Corticosteroids: Corticosteroids are powerful anti-inflammatory hormones made naturally in the body or man-made for use as medicine. They may be injected into the affected joints to temporarily relieve pain. This is a short-term measure, generally not recommended for more than two to four treatments per year. Oral corticosteroids are not routinely used to treat osteoarthritis. They are occasionally used for inflammatory flares.

Hyaluronic acid substitutes: Sometimes called viscosupplements, hyaluronic acid substitutes are designed to replace a normal component of the joint involved in joint lubrication and nutrition. Depending on the particular product your doctor prescribes, it will be given in a series of three to five injections. These products are approved only for osteoarthritis of the knee.

Other medications: Doctors may prescribe several other medicines for osteoarthritis. They include topical pain-relieving creams, rubs, and sprays, which are applied directly to the skin over painful joints.

Surgery

For many people, surgery helps relieve the pain and disability of osteoarthritis. Surgery may be performed to achieve one or more of the following:

- Removal of loose pieces of bone and cartilage from the joint if they are causing symptoms of buckling or locking (arthroscopic debridement).
- Repositioning of bones (osteotomy).
- Resurfacing (smoothing out) bones (joint resurfacing).

Surgeons may replace affected joints with artificial joints called prostheses. These joints can be made from metal alloys, high-density plastic, and ceramic material. Some prostheses are joined to bone surfaces with special cements. Others have porous surfaces and rely on the growth of bone into that surface (a process called biologic fixation) to hold them in place. Artificial joints can last 10 to 15 years or longer. Surgeons choose the design and components of prostheses according to their patient's weight, sex, age, activity level, and other medical conditions.

Joint replacement advances have included the ability, in some cases, to replace only the damaged part of the knee joint, leaving undamaged parts of the joint intact, and the ability to perform hip replacement through much smaller incisions than previously possible.

The decision to use surgery depends on several factors, including the patient's age, occupation, level of disability, pain intensity, and the degree to which arthritis interferes with his or her lifestyle. After surgery and rehabilitation, the patient usually feels less pain and swelling and can move more easily.

Who Provides Care for People with Osteoarthritis?

Treating arthritis often requires a multidisciplinary or team approach. Many types of health professionals care for people with arthritis. You may choose a few or more of the following professionals to be part of your healthcare team:

Primary care physicians: Doctors who treat patients before they are referred to other specialists in the healthcare system. Often a primary care physician will be the main doctor to treat your arthritis. Primary care physicians also handle other medical problems and coordinate the care you receive from other physicians and healthcare providers.

Rheumatologists: Doctors who specialize in treating arthritis and related conditions that affect joints, muscles, and bones.

Orthopaedists: Surgeons who specialize in the treatment of, and surgery for, bone and joint diseases.

Physical therapists: Health professionals who work with patients to improve joint function.

Occupational therapists: Health professionals who teach ways to protect joints, minimize pain, perform activities of daily living, and conserve energy.

Dietitians: Health professionals who teach ways to use a good diet to improve health and maintain a healthy weight.

Nurse educators: Nurses who specialize in helping patients understand their overall condition and implement their treatment plans.

Physiatrists (rehabilitation specialists): Medical doctors who help patients make the most of their physical potential.

Licensed acupuncture therapists: Health professionals who reduce pain and improve physical functioning by inserting fine needles into the skin at specific points on the body.

Psychologists: Health professionals who seek to help patients cope with difficulties in the home and workplace resulting from their medical conditions.

Social workers: Professionals who assist patients with social challenges caused by disability, unemployment, financial hardships, home healthcare, and other needs resulting from their medical conditions.

Chiropractors: Health professionals who focus treatment on the relationship between the body's structure—mainly the spine—and its functioning.

Massage therapists: Health professionals who press, rub, and otherwise manipulate the muscles and other soft tissues of the body. They most often use their hands and fingers, but may use their forearms, elbows, or feet.

Section 22.3

Osteoporosis

This section includes text excerpted from "Osteoporosis," National Institute on Aging (NIA), National Institutes of Health (NIH), August 21, 2017.

Osteoporosis is a disease that weakens bones to the point where they break easily—most often, bones in the hip, backbone (spine), and wrist. Osteoporosis is called a "silent disease" because you may not notice any changes until a bone breaks. All the while, though, your bones had been losing strength for many years.

Bone is living tissue. To keep bones strong, your body breaks down old bone and replaces it with new bone tissue. Sometime around age 30, bone mass stops increasing, and the goal for bone health is to keep as much bone as possible for as long as you can. As people enter their 40s and 50s, more bone may be broken down than is replaced. A close look at the inside of bone shows something like a honeycomb. When you have osteoporosis, the spaces in this honeycomb grow larger, and the bone that forms the honeycomb gets smaller. The outer shell of your bones also gets thinner. All of this makes your bones weaker.

Who Has Osteoporosis? Risk Factors and Causes

Although osteoporosis can strike at any age, it is most common among older people, especially older women. Men also have this disease. White and Asian women are most likely to have osteoporosis. Other women at great risk include those who:

- Have a family history of broken bones or osteoporosis

- Have broken a bone after age 50

- Had surgery to remove their ovaries before their periods stopped

- Had early menopause

- Have not gotten enough calcium and/or vitamin D throughout their lives

- Had extended bed rest or were physically inactive

- Smoke (smokers may absorb less calcium from their diets)

- Take certain medications, including medicines for arthritis and asthma and some cancer drugs

- Used certain medicines for a long time

- Have a small body frame

The risk of osteoporosis grows as you get older. At the time of menopause, women may lose bone quickly for several years. After that, the loss slows down but continues. In men, the loss of bone mass is slower. But, by age 65 or 70, men and women are losing bone at the same rate.

What Is Osteopenia?

Whether your doctor calls it osteopenia or low bone mass, consider it a warning. Bone loss has started, but you can still take action to keep your bones strong and maybe prevent osteoporosis later in life. That way you will be less likely to break a wrist, hip, or vertebrae (bone in your spine) when you are older.

Can My Bones Be Tested?

For some people, the first sign of osteoporosis is to realize they are getting shorter or to break a bone easily. Don't wait until that happens to see if you have osteoporosis. You can have a bone density test to find out how strong your bones are.

How Can I Keep My Bones Strong? Preventing Osteoporosis

There are things you should do at any age to prevent weakened bones. Eating foods that are rich in calcium and vitamin D is important. So is regular weight-bearing exercise, such as weight training, walking, hiking, jogging, climbing stairs, tennis, and dancing. If you have osteoporosis, avoid activities that involve twisting your spine or bending forward from the waist, such as conventional sit-ups, toe touches, or swinging a golf club.

What Can I Do for My Osteoporosis?

Treating osteoporosis means stopping the bone loss and rebuilding bone to prevent breaks. Healthy lifestyle choices such as proper diet, exercise, and medications can help prevent further bone loss and reduce the risk of fractures.

But, lifestyle changes may not be enough if you have lost a lot of bone density. There are also several medicines to think about. Some will slow your bone loss, and others can help rebuild bone. Talk with your doctor to see if medicines might work to treat your osteoporosis. In addition, you'll want to learn how to fall-proof your home and change your lifestyle to avoid fracturing fragile bones.

Can I Avoid Falling?

When your bones are weak, a simple fall can cause a broken bone. This can mean a trip to the hospital and maybe surgery. It might also mean being laid up for a long time, especially in the case of a hip fracture. So, it is important to prevent falls.

Do Men Have Osteoporosis?

Osteoporosis is not just a woman's disease. Not as many men have it as women do, maybe because most men start with more bone density. As they age, men lose bone density more slowly than women. But, men need to be aware of osteoporosis.

Experts don't know as much about this disease in men as they do in women. However, many of the things that put men at risk are the same as those for women, including family history, not enough calcium or vitamin D, and too little exercise. Low levels of testosterone, too much alcohol, taking certain drugs, and smoking are other risk factors. Older men who break a bone easily or are at risk for osteoporosis should talk with their doctors about testing and treatment.

Chapter 23

Neurodegenerative Disorders

Chapter Contents

Section 23.1

Alzheimer Disease

This section includes text excerpted from "Alzheimer Disease and
Related Dementias—Alzheimer's Disease Fact Sheet," National
Institute on Aging (NIA), National Institutes of Health (NIH), July
25, 2017.

Alzheimer disease (AD) is an irreversible, progressive brain disorder that slowly destroys memory and thinking skills, and eventually
the ability to carry out the simplest tasks. In most people with Alzheimer disease, symptoms first appear in their mid-60s. Estimates
vary, but experts suggest that more than 5 million Americans may
have Alzheimer disease.

Alzheimer disease is currently ranked as the sixth leading cause
of death in the United States, but recent estimates indicate that the
disorder may rank third, just behind heart disease and cancer, as a
cause of death for older people.

Alzheimer disease is named after Dr. Alois Alzheimer. In 1906, Dr.
Alzheimer noticed changes in the brain tissue of a woman who had
died of an unusual mental illness. Her symptoms included memory
loss, language problems, and unpredictable behavior. After she died,
he examined her brain and found many abnormal clumps (now called
amyloid plaques) and tangled bundles of fibers (now called neurofibril-
lary, or tau, tangles).

These plaques and tangles in the brain are still considered some
of the main features of Alzheimer disease. Another feature is the loss
of connections between nerve cells (neurons) in the brain. Neurons
transmit messages between different parts of the brain, and from the
brain to muscles and organs in the body.

Changes in the Brain

Scientists continue to unravel the complex brain changes involved
in the onset and progression of Alzheimer disease. It seems likely
that damage to the brain starts a decade or more before memory
and other cognitive problems appear. During this preclinical stage

of Alzheimer disease, people seem to be symptom-free, but toxic changes are taking place in the brain. Abnormal deposits of proteins form amyloid plaques and tau tangles throughout the brain, and once-healthy neurons stop functioning, lose connections with other neurons, and die.

The damage initially appears to take place in the hippocampus, the part of the brain essential in forming memories. As more neurons die, additional parts of the brain are affected, and they begin to shrink. By the final stage of Alzheimer disease, damage is widespread, and brain tissue has shrunk significantly.

Signs and Symptoms

Memory problems are typically one of the first signs of cognitive impairment related to Alzheimer disease. Some people with memory problems have a condition called mild cognitive impairment (MCI). In MCI, people have more memory problems than normal for their age, but their symptoms do not interfere with their everyday lives. Movement difficulties and problems with the sense of smell have also been linked to MCI. Older people with MCI are at greater risk for developing Alzheimer disease, but not all of them do. Some may even go back to normal cognition.

The first symptoms of Alzheimer disease vary from person to person. For many, decline in nonmemory aspects of cognition, such as word-finding, vision/spatial issues, and impaired reasoning or judgment, may signal the very early stages of Alzheimer disease. Researchers are studying biomarkers (biological signs of disease found in brain images, cerebrospinal fluid, and blood) to see if they can detect early changes in the brains of people with MCI and in cognitively normal people who may be at greater risk for Alzheimer disease. Studies indicate that such early detection may be possible, but more research is needed before these techniques can be relied upon to diagnose Alzheimer disease in everyday medical practice.

Mild Alzheimer Disease

As Alzheimer disease progresses, people experience greater memory loss and other cognitive difficulties. Problems can include wandering and getting lost, trouble handling money and paying bills, repeating questions, taking longer to complete normal daily tasks, and personality and behavior changes. People are often diagnosed in this stage.

Moderate Alzheimer Disease

In this stage, damage occurs in areas of the brain that control language, reasoning, sensory processing, and conscious thought. Memory loss and confusion grow worse, and people begin to have problems recognizing family and friends. They may be unable to learn new things, carry out multistep tasks such as getting dressed, or cope with new situations. In addition, people at this stage may have hallucinations, delusions, and paranoia and may behave impulsively.

Severe Alzheimer Disease

Ultimately, plaques and tangles spread throughout the brain, and brain tissue shrinks significantly. People with severe Alzheimer disease cannot communicate and are completely dependent on others for their care. Near the end, the person may be in bed most or all of the time as the body shuts down.

What Causes Alzheimer Disease

Scientists don't yet fully understand what causes Alzheimer disease in most people. There is a genetic component to some cases of early-onset Alzheimer disease. Late-onset Alzheimer disease arises from a complex series of brain changes that occur over decades. The causes probably include a combination of genetic, environmental, and lifestyle factors. The importance of any one of these factors in increasing or decreasing the risk of developing Alzheimer disease may differ from person to person.

The Basics of Alzheimer

Scientists are conducting studies to learn more about plaques, tangles, and other biological features of Alzheimer disease. Advances in brain imaging techniques allow researchers to see the development and spread of abnormal amyloid and tau proteins in the living brain, as well as changes in brain structure and function. Scientists are also exploring the very earliest steps in the disease process by studying changes in the brain and body fluids that can be detected years before Alzheimer disease symptoms appear. Findings from these studies will help in understanding the causes of Alzheimer disease and make diagnosis easier.

One of the great mysteries of Alzheimer disease is why it largely strikes older adults. Research on normal brain aging is shedding light on this question. For example, scientists are learning how age-related changes in the brain may harm neurons and contribute to Alzheimer disease damage. These age-related changes include atrophy (shrinking) of certain parts of the brain, inflammation, production of unstable molecules called free radicals, and mitochondrial dysfunction (a breakdown of energy production within a cell).

Genetics

Most people with Alzheimer disease have the late-onset form of the disease, in which symptoms become apparent in their mid-60s. The apolipoprotein E *(APOE)* gene is involved in late-onset Alzheimer disease. This gene has several forms. One of them, *APOE ε4*, increases a person's risk of developing the disease and is also associated with an earlier age of disease onset. However, carrying the *APOE ε4* form of the gene does not mean that a person will definitely develop Alzheimer disease, and some people with no *APOE ε4* may also develop the disease.

Also, scientists have identified a number of regions of interest in the genome (an organism's complete set of deoxyribonucleic acid (DNA)) that may increase a person's risk for late-onset Alzheimer to varying degrees.

Early-onset Alzheimer disease occurs between a person's 30s to mid-60s and represents less than 10 percent of all people with Alzheimer disease. Some cases are caused by an inherited change in one of three genes, resulting in a type known as early-onset familial Alzheimer disease, or FAD. For other cases of early-onset Alzheimer disease, research suggests there may be a genetic component related to factors other than these three genes.

Most people with Down syndrome develop Alzheimer disease. This may be because people with Down syndrome have an extra copy of chromosome 21, which contains the gene that generates harmful amyloid.

Health, Environmental, and Lifestyle Factors

Research suggests that a host of factors beyond genetics may play a role in the development and course of Alzheimer disease. There is a great deal of interest, for example, in the relationship between cognitive decline and vascular conditions such as heart disease, stroke, and high blood pressure, as well as metabolic conditions such as diabetes and obesity. Ongoing research will help us understand whether and how reducing risk factors for these conditions may also reduce the risk of Alzheimer disease.

A nutritious diet, physical activity, social engagement, and mentally stimulating pursuits have all been associated with helping people stay healthy as they age. These factors might also help reduce the risk of cognitive decline and Alzheimer disease.

Diagnosis of Alzheimer Disease

Doctors use several methods and tools to help determine whether a person who is having memory problems has "possible Alzheimer dementia" (dementia may be due to another cause) or "probable Alzheimer dementia" (no other cause for dementia can be found).

To diagnose Alzheimer disease, doctors may:

- Ask the person and a family member or friend questions about overall health, past medical problems, ability to carry out daily activities, and changes in behavior and personality

- Conduct tests of memory, problem solving, attention, counting, and language

- Carry out standard medical tests, such as blood and urine tests, to identify other possible causes of the problem

- Perform brain scans, such as computed tomography (CT), magnetic resonance imaging (MRI), or positron emission tomography (PET), to rule out other possible causes for symptoms.

These tests may be repeated to give doctors information about how the person's memory and other cognitive functions are changing over time.

Alzheimer disease can be definitely diagnosed only after death, by linking clinical measures with an examination of brain tissue in an autopsy.

People with memory and thinking concerns should talk to their doctor to find out whether their symptoms are due to Alzheimer disease or another cause, such as stroke, tumor, Parkinson disease, sleep disturbances, side effects of medication, an infection, or a non-Alzheimer dementia. Some of these conditions may be treatable and possibly reversible.

If the diagnosis is Alzheimer disease, beginning treatment early in the disease process may help preserve daily functioning for some time, even though the underlying disease process cannot be stopped or reversed. An early diagnosis also helps families plan for the future. They can take care of financial and legal matters, address potential safety issues, learn about living arrangements, and develop support networks.

Treatment of Alzheimer Disease

Alzheimer disease is complex, and it is unlikely that any one drug or other intervention can successfully treat it. Current approaches focus on helping people maintain mental function, manage behavioral symptoms, and slow or delay the symptoms of disease. Researchers hope to develop therapies targeting specific genetic, molecular, and cellular mechanisms so that the actual underlying cause of the disease can be stopped or prevented.

Maintaining Mental Function

Several medications are approved by the U.S. Food and Drug Administration (FDA) to treat symptoms of Alzheimer disease. Donepezil (Aricept®), rivastigmine (Exelon®), and galantamine (Razadyne®) are used to treat mild to moderate Alzheimer disease (donepezil can be used for severe Alzheimer disease as well). Memantine (Namenda®) is used to treat moderate to severe Alzheimer disease. These drugs work by regulating neurotransmitters, the chemicals that transmit messages between neurons. They may help maintain thinking, memory, and communication skills, and help with certain behavioral problems. However, these drugs don't change the underlying disease process. They are effective for some but not all people, and may help only for a limited time. The FDA has also approved Aricept® and Namzaric®, a combination of Namenda® and Aricept®, for the treatment of moderate to severe Alzheimer disease.

Managing Behavior

Common behavioral symptoms of Alzheimer disease include sleeplessness, wandering, agitation, anxiety, and aggression. Scientists are learning why these symptoms occur and are studying new treatments—drug and nondrug—to manage them. Research has shown that treating behavioral symptoms can make people with Alzheimer disease more comfortable and makes things easier for caregivers.

Looking for New Treatments

Alzheimer disease research has developed to a point where scientists can look beyond treating symptoms to think about addressing underlying disease processes. In ongoing clinical trials, scientists are developing and testing several possible interventions, including immunization therapy, drug therapies, cognitive training, physical activity, and treatments used for cardiovascular disease and diabetes.

Support for Families and Caregivers

Caring for a person with Alzheimer disease can have high physical, emotional, and financial costs. The demands of day-to-day care, changes in family roles, and decisions about placement in a care facility can be difficult. There are several evidence-based approaches and programs that can help, and researchers are continuing to look for new and better ways to support caregivers.

Becoming well-informed about the disease is one important long-term strategy. Programs that teach families about the various stages of Alzheimer disease and about ways to deal with difficult behaviors and other caregiving challenges can help.

Good coping skills, a strong support network, and respite care are other ways that help caregivers handle the stress of caring for a loved one with Alzheimer disease. For example, staying physically active provides physical and emotional benefits.

Some caregivers have found that joining a support group is a critical lifeline. These support groups allow caregivers to find respite, express concerns, share experiences, get tips, and receive emotional comfort. Many organizations sponsor in-person and online support groups, including groups for people with early-stage Alzheimer disease and their families.

Section 23.2

Lewy Body Dementia

This section includes text excerpted from "Related Dementias—
What Is Lewy Body Dementia?" National Institute on Aging (NIA),
National Institutes of Health (NIH), July 25, 2017.

What Is Lewy Body Dementia (LBD)?

LBD is a disease associated with abnormal deposits of a protein
called alpha-synuclein in the brain. These deposits, called Lewy bodies, affect chemicals in the brain whose changes, in turn, can lead to
problems with thinking, movement, behavior, and mood. LBD is one
of the most common causes of dementia, after Alzheimer disease and
vascular disease.

Diagnosing LBD can be challenging for a number of reasons. Early
LBD symptoms are often confused with similar symptoms found in
other brain diseases like Alzheimer. Also, LBD can occur alone or along
with Alzheimer or Parkinson disease.

There are two types of LBD—dementia with Lewy bodies and Parkinson disease dementia. The earliest signs of these two diseases differ
but reflect the same biological changes in the brain. Over time, people
with dementia with Lewy bodies or Parkinson disease dementia may
develop similar symptoms.

Who Is Affected by LBD?

LBD affects more than 1 million individuals in the United States.
LBD typically begins at age 50 or older, although sometimes younger
people have it. LBD appears to affect slightly more men than women.

LBD is a progressive disease, meaning symptoms start slowly and
worsen over time. The disease lasts an average of 5 to 7 years from the
time of diagnosis to death, but the time span can range from 2 to 20 years.
How quickly symptoms develop and change varies greatly from person
to person, depending on overall health, age, and severity of symptoms.

In the early stages of LBD, usually before a diagnosis is made,
symptoms can be mild, and people can function fairly normally. As the

disease advances, people with LBD require more and more help due to a decline in thinking and movement abilities. In the later stages of the disease, they may depend entirely on others for assistance and care.

Some LBD symptoms may respond to treatment for a period of time. Currently, there is no cure for the disease. Research is improving researchers understanding of this challenging condition, and advances in science may one day lead to better diagnosis, improved care, and new treatments.

What Are Lewy Bodies?

Lewy bodies are named for Dr. Friederich Lewy, a German neurologist. In 1912, he discovered abnormal protein deposits that disrupt the brain's normal functioning in people with Parkinson disease. These abnormal deposits are now called "Lewy bodies."

Lewy bodies are made of a protein called alpha-synuclein. In the healthy brain, alpha-synuclein plays a number of important roles in neurons (nerve cells) in the brain, especially at synapses, where brain cells communicate with each other. In LBD, alpha-synuclein forms into clumps inside neurons, starting in particular regions of the brain. This process causes neurons to work less effectively and, eventually, to die. The activities of brain chemicals important to brain function are also affected. The result is widespread damage to certain parts of the brain and a decline in abilities affected by those brain regions.

Lewy bodies affect several different brain regions in LBD:

- The cerebral cortex, which controls many functions, including information processing, perception, thought, and language.

- The limbic cortex, which plays a major role in emotions and behavior.

- The hippocampus, which is essential to forming new memories.

- The midbrain, including the substantia nigra, which is involved in movement.

- The brain stem, which is important in regulating sleep and maintaining alertness

- Brain regions important in recognizing smells (olfactory pathways).

Section 23.3

Parkinson Disease

This section includes text excerpted from "Parkinson
Disease," National Institute on Aging (NIA), National
Institutes of Health (NIH), July 24, 2017.

Parkinson disease is a brain disorder that leads to shaking, stiffness, and difficulty with walking, balance, and coordination.

Parkinson symptoms usually begin gradually and get worse over
time. As the disease progresses, people may have difficulty walking
and talking. They may also have mental and behavioral changes, sleep
problems, depression, memory difficulties, and fatigue.

Both men and women can have Parkinson disease. However, the
disease affects about 50 percent more men than women.

One clear risk factor for Parkinson is age. Although most people
with Parkinson first develop the disease at about age 60, about 5 to
10 percent of people with Parkinson have "early-onset" disease, which
begins before the age of 50. Early-onset forms of Parkinson are often,
but not always, inherited, and some forms have been linked to specific
gene mutations.

What Causes Parkinson Disease?

Parkinson disease occurs when nerve cells, or neurons, in an area
of the brain that controls movement become impaired and/or die. Normally, these neurons produce an important brain chemical known as
dopamine. When the neurons die or become impaired, they produce
less dopamine, which causes the movement problems of Parkinson.
Scientists still do not know what causes cells that produce dopamine
to die.

People with Parkinson also lose the nerve endings that produce norepinephrine, the main chemical messenger of the sympathetic nervous
system, which controls many automatic functions of the body, such
as heart rate and blood pressure. The loss of norepinephrine might
help explain some of the nonmovement features of Parkinson, such as
fatigue, irregular blood pressure, decreased movement of food through

the digestive tract, and sudden drop in blood pressure when a person stands up from a sitting or lying-down position.

Many brain cells of people with Parkinson contain Lewy bodies, unusual clumps of the protein alpha-synuclein. Scientists are trying to better understand the normal and abnormal functions of alpha-synuclein and its relationship to genetic mutations that impact Parkinson disease and Lewy body dementia.

Although some cases of Parkinson appear to be hereditary, and a few can be traced to specific genetic mutations, in most cases the disease occurs randomly and does not seem to run in families. Many researchers now believe that Parkinson disease results from a combination of genetic factors and environmental factors such as exposure to toxins.

Symptoms of Parkinson Disease

Parkinson disease has four main symptoms:

• Tremor (trembling) in hands, arms, legs, jaw, or head

• Stiffness of the limbs and trunk

• Slowness of movement

• Impaired balance and coordination, sometimes leading to falls

Other symptoms may include depression and other emotional changes; difficulty swallowing, chewing, and speaking; urinary problems or constipation; skin problems; and sleep disruptions.

Symptoms of Parkinson and the rate of progression differ among individuals. Sometimes people dismiss early symptoms of Parkinson as the effects of normal aging. In most cases, there are no medical tests to definitively detect the disease, so it can be difficult to diagnose accurately.

Early symptoms of Parkinson disease are subtle and occur gradually. For example, affected people may feel mild tremors or have difficulty getting out of a chair. They may notice that they speak too softly, or that their handwriting is slow and looks cramped or small. Friends or family members may be the first to notice changes in someone with early Parkinson. They may see that the person's face lacks expression and animation, or that the person does not move an arm or leg normally.

People with Parkinson often develop a parkinsonian gait that includes a tendency to lean forward, small quick steps as if hurrying forward, and reduced swinging of the arms. They also may have trouble initiating or continuing movement.

Symptoms often begin on one side of the body or even in one limb on one side of the body. As the disease progresses, it eventually affects both sides. However, the symptoms may still be more severe on one side than on the other.

Many people with Parkinson note that prior to experiencing stiffness and tremor, they had sleep problems, constipation, decreased ability to smell, and restless legs.

Diagnosis of Parkinson Disease

A number of disorders can cause symptoms similar to those of Parkinson disease. People with Parkinson-like symptoms that result from other causes are sometimes said to have parkinsonism. While these disorders initially may be misdiagnosed as Parkinson, certain medical tests, as well as response to drug treatment, may help to distinguish them from Parkinson. Since many other diseases have similar features but require different treatments, it is important to make an exact diagnosis as soon as possible.

There are currently no blood or laboratory tests to diagnose non-genetic cases of Parkinson disease. Diagnosis is based on a person's medical history and a neurological examination. Improvement after initiating medication is another important hallmark of Parkinson disease.

Treatment of Parkinson Disease

Although there is no cure for Parkinson disease, medicines, surgical treatment, and other therapies can often relieve some symptoms.

Medicines for Parkinson Disease

Medicines prescribed for Parkinson include:

- Drugs that increase the level of dopamine in the brain

- Drugs that affect other brain chemicals in the body

- Drugs that help control nonmotor symptoms

The main therapy for Parkinson is levodopa, also called L-dopa. Nerve cells use levodopa to make dopamine to replenish the brain's dwindling supply. Usually, people take levodopa along with another medication called carbidopa. Carbidopa prevents or reduces some of the side effects of levodopa therapy—such as nausea, vomiting, low blood pressure, and restlessness—and reduces the amount of levodopa needed to improve symptoms.

People with Parkinson should never stop taking levodopa without telling their doctor. Suddenly stopping the drug may have serious side effects, such as being unable to move or having difficulty breathing.

Other medicines used to treat Parkinson symptoms include:

- Dopamine agonists to mimic the role of dopamine in the brain

- Monoamine Oxidase B (MAO-B) inhibitors to slow down an enzyme that breaks down dopamine in the brain

- Catechol-O-methyl transferase (COMT) inhibitors to help break down dopamine

- Amantadine, an old antiviral drug, to reduce involuntary movements

- Anticholinergic drugs to reduce tremors and muscle rigidity

Deep Brain Stimulation (DBS)

For people with Parkinson who do not respond well to medications, deep brain stimulation, or DBS, may be appropriate. DBS is a surgical procedure that surgically implants electrodes into part of the brain and connects them to a small electrical device implanted in the chest. The device and electrodes painlessly stimulate the brain in a way that helps stop many of the movement-related symptoms of Parkinson, such as tremor, slowness of movement, and rigidity.

Other Therapies

Other therapies may be used to help with Parkinson disease symptoms. They include physical, occupational, and speech therapies, which help with gait and voice disorders, tremors and rigidity, and decline in mental functions. Other supportive therapies include a healthy diet and exercises to strengthen muscles and improve balance.

Chapter 24

Respiratory Disorders

Every day you breathe in and out nearly 20,000 times. That's a lot of work for your lungs. Over time your likelihood of having a serious lung problem increases, especially if you smoke.

Lung problems that are more common among older people include:

- Chronic obstructive pulmonary disease

- Pneumonia

- Lung cancer

Chronic Obstructive Pulmonary Disease (COPD)

Chronic obstructive pulmonary disease (COPD) is a disease that makes it hard to breathe. There are two main types of COPD: emphysema and chronic bronchitis.

Symptoms of COPD

Shortness of breath is one of the most common symptoms of COPD. People who have COPD may feel like their chest is so tight that they

This chapter contains text excerpted from the following sources: Text in this chapter begins with excerpts from "Understanding Lung Problems," National Institute of Aging (NIA), National Institutes of Health (NIH), July 24, 2017; Text beginning with the heading "Asthma" is excerpted from "What Is Asthma?" U.S. Environmental Protection Agency (EPA), February 3, 2017; Text beginning with the heading "Influenza (Flu)" is excerpted from "Key Facts about Influenza (Flu)," Centers for Disease Control and Prevention (CDC), August 25, 2016.

cannot breathe. They may cough a lot. The coughing may or may not produce sticky, slimy mucus. COPD can also cause wheezing.

These problems develop slowly and get worse over time. For example, at first someone with COPD might only have trouble catching his or her breath when being physically active. But over time, the shortness of breath may occur even when resting. COPD can lead to other problems like creating strain on the heart, which can result in swollen ankles, feet, or legs. In advanced stages of COPD, people can have blue lips because they do not have enough oxygen in their blood.

In older adults, COPD can sometimes be confused with asthma. If you have shortness of breath, wheezing, or other problems breathing, your doctor will be able to tell if you have COPD, asthma, or another condition.

Causes of COPD

COPD is often caused by smoking. Breathing secondhand smoke (someone else's smoke), air pollution, chemical fumes, a lot of dust, or other things that bother the lungs and airways over time can also cause COPD. Some people may have a genetic condition that increases their chance of getting COPD.

Tests for COPD

If you have symptoms of COPD, see your doctor right away. Your doctor may test your lungs and how well you breathe, look at your lungs, or do other exams. Your doctor might also send you to a pulmonologist, a doctor who specializes in lung problems.

Treatment for COPD

There is no cure for COPD. But, there are things people with COPD can do to feel better. Most important, do not smoke. Smoking is the leading cause of COPD. If you stop smoking, you may breathe more easily and could add years to your life. It's never too late to quit smoking!

If you have COPD, your doctor might prescribe an inhaler. This is a device that gets medicine right into your lungs. Your doctor might suggest a special exercise program. Also, you can learn breathing techniques and other tricks to help you stay active. If your COPD gets worse, you might need to receive extra oxygen. In rare cases, surgery may help. People with COPD can protect themselves by getting shots to prevent the flu and pneumonia.

Pneumonia

Pneumonia is an infection of one or both of your lungs.

Symptoms of Pneumonia

People who have pneumonia may have a fever, chills, trouble breathing, and a cough with mucus. They may feel sick to their stomach. Pneumonia can make people feel very tired, even after other symptoms go away.

Pneumonia can be mild or severe. For some older people, pneumonia can be a serious problem. It can take 3 weeks or longer before they feel better and over a month before they stop feeling tired.

Causes of Pneumonia

Pneumonia is caused by germs like bacteria, viruses, and fungi. It is most common in the winter months. Your chance of getting pneumonia goes up if you smoke or drink a lot of alcohol. Some people come in contact with germs that cause pneumonia during a hospital stay or at their nursing home. These people may already have health problems, so pneumonia can be very serious.

Tests for Pneumonia

Your doctor may be able to tell if you have pneumonia by doing a physical exam, taking an X-ray of your chest, collecting a blood sample, or doing other tests.

Treatment for Pneumonia

Mild cases of pneumonia can sometimes be treated at home. If you have a mild case of pneumonia, your doctor will likely prescribe pills to fight the germs causing the infection. Take the medicine exactly as your doctor tells you, even if you are feeling better.

Sometimes pneumonia must be treated in the hospital. Along with medication, you may receive oxygen and other treatments to help you breathe.

Prevent Pneumonia

Pneumonia can be very serious and even life-threatening. Take steps to prevent pneumonia:

- Talk to your doctor about shots for the flu and pneumonia.

- Wash your hands with soap and water.

- Cover your nose and mouth when you sneeze or cough; throw out tissues and wash your hands right away.

- Keep yourself healthy by getting plenty of rest, making healthy food choices, and being active.

- Don't smoke.

Asthma

Asthma is a serious, sometimes life-threatening chronic respiratory disease that affects the quality of life for more than 23 million Americans, including an estimated 6 million children. Although there is no cure for asthma yet, asthma can be controlled through medical treatment and management of environmental triggers.

Risk of Asthma

Anyone can get asthma—people of all ethnic groups, male and female, young and old, city dwellers and rural dwellers. In the United States, more than 20 million people have asthma. While no one knows for sure why some people develop asthma and others don't, we do know that it is a combination of your family history and your environment.

There is no cure for asthma. Once you have asthma, you will have the disease for the rest of your life. But with proper care, you can lead a healthy, productive, fully active life.

Asthma Triggers

Learn more about factors found in the indoor and outdoor environment that can cause, trigger or exacerbate asthma symptoms and what you can do to reduce their impact. You might be surprised by the list of common environmental asthma triggers and how simple it can be to eliminate them from your environment.

Preventing Asthma Attacks

Step One: Talk to a doctor

If you think that you or your child may have asthma, talk to a doctor. Your doctor will work with you to diagnose asthma and keep you or your child from having asthma attacks.

- Learn what triggers asthma attacks.

- Identify asthma triggers in your home.

- Talk about ways to get rid of triggers in your home.

- Find out what medicine(s) to take.

Step Two: Make a Plan

Ask your doctor to help you create an Asthma Action Plan (AAP) to prevent asthma attacks. An AAP will help you control asthma on a regular basis. Use this plan together with your doctor to write down how to manage asthma; routinely on a daily basis and during an attack. Look on the back for a list of possible asthma triggers and ways to avoid them.

Step Three: Asthma-Proof Your Home

Triggers are a part of everyday life. Asthma attacks can be triggered by things like mold growing on your shower curtain, or tiny dust mites that live in blankets, pillows, or your child's stuffed animals. Learn more about things that might trigger an asthma attack and what you can do to get rid of them and to stay healthy.

Influenza (Flu)

The flu is a contagious respiratory illness caused by influenza viruses that infect the nose, throat, and lungs. It can cause mild to severe illness, and at times can lead to death. The best way to prevent the flu is by getting a flu vaccine each year.

Signs and Symptoms of Flu

People who have the flu often feel some or all of these signs and symptoms:

- Fever* or feeling feverish/chills

- Cough

- Sore throat

- Runny or stuffy nose

- Muscle or body aches

* It's important to note that not everyone with flu will have a fever.

- Headaches
- Fatigue (very tired)

Some people may have vomiting and diarrhea, though this is more common in children than adults.

How Flu Spreads

Most experts believe that flu viruses spread mainly by droplets made when people with flu cough, sneeze or talk. These droplets can land in the mouths or noses of people who are nearby. Less often, a person might also get flu by touching a surface or object that has flu virus on it and then touching their own mouth, eyes or possibly their nose.

Period of Contagiousness

You may be able to pass on the flu to someone else before you know you are sick, as well as while you are sick. Most healthy adults may be able to infect others beginning 1 day before symptoms develop and up to 5 to 7 days after becoming sick. Some people, especially young children and people with weakened immune systems, might be able to infect others for an even longer time.

Onset of Symptoms

The time from when a person is exposed to flu virus to when symptoms begin is about 1 to 4 days, with an average of about 2 days.

Complications of Flu

Complications of flu can include bacterial pneumonia, ear infections, sinus infections, dehydration, and worsening of chronic medical conditions, such as congestive heart failure, asthma, or diabetes.

People at High Risk from Flu

Anyone can get the flu (even healthy people), and serious problems related to the flu can happen at any age, but some people are at high risk of developing serious flu-related complications if they get sick. This includes people 65 years and older, people of any age with certain chronic medical conditions (such as asthma, diabetes, or heart disease), pregnant women, and young children.

Preventing Flu

The first and most important step in preventing flu is to get a flu vaccination each year. Centers for Disease Control and Prevention (CDC) also recommends everyday preventive actions (like staying away from people who are sick, covering coughs and sneezes and frequent handwashing) to help slow the spread of germs that cause respiratory (nose, throat, and lungs) illnesses, like flu.

Diagnosing Flu

It is very difficult to distinguish the flu from other viral or bacterial causes of respiratory illnesses on the basis of symptoms alone. There are tests available to diagnose flu.

Treating

There are influenza antiviral drugs that can be used to treat flu illness.

Chapter 25

Renal Disorders

Chapter Contents

Section 25.1

Chronic Kidney Disease

This section includes text excerpted from "Chronic
Kidney Disease (CKD)," National Institute of Diabetes and
Digestive and Kidney Diseases (NIDDK), June 2017.

What Is Chronic Kidney Disease?

Chronic kidney disease (CKD) means your kidneys are damaged and
can't filter blood the way they should. The disease is called "chronic"
because the damage to your kidneys happens slowly over a long period
of time. This damage can cause wastes to build up in your body. CKD
can also cause other health problems.

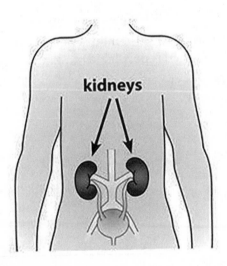

Figure 25.1. *The Kidneys*

Your kidneys are located in the middle of your back, just below your ribcage.

The kidneys' main job is to filter extra water and wastes out of your
blood to make urine. To keep your body working properly, the kidneys

balance the salts and minerals—such as calcium, phosphorus, sodium, and potassium—that circulate in the blood. Your kidneys also make hormones that help control blood pressure, make red blood cells, and keep your bones strong.

Kidney disease often can get worse over time and may lead to kidney failure. If your kidneys fail, you will need dialysis or a kidney transplant to maintain your health. The sooner you know you have kidney disease, the sooner you can make changes to protect your kidneys.

How Common Is CKD?

CKD is common among adults in the United States. More than 30 million American adults may have CKD.

Who Is More Likely to Develop CKD?

You are at risk for kidney disease if you have:

- **Diabetes.** Diabetes is the leading cause of CKD. High blood glucose, also called blood sugar, from diabetes can damage the blood vessels in your kidneys. Almost 1 in 3 people with diabetes has CKD.

- **High blood pressure.** High blood pressure is the second leading cause of CKD. Like high blood glucose, high blood pressure also can damage the blood vessels in your kidneys. Almost 1 in 5 adults with high blood pressure has CKD.

- **Heart disease.** Research shows a link between kidney disease and heart disease. People with heart disease are at higher risk for kidney disease, and people with kidney disease are at higher risk for heart disease. Researchers are working to better understand the relationship between kidney disease and heart disease.

- **Family history of kidney failure.** If your mother, father, sister, or brother has kidney failure, you are at risk for CKD. Kidney disease tends to run in families. If you have kidney disease, encourage family members to get tested. Use tips from the family health reunion guide and speak with your family during special gatherings.

Your chances of having kidney disease increase with age. The longer you have had diabetes, high blood pressure, or heart disease, the more likely that you will have kidney disease.

345

African Americans, Hispanics, and American Indians tend to have a greater risk for CKD. The greater risk is due mostly to higher rates of diabetes and high blood pressure among these groups. Scientists are studying other possible reasons for this increased risk.

What Are the Symptoms of CKD?

Early CKD May Not Have Any Symptoms

You may wonder how you can have CKD and feel fine. Our kidneys have a greater capacity to do their job than is needed to keep us healthy. For example, you can donate one kidney and remain healthy. You can also have kidney damage without any symptoms because, despite the damage, your kidneys are still doing enough work to keep you feeling well. For many people, the only way to know if you have kidney disease is to get your kidneys checked with blood and urine tests.

As kidney disease gets worse, a person may have swelling, called edema. Edema happens when the kidneys can't get rid of extra fluid and salt. Edema can occur in the legs, feet, or ankles, and less often in the hands or face.

Symptoms of Advanced CKD

- chest pain
- dry skin
- itching or numbness
- feeling tired
- headaches
- increased or decreased urination
- loss of appetite
- muscle cramps
- nausea
- shortness of breath
- sleep problems
- trouble concentrating
- vomiting
- weight loss

People with CKD can also develop anemia, bone disease, and malnutrition.

Does CKD Cause Other Health Problems?

Kidney disease can lead to other health problems, such as heart disease. If you have kidney disease, it increases your chances of having a stroke or heart attack. High blood pressure can be both a cause and a result of kidney disease. High blood pressure damages your kidneys, and damaged kidneys don't work as well to help control your blood pressure. If you have CKD, you also have a higher chance of having a sudden change in kidney function caused by illness, injury, or certain medicines. This is called acute kidney injury (AKI).

How Can CKD Affect My Day-to-Day Life?

Many people are afraid to learn that they have kidney disease because they think that all kidney disease leads to dialysis. However, most people with kidney disease will not need dialysis. If you have kidney disease, you can continue to live a productive life, work, spend time with friends and family, stay physically active, and do other things you enjoy. You may need to change what you eat and add healthy habits to your daily routine to help you protect your kidneys.

Will My Kidneys Get Better?

Kidney disease is often "progressive," which means it gets worse over time. The damage to your kidneys causes scars and is permanent.

You can take steps to protect your kidneys, such as managing your blood pressure and your blood glucose, if you have diabetes.

What Happens If My Kidneys Fail?

Kidney failure means that your kidneys have lost most of their ability to function—less than 15 percent of normal kidney function. If you have kidney failure, you will need treatment to maintain your health. Learn more about what happens if your kidneys fail.

Section 25.2

Polycystic Kidney Disease

This section includes text excerpted from "Polycystic Kidney Disease (PKD)," National Institute of Diabetes and Digestive and Kidney Diseases (NIDDK), January 2017.

What Is Polycystic Kidney Disease?

Polycystic kidney disease (PKD) is a genetic disorder that causes many fluid-filled cysts to grow in your kidneys. Unlike the usually harmless simple kidney cysts that can form in the kidneys later in life, PKD cysts can change the shape of your kidneys, including making them much larger. PKD is a form of chronic kidney disease (CKD) that reduces kidney function and may lead to kidney failure. PKD also can cause other complications, or problems, such as high blood pressure, cysts in the liver, and problems with blood vessels in your brain and heart.

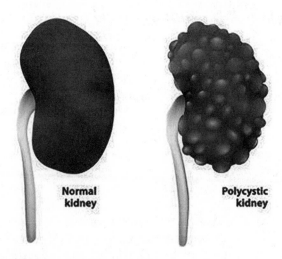

Normal kidney   **Polycystic kidney**

Figure 25.2. *Polycystic Kidney Disease*

Polycystic kidney disease is a genetic disorder that causes many fluid-filled cysts to grow in your kidneys.

What Are the Types of PKD?

The two main types of PKD are:

* autosomal dominant PKD (ADPKD), which is usually diagnosed in adulthood

* autosomal recessive PKD (ARPKD), which can be diagnosed in the womb or shortly after a baby is born

How Common Is PKD?

PKD is one of the most common genetic disorders. PKD affects about 500,000 people in the United States. ADPKD affects 1 in every 400 to 1,000 people in the world, and ARPKD affects 1 in 20,000 children.

Who Is More Likely to Have PKD?

PKD affects people of all ages, races, and ethnicities worldwide. The disorder occurs equally in women and men.

What Causes PKD?

A gene mutation, or defect, causes PKD. In most PKD cases, a child got the gene mutation from a parent. In a small number of PKD cases, the gene mutation developed on its own, without either parent carrying a copy of the mutated gene. This type of mutation is called "spontaneous."

What Are the Signs and Symptoms of PKD?

The signs and symptoms of ADPKD, such as pain, high blood pressure, and kidney failure, are also PKD complications. In many cases, ADPKD does not cause signs or symptoms until your kidney cysts are a half inch or larger in size.

Early signs of ARPKD in the womb are larger-than-normal kidneys and a smaller-than-average size baby, a condition called growth failure. The early signs of ARPKD are also complications. However, some people with ARPKD do not develop signs or symptoms until later in childhood or even adulthood.

Can I Prevent PKD?

Researchers have not yet found a way to prevent PKD. However, you may be able to slow PKD problems caused by high blood pressure, such as kidney damage. Aim for a blood pressure goal of less than 120/80. Work with a healthcare team to help manage your or your child's PKD. The healthcare team will probably include a general practitioner and a nephrologist, a healthcare provider specializing in kidney health.

What Can I Do to Slow Down PKD?

The sooner you know you or your child has PKD, the sooner you can keep the condition from getting worse. Getting tested if you or your child are at risk for PKD can help you take early action.

You also can take steps to help delay or prevent kidney failure. Healthy lifestyle practices such as being active, reducing stress, and quitting smoking can help.

Make Lifestyle Changes

Be active for 30 minutes or more on most days. Regular physical activity can help you reduce stress, manage your weight, and control your blood pressure. If you are not active now, ask your healthcare provider about how much and what type of physical activity is right for you.

If you play contact sports, such as football or hockey, a healthcare provider should do a magnetic resonance imaging (MRI) test to see whether these sports are safe for you. Trauma to your body, especially to your back and sides, may cause kidney cysts to burst.

Lose weight. Being overweight makes your kidneys work harder. Losing weight helps protect your kidneys.

Aim for 7 to 8 hours of sleep each night. Getting enough sleep is important to your overall physical and mental health and can help you manage your blood pressure and blood glucose, or blood sugar.

Reduce stress. Long-term stress can raise your blood pressure and even lead to depression. Some of the steps you take to manage your PKD are also healthy ways to cope with stress. For example, getting enough physical activity and sleep helps reduce stress.

Quit smoking. Cigarette smoking can raise your blood pressure, making your kidney damage worse. Quitting smoking may help you meet your blood pressure goals, which is good for your kidneys and can lower your chances of having a heart attack or stroke. Quitting smoking is even more important for people with PKD who have aneurysms. An aneurysm is a bulge in the wall of a blood vessel.

Change What You Eat and Drink

You may need to change what you eat and drink to help control your blood pressure and protect your kidneys. People with any kind of kidney disease, including PKD, should talk with a dietitian about which foods and drinks to include in their healthy eating plan and which may be harmful. Staying hydrated by drinking the right amount of fluid may help slow PKD's progress toward kidney failure.

Take Blood Pressure Medicines

If lifestyle and diet changes don't help control your blood pressure, a healthcare provider may prescribe one or more blood pressure medicines. Two types of blood pressure medicines, angiotensin converting enzyme (ACE) inhibitors and angiotensin receptor blockers (ARBs), may slow kidney disease and delay kidney failure. The names of these medicines end in –pril or –sartan.

Section 25.3

Kidney Failure

This section includes text excerpted from "Kidney Failure," National Institute of Diabetes and Digestive and Kidney Diseases (NIDDK), May 2014. Reviewed September 2017.

What Is Kidney Failure and How Is It Treated?

Kidney failure means your kidneys no longer work well enough to do their job. You need treatment to replace the work your damaged kidneys have stopped doing. The treatments for kidney failure are:

- hemodialysis
- peritoneal dialysis
- a kidney transplant

Your kidneys filter wastes and extra fluid from your blood to keep you healthy. The wastes and extra fluid become urine that is stored in your bladder until you urinate. When your kidneys fail, dialysis can take over a small part of the work your damaged kidneys can no longer do. You can make treatments work better by:

- sticking to your treatment schedule

- taking all medicines your doctor prescribes

- following a special diet that keeps wastes from building up in your blood

- being active most days of the week

Hemodialysis

Hemodialysis is a treatment for kidney failure. Hemodialysis uses a machine to filter your blood outside your body. First, a dialysis nurse places two needles into your arm. A pump on the hemodialysis machine draws your blood through one of the needles into a tube. The tube takes the blood to a filter, called a dialyzer. Inside the dialyzer, your blood flows through thin fibers that are like straws. The wastes and extra fluid leave the blood through tiny holes in the fibers. Then, a different tube carries the filtered blood back to your body through the second needle.

Peritoneal Dialysis

The other form of dialysis, called peritoneal dialysis, uses the lining of your abdomen, or belly, to filter your blood inside your body. A doctor places a soft tube called a catheter in your belly a few weeks before you start peritoneal dialysis. You empty dialysis solution from a plastic bag through the catheter into the empty space inside your belly. The dialysis solution soaks up wastes and extra fluid from your body. After a few hours, you drain the used dialysis solution into another bag. Then you start over with a fresh bag of dialysis solution.

Kidney Transplant

A kidney transplant places a healthy kidney from another person into your body. The kidney may come from someone who has just died. Your doctor will place your name on a waiting list for a kidney. A family member or friend might be able to give you a kidney. Then you don't have to wait.

The new kidney takes over filtering your blood. The damaged kidneys usually stay where they are. The new kidney is placed in the front lower abdomen, on one side of the bladder. Your body normally attacks anything that shouldn't be there, such as bacteria. Your body will think the new kidney shouldn't be there. You will take medicines called immunosuppressants to keep your body from attacking the new kidney.

How Should I Choose the Treatment That's Right for Me?

Learning about different treatments for kidney failure will help you choose the one that best fits your lifestyle. Talk with your doctor and people on hemodialysis or peritoneal dialysis to learn about the pros and cons of each treatment. Ask your doctor about the transplant waiting list and about medicines required after a transplant. Talk with people who have had kidney transplants and ask how it has changed their lives.

If you plan to keep working, think about which treatment can help make that easier. If spending time with family and friends means a lot to you, learn about which treatment may give you the most free time. Find out which treatment will give you the best chance to be healthy and live longer.

Talking with your doctor ahead of time about your options can help you take control of your care. Understanding the treatment you choose and getting used to the idea that you will be receiving this treatment takes time. If you choose one type of dialysis treatment and find it is not a good fit for your life, talk with your doctor about selecting another type of dialysis treatment that better meets your needs.

While kidney failure can make your life harder, treatments can help improve your life.

How Will Kidney Failure Affect My Life?

Kidney failure will affect your life in many ways. You may find you cannot do all the things you used to do at home or at work. You may have less energy and may feel depressed. Physical problems may include:

- ankle or belly swelling

- stomach sickness

- throwing up

- loss of appetite
- feeling tired
- weakness
- confusion
- headaches

Having kidney failure does not have to take over your life. Having kidney failure does not have to mean giving up hobbies, work, social activities, or time with family.

Can I Continue to Work with Kidney Failure?

Yes, many people with kidney failure continue to work. Your employer may give you lighter physical jobs or schedule your work hours around your hemodialysis sessions. If you are on peritoneal dialysis, you will need space and time to change the dialysis solution in the middle of the work day. Most employers are happy to make these changes.

As a result of the Americans with Disabilities Act (ADA), an employer cannot fire you because you are on dialysis or had a kidney transplant. The law requires an employer to make reasonable adjustments to the workplace for a person with a disability. If your employer is not willing to meet your needs, your dialysis clinic's renal social worker may be able to help find a way to satisfy both you and your employer. As a last resort, you may need to file a complaint with the Equal Employment Opportunity Commission (EEOC). Your renal social worker may be able to help you with this complaint, or you may need the help of a lawyer. Many times, just the mention of legal action is enough to cause an employer to make reasonable changes in the workplace.

Can I Be Active with Kidney Failure?

Yes. Physical activity is an important part of staying healthy when you have kidney failure. Being active makes your muscles, bones, and heart stronger. Physical activity also makes your blood circulate faster so your body gets more oxygen. Your body needs oxygen to use the energy from food. If you are on dialysis, physical activity can help more wastes move into your blood for dialysis to remove them. You will find that physical activity can also improve your mood and give you a sense of wellbeing.

Talk with your doctor before you start an exercise routine. Start slow, with easier activities such as walking at a normal pace or gardening. Work up to harder activities such as walking briskly or swimming. Aim for at least 30 minutes of exercise most days of the week.

Where Can I Find Help for Coping with Kidney Failure?

When you start dialysis or are referred to a transplant center, you will meet many people who can help you. These people make up your healthcare team. Your healthcare team can help you with the emotional and physical problems and changes caused by kidney failure. Asking for help is not a sign of weakness. Talk with your family, friends, and healthcare team about your concerns.

Doctor. Your doctor can help you with many of the physical and emotional health problems caused by kidney failure. You will see your doctor often as you start dialysis or recover from transplant surgery. After a while, you will see your doctor regularly, though less often than at the beginning of treatment. If you have a transplant, you will see your doctor once or twice a month during the first 6 months after your transplant surgery. Then, if everything goes well with your new kidney, you only need to see your doctor once every 6 months.

Dialysis nurse. If you receive hemodialysis at a dialysis center, your dialysis nurse will oversee your treatment. The nurse will take your blood pressure, pulse, and temperature; watch your breathing; and explain your lab results. Your dialysis nurse will also make sure you are taking your medicines correctly and can help you find ways to lessen the side effects of dialysis. If you do home hemodialysis or peritoneal dialysis, your dialysis nurse will teach you how to set up your treatment, take care of the equipment, and watch for infections or other problems.

Transplant coordinator. Transplant coordinators work with people who need a transplant. They are usually nurses with special training in transplantation. Your transplant coordinator guides you through the transplant process, from setting up your first physical exam and getting you on the kidney transplant waiting list to calling you when a matching kidney has been found and preparing you for transplant surgery. The transplant coordinator also works with you after transplant surgery by:

- scheduling your follow-up care

- teaching you how to care for and protect your new kidney
- helping you find ways to cope with the side effects of medicines

Renal dietitian. Renal dietitians help you learn about your nutrition needs and why you must avoid or limit certain foods. A renal dietitian will help you plan healthy meals you will enjoy.

Renal social worker. Dialysis centers have a social worker, called a renal social worker, who works with people on dialysis or who have transplants. Your renal social worker can help you find answers to problems such as:

- keeping a job or changing jobs
- getting help with financial issues
- finding services to help with transportation or chores around the house
- finding counseling services to deal with family or couples' problems

Mental health counselor/psychiatrist. Your healthcare team may recommend you see a mental health counselor or a psychiatrist. A mental health counselor can help with depression and other mental health issues by talking with you and suggesting ways to deal with stress and unhealthy thoughts and behaviors. A psychiatrist is a doctor trained to help people with mental health issues such as depression and to prescribe medicines, if needed.

Family and friends. Your healthcare team members are not the only people who can help you cope with the problems and changes caused by kidney failure. Having a strong support system of family and friends can make it easier to deal with problems and life changes. Now is not the time to stop seeing your friends. Make a point to spend time with friends or keep in touch with them by phone or email. Attend social functions and community events.

You. You can improve the quality of your healthcare by letting your healthcare team know how you want to be treated. Don't hesitate to ask questions when your doctor or nurse tells you something you don't understand. Let your dialysis nurse know if you feel light-headed or sick to your stomach during dialysis. If you do home hemodialysis or peritoneal dialysis, tell your dialysis nurse about any problems you have with equipment or supplies. If you have a transplant, talk with your transplant coordinator if your medicines cause digestion problems or other side effects. You are responsible for taking your medicines and keeping your appointments. Taking charge of your own medical care will help you feel more in control of your life.

Does Kidney Failure Run in Families?

Yes, kidney failure runs in families, so your blood relatives are at risk. You can help prevent relatives from having kidney failure by talking with them about their risk. Members of your family may already have chronic kidney disease (CKD), which means their kidneys are damaged and do not work as well as they should. CKD tends to get worse over time. CKD often, though not always, leads to kidney failure. CKD most often has no symptoms, so the only way for your family members to know whether they have CKD is to get tested. Simple urine and blood tests can show if they have CKD. The earlier CKD is found, the sooner your family members can take steps to keep their kidneys healthy longer, including taking medicines that help control blood pressure and prevent further kidney damage. Exercising and eating a better diet can also keep CKD from getting worse.

Eating, Diet, and Nutrition

Eating the right foods can help you feel better when you are on dialysis or have a kidney transplant. Staying healthy with kidney failure requires watching how much of these elements are included in your diet:

- **Protein** is in many foods you eat. Protein is in foods from animals and plants. Most diets include both types of protein. Protein provides the building blocks that maintain and repair muscles, organs, and other parts of the body. Too much protein can cause waste to build up in your blood, making your kidneys work harder. However, if you are on hemodialysis or peritoneal dialysis, you need lots of protein to replace the protein that dialysis removes.

- **Phosphorus** is a mineral that keeps your bones healthy. Phosphorus also keeps blood vessels and muscles working. This mineral is found naturally in foods rich in protein, such as meat, poultry, fish, nuts, beans, and dairy products. Phosphorus is also added to many processed foods. You need phosphorus to turn food into energy; however, too much can cause your bones to weaken.

- **Water** is in drinks and in foods such as fruits, vegetables, ice cream, gelatin, soup, and popsicles. Your body needs water; however, too much can cause fluid to build up in your body and make your heart work harder.

- **Sodium** is a part of salt. You can find sodium in many canned, packaged, and fast foods and in seasonings and meats. You need sodium to help control the amount of fluid in your body; however, too much can cause high blood pressure.

- **Potassium** is a mineral that helps your nerves and muscles work the right way. Potassium is found in fruits and vegetables such as oranges, bananas, tomatoes, and potatoes. You need potassium for healthy nerves and brain cells; however, too much can make your heartbeat irregular.

- **Calories** are found in all foods and are especially high in oils and sugary foods. You need calories for energy; however, too many can cause weight gain and high blood sugar.

Talk with your clinic's renal dietitian to find a meal plan that works for you. Each treatment requires a different diet. If you are on hemodialysis, you have to stay away from foods such as potatoes and oranges because they have lots of potassium. If you are on peritoneal dialysis, eating potassium is fine. Instead, you may need to watch your calories. Your food needs will also depend on your weight and activity level.

Changing your diet may be hard at first. Eating the right foods will help you feel better. You will have more strength and energy. Having more energy will help you live a fuller, healthier life.

Section 25.4

Prostate Enlargement (Benign Prostatic Hyperplasia)

This section includes text excerpted from "Prostate Enlargement (Benign Prostatic Hyperplasia)," National Institute of Diabetes and Digestive and Kidney Diseases (NIDDK), September 2014. Reviewed September 2017.

What Is Benign Prostatic Hyperplasia?

Benign prostatic hyperplasia—also called BPH—is a condition in men in which the prostate gland is enlarged and not cancerous. Benign prostatic hyperplasia is also called benign prostatic hypertrophy or benign prostatic obstruction.

The prostate goes through two main growth periods as a man ages. The first occurs early in puberty, when the prostate doubles in size. The second phase of growth begins around age 25 and continues during most of a man's life. Benign prostatic hyperplasia often occurs with the second growth phase.

As the prostate enlarges, the gland presses against and pinches the urethra. The bladder wall becomes thicker. Eventually, the bladder may weaken and lose the ability to empty completely, leaving some urine in the bladder. The narrowing of the urethra and urinary retention—the inability to empty the bladder completely—cause many of the problems associated with benign prostatic hyperplasia.

What Is the Prostate?

The prostate is a walnut-shaped gland that is part of the male reproductive system. The main function of the prostate is to make a fluid that goes into semen. Prostate fluid is essential for a man's fertility. The gland surrounds the urethra at the neck of the bladder. The bladder neck is the area where the urethra joins the bladder. The bladder and urethra are parts of the lower urinary tract. The prostate has two or more lobes, or sections, enclosed by an outer layer of tissue, and it is in front of the rectum, just below the bladder. The urethra is the tube that carries urine from the bladder to the outside of the body. In men, the urethra also carries semen out through the penis.

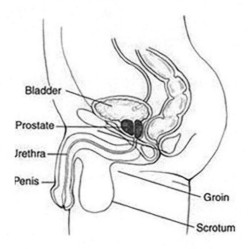

Figure 25.3. *The Prostate Gland*

The prostate is a walnut-shaped gland that is part of the male reproductive system.

What Causes Benign Prostatic Hyperplasia?

The cause of benign prostatic hyperplasia is not well understood; however, it occurs mainly in older men. Benign prostatic hyperplasia does not develop in men whose testicles were removed before puberty. For this reason, some researchers believe factors related to aging and the testicles may cause benign prostatic hyperplasia.

Throughout their lives, men produce testosterone, a male hormone, and small amounts of estrogen, a female hormone. As men age, the amount of active testosterone in their blood decreases, which leaves a higher proportion of estrogen. Scientific studies have suggested that benign prostatic hyperplasia may occur because the higher proportion of estrogen within the prostate increases the activity of substances that promote prostate cell growth.

Another theory focuses on dihydrotestosterone (DHT), a male hormone that plays a role in prostate development and growth. Some research has indicated that even with a drop in blood testosterone levels, older men continue to produce and accumulate high levels of DHT in the prostate. This accumulation of DHT may encourage prostate cells to continue to grow. Scientists have noted that men who do not produce DHT do not develop benign prostatic hyperplasia.

How Common Is Benign Prostatic Hyperplasia?

Benign prostatic hyperplasia is the most common prostate problem for men older than age 50. In 2010, as many as 14 million men in the United States had lower urinary tract symptoms suggestive of benign prostatic hyperplasia. Although benign prostatic hyperplasia rarely causes symptoms before age 40, the occurrence and symptoms increase with age. Benign prostatic hyperplasia affects about 50 percent of men between the ages of 51 and 60 and up to 90 percent of men older than 80.

Who Is More Likely to Develop Benign Prostatic Hyperplasia?

Men with the following factors are more likely to develop benign prostatic hyperplasia:

- age 40 years and older
- family history of benign prostatic hyperplasia
- medical conditions such as obesity, heart and circulatory disease, and type 2
- diabetes
- lack of physical exercise
- erectile dysfunction

What Are the Symptoms of Benign Prostatic Hyperplasia?

Lower urinary tract symptoms suggestive of benign prostatic hyperplasia may include:

- urinary frequency—urination eight or more times a day
- urinary urgency—the inability to delay urination
- trouble starting a urine stream
- a weak or an interrupted urine stream
- dribbling at the end of urination
- nocturia—frequent urination during periods of sleep
- urinary retention

361

- urinary incontinence—the accidental loss of urine
- pain after ejaculation or during urination
- urine that has an unusual color or smell

Symptoms of benign prostatic hyperplasia most often come from:
- a blocked urethra
- a bladder that is overworked from trying to pass urine through the blockage

The size of the prostate does not always determine the severity of the blockage or symptoms. Some men with greatly enlarged prostates have little blockage and few symptoms, while other men who have minimally enlarged prostates have greater blockage and more symptoms. Less than half of all men with benign prostatic hyperplasia have lower urinary tract symptoms.

Sometimes men may not know they have a blockage until they cannot urinate. This condition, called acute urinary retention, can result from taking over-the-counter cold or allergy medications that contain decongestants, such as pseudoephedrine and oxymetazoline. A potential side effect of these medications may prevent the bladder neck from relaxing and releasing urine. Medications that contain antihistamines, such as diphenhydramine, can weaken the contraction of bladder muscles and cause urinary retention, difficulty urinating, and painful urination. When men have partial urethra blockage, urinary retention also can occur as a result of alcohol consumption, cold temperatures, or a long period of inactivity.

What Are the Complications of Benign Prostatic Hyperplasia?

The complications of benign prostatic hyperplasia may include:
- acute urinary retention
- chronic, or long lasting, urinary retention
- blood in the urine
- urinary tract infections (UTIs)
- bladder damage
- kidney damage
- bladder stones

Most men with benign prostatic hyperplasia do not develop these complications. However, kidney damage in particular can be a serious health threat when it occurs.

When to Seek Medical Care

A person may have urinary symptoms unrelated to benign prostatic hyperplasia that are caused by bladder problems, UTIs, or prostatitis— inflammation of the prostate. Symptoms of benign prostatic hyperplasia also can signal more serious conditions, including prostate cancer.

Men with symptoms of benign prostatic hyperplasia should see a healthcare provider.

Men with the following symptoms should seek immediate medical care:

- complete inability to urinate

- painful, frequent, and urgent need to urinate, with fever and chills

- blood in the urine

- great discomfort or pain in the lower abdomen and urinary tract

How Is Benign Prostatic Hyperplasia Diagnosed?

A healthcare provider diagnoses benign prostatic hyperplasia based on:

- a personal and family medical history

- a physical exam

- medical tests

Personal and Family Medical History

Taking a personal and family medical history is one of the first things a healthcare provider may do to help diagnose benign prostatic hyperplasia. A healthcare provider may ask a man:

- what symptoms are present

- when the symptoms began and how often they occur

- whether he has a history of recurrent UTIs

- what medications he takes, both prescription and over the counter

- how much liquid he typically drinks each day
- whether he consumes caffeine and alcohol
- about his general medical history, including any significant illnesses or surgeries

Physical Exam

A physical exam may help diagnose benign prostatic hyperplasia. During a physical exam, a healthcare provider most often

- examines a patient's body, which can include checking for:
  - discharge from the urethra
  - enlarged or tender lymph nodes in the groin
  - a swollen or tender scrotum
- taps on specific areas of the patient's body
- performs a digital rectal exam

Medical Tests

A healthcare provider may refer men to a urologist—a doctor who specializes in urinary problems and the male reproductive system— though the healthcare provider most often diagnoses benign prostatic hyperplasia on the basis of symptoms and a digital rectal exam. A urologist uses medical tests to help diagnose lower urinary tract problems related to benign prostatic hyperplasia and recommend treatment. Medical tests may include:

- urinalysis
- a prostate-specific antigen (PSA) blood test
- urodynamic tests
- cystoscopy
- transrectal ultrasound
- biopsy

How Is Benign Prostatic Hyperplasia Treated?

Treatment options for benign prostatic hyperplasia may include:

- lifestyle changes

- Medications

- minimally invasive procedures

- surgery

A healthcare provider treats benign prostatic hyperplasia based on the severity of symptoms, how much the symptoms affect a man's daily life, and a man's preferences.

Men may not need treatment for a mildly enlarged prostate unless their symptoms are bothersome and affecting their quality of life. In these cases, instead of treatment, a urologist may recommend regular checkups. If benign prostatic hyperplasia symptoms become bothersome or present a health risk, a urologist most often recommends treatment.

Lifestyle Changes

A healthcare provider may recommend lifestyle changes for men whose symptoms are mild or slightly bothersome. Lifestyle changes can include:

- reducing intake of liquids, particularly before going out in public or before periods of sleep

- avoiding or reducing intake of caffeinated beverages and alcohol

- avoiding or monitoring the use of medications such as decongestants, antihistamines, antidepressants, and diuretics

- training the bladder to hold more urine for longer periods

- exercising pelvic floor muscles

- preventing or treating constipation

Medications

A healthcare provider or urologist may prescribe medications that stop the growth of or shrink the prostate or reduce symptoms associated with benign prostatic hyperplasia:

- alpha blockers

- phosphodiesterase-5 inhibitors

- 5-alpha reductase inhibitors

• combination medications

Alpha blockers. These medications relax the smooth muscles of the prostate and bladder neck to improve urine flow and reduce bladder blockage:

• terazosin (Hytrin)

• doxazosin (Cardura)

• tamsulosin (Flomax)

• alfuzosin (Uroxatral)

• silodosin (Rapaflo)

Phosphodiesterase-5 inhibitors. Urologists prescribe these medications mainly for erectile dysfunction. Tadalafil (Cialis) belongs to this class of medications and can reduce lower urinary tract symptoms by relaxing smooth muscles in the lower urinary tract. Researchers are working to determine the role of erectile dysfunction drugs in the long-term treatment of benign prostatic hyperplasia.

5-alpha reductase inhibitors. These medications block the production of DHT, which accumulates in the prostate and may cause prostate growth.

Minimally Invasive Procedures

Researchers have developed a number of minimally invasive procedures that relieve benign prostatic hyperplasia symptoms when medications prove ineffective. These procedures include:

• transurethral needle ablation

• transurethral microwave thermotherapy

• high intensity focused ultrasound

• transurethral electrovaporization

• water induced thermotherapy

• prostatic stent insertion

Minimally invasive procedures can destroy enlarged prostate tissue or widen the urethra, which can help relieve blockage and urinary retention caused by benign prostatic hyperplasia.

Surgery

For long-term treatment of benign prostatic hyperplasia, a urologist may recommend removing enlarged prostate tissue or making cuts in the prostate to widen the urethra. Urologists recommend surgery when:

- medications and minimally invasive procedures are ineffective
- symptoms are particularly bothersome or severe
- complications arise

Although removing troublesome prostate tissue relieves many benign prostatic hyperplasia symptoms, tissue removal does not cure benign prostatic hyperplasia.

Surgery to remove enlarged prostate tissue includes:

- transurethral resection of the prostate (TURP)
- laser surgery
- open prostatectomy
- transurethral incision of the prostate (TUIP)

What Are the Complications of Benign Prostatic Hyperplasia Treatment?

The complications of benign prostatic hyperplasia treatment depend on the type of treatment.

Medications

Medications used to treat benign prostatic hyperplasia may have side effects that sometimes can be serious. Men who are prescribed medications to treat benign prostatic hyperplasia should discuss possible side effects with a healthcare provider before taking the medications. Men who experience the following side effects should contact a healthcare provider right away or get emergency medical care:

- Hives
- Rash
- Itching
- shortness of breath

- rapid, pounding, or irregular heartbeat
- painful erection of the penis that lasts for hours
- swelling of the eyes, face, tongue, lips, throat, arms, hands, feet, ankles, or lower legs
- difficulty breathing or swallowing
- chest pain
- dizziness or fainting when standing up suddenly
- sudden decrease or loss of vision
- blurred vision
- sudden decrease or loss of hearing
- chest pain, dizziness, or nausea during sexual activity

These side effects are mostly related to phosphodiesterase-5 inhibitors. Side effects related to alpha blockers include:

- dizziness or fainting when standing up suddenly
- decreased sexual drive
- problems with ejaculation

Minimally Invasive Procedures

Complications after minimally invasive procedures may include:

- UTIs
- painful urination
- difficulty urinating
- an urgent or a frequent need to urinate
- urinary incontinence
- blood in the urine for several days after the procedure
- sexual dysfunction
- chronic prostatitis—long-lasting inflammation of the prostate
- recurring problems such as urinary retention and UTIs

Most of the complications of minimally invasive procedures go away within a few days or weeks. Minimally invasive procedures are less likely to have complications than surgery.

Surgery

Complications after surgery may include:

- problems urinating
- urinary incontinence
- bleeding and blood clots
- Infection
- scar tissue
- sexual dysfunction
- recurring problems such as urinary retention and UTIs

Problems urinating. Men may initially have painful urination or difficulty urinating. They may experience urinary frequency, urgency, or retention. These problems will gradually lessen and, after a couple of months, urination will be easier and less frequent.

Urinary incontinence. As the bladder returns to normal, men may have some temporary problems controlling urination. However, long-term urinary incontinence rarely occurs. The longer urinary problems existed before surgery, the longer it takes for the bladder to regain its full function after surgery.

Bleeding and blood clots. After benign prostatic hyperplasia surgery, the prostate or tissues around it may bleed. Blood or blood clots may appear in urine. Some bleeding is normal and should clear up within several days. However, men should contact a healthcare provider right away if:

- they experience pain or discomfort
- their urine contains large clots
- their urine is so red it is difficult to see through

Blood clots from benign prostatic hyperplasia surgery can pass into the bloodstream and lodge in other parts of the body—most often the legs. Men should contact a healthcare provider right away if they experience swelling or discomfort in their legs.

Infection. Use of a Foley catheter after benign prostatic hyperplasia surgery may increase the risk of a UTI. Anesthesia during surgery may cause urinary retention and also increase the risk of a UTI. In addition, the incision site of an open prostatectomy may become infected. A healthcare provider will prescribe antibiotics to treat infections.

Scar tissue. In the year after the original surgery, scar tissue sometimes forms and requires surgical treatment. Scar tissue may form in the urethra and cause it to narrow. A urologist can solve this problem during an office visit by stretching the urethra. Rarely, the opening of the bladder becomes scarred and shrinks, causing blockage. This problem may require a surgical procedure similar to TUIP.

Sexual dysfunction. Some men may experience temporary problems with sexual function after benign prostatic hyperplasia surgery. The length of time for restored sexual function depends on the type of benign prostatic hyperplasia surgery performed and how long symptoms were present before surgery. Many men have found that concerns about sexual function can interfere with sex as much as the benign prostatic hyperplasia surgery itself. Understanding the surgical procedure and talking about concerns with a healthcare provider before surgery often help men regain sexual function earlier. Many men find it helpful to talk with a counselor during the adjustment period after surgery. Even though it can take a while for sexual function to fully return, with time, most men can enjoy sex again.

Most healthcare providers agree that if men with benign prostatic hyperplasia were able to maintain an erection before surgery, they will probably be able to have erections afterward. Surgery rarely causes a loss of erectile function. However, benign prostatic hyperplasia surgery most often cannot restore function that was lost before the procedure. Some men find a slight difference in the quality of orgasm after surgery. However, most report no difference.

How Can Benign Prostatic Hyperplasia Be Prevented?

Researchers have not found a way to prevent benign prostatic hyperplasia. Men with risk factors for benign prostatic hyperplasia should talk with a healthcare provider about any lower urinary tract symptoms and the need for regular prostate exams. Men can get early treatment and minimize benign prostatic hyperplasia effects by recognizing lower urinary tract symptoms and identifying an enlarged prostate.

Eating, Diet, and Nutrition

Researchers have not found that eating, diet, and nutrition play a role in causing or preventing benign prostatic hyperplasia. However, a healthcare provider can give information about how changes in eating, diet, or nutrition could help with treatment. Men should talk with a healthcare provider or dietitian about what diet is right for them.

Section 25.5

Urinary Incontinence

This section includes text excerpted from "Urinary Incontinence in Older Adults," National Institute on Aging (NIA), National Institutes of Health (NIH), August 21, 2017.

Urinary incontinence means a person leaks urine by accident. While it may happen to anyone, urinary incontinence is more common in older people, especially women. Incontinence can often be cured or controlled. Talk to your healthcare provider about what you can do.

What happens in the body to cause bladder control problems? The body stores urine in the bladder. During urination, muscles in the bladder tighten to move urine into a tube called the urethra. At the same time, the muscles around the urethra relax and let the urine pass out of the body. When the muscles in and around the bladder don't work the way they should, urine can leak. Incontinence typically occurs if the muscles relax without warning.

Causes of Urinary Incontinence

Incontinence can happen for many reasons. For example, urinary tract infections, vaginal infection or irritation, constipation. Some medicines can cause bladder control problems that last a short time. When incontinence lasts longer, it may be due to:

- Weak bladder muscles

- Overactive bladder muscles

- Weak pelvic floor muscles

- Damage to nerves that control the bladder from diseases such as multiple sclerosis, diabetes, or Parkinson disease

- Blockage from an enlarged prostate in men

- Diseases such as arthritis that may make it difficult to get to the bathroom in time

- Pelvic organ prolapse, which is when pelvic organs (such as the bladder, rectum, or uterus) shift out of their normal place into the vagina. When pelvic organs are out of place, the bladder and urethra are not able to work normally, which may cause urine to leak.

Most incontinence in men is related to the prostate gland. Male incontinence may be caused by:

- Prostatitis—a painful inflammation of the prostate gland

- Injury, or damage to nerves or muscles from surgery

- An enlarged prostate gland, which can lead to benign prostate hyperplasia (BPH), a condition where the prostate grows as men age.

Diagnosis of Urinary Incontinence

The first step in treating incontinence is to see a doctor. He or she will give you a physical exam and take your medical history. The doctor will ask about your symptoms and the medicines you use. He or she will want to know if you have been sick recently or had surgery. Your doctor also may do a number of tests. These might include:

- Urine and blood tests

- Tests that measure how well you empty your bladder

In addition, your doctor may ask you to keep a daily diary of when you urinate and when you leak urine. Your family doctor may also send you to a urologist, a doctor who specializes in urinary tract problems.

Types of Urinary Incontinence

There are different types of incontinence:

- **Stress incontinence** occurs when urine leaks as pressure is put on the bladder, for example, during exercise, coughing, sneezing, laughing, or lifting heavy objects. It's the most common type of bladder control problem in younger and middle-age women. It may begin around the time of menopause.

- **Urge incontinence** happens when people have a sudden need to urinate and cannot hold their urine long enough to get to the toilet. It may be a problem for people who have diabetes, Alzheimer disease, Parkinson disease, multiple sclerosis, or stroke.

- **Overflow incontinence** happens when small amounts of urine leak from a bladder that is always full. A man can have trouble emptying his bladder if an enlarged prostate is blocking the urethra. Diabetes and spinal cord injuries can also cause this type of incontinence.

- **Functional incontinence** occurs in many older people who have normal bladder control. They just have a problem getting to the toilet because of arthritis or other disorders that make it hard to move quickly.

Treatment for Urinary Incontinence

Today, there are more treatments for urinary incontinence than ever before. The choice of treatment depends on the type of bladder control problem you have, how serious it is, and what best fits your lifestyle. As a general rule, the simplest and safest treatments should be tried first.

Bladder control training may help you get better control of your bladder. Your doctor may suggest you try the following:

- **Pelvic muscle exercises** (also known as Kegel exercises) work the muscles that you use to stop urinating. Making these muscles stronger helps you hold urine in your bladder longer. Learn more about pelvic floor exercises and how to do them.

- **Biofeedback** uses sensors to make you aware of signals from your body. This may help you regain control over the muscles in your bladder and urethra. Biofeedback can be helpful when learning pelvic muscle exercises.

- **Timed voiding** may help you control your bladder. In timed voiding, you urinate on a set schedule, for example, every hour. You can slowly extend the time between bathroom trips. When timed voiding is combined with biofeedback and pelvic muscle exercises, you may find it easier to control urge and overflow incontinence.

- **Lifestyle changes** may help with incontinence. Losing weight, quitting smoking, saying "no" to alcohol, drinking less caffeine

373

(found in coffee, tea, and many sodas), preventing constipation and avoiding lifting heavy objects may help with incontinence. Choosing water instead of other drinks and limiting drinks before bedtime may also help.

Incontinence and Alzheimer Disease

People in the later stages of Alzheimer disease often have problems with urinary incontinence. This can be a result of not realizing they need to urinate, forgetting to go to the bathroom, or not being able to find the toilet. To minimize the chance of accidents, the caregiver can:

- Avoid giving drinks like caffeinated coffee, tea, and sodas, which may increase urination. But don't limit water.

- Keep pathways clear and the bathroom clutter-free, with a light on at all times.

- Make sure you provide regular bathroom breaks.

- Supply underwear that is easy to get on and off.

- Use absorbent underclothes for trips away from home.

Managing Urinary Incontinence

Besides bladder control training, you may want to talk with your doctor about other ways to help manage incontinence:

- Medicines can help the bladder empty more fully during urination. Other drugs tighten muscles and can lessen leakage.

- Some women find that using an estrogen vaginal cream may help relieve stress or urge incontinence. A low dose of estrogen cream is applied directly to the vaginal walls and urethral tissue.

- A doctor may inject a substance that thickens the area around the urethra to help close the bladder opening. This can reduce stress incontinence in women. This treatment may need to be repeated.

- Some women may be able to use a medical device, such as a urethral insert, a small disposable device inserted into the urethra. A pessary, a stiff ring inserted into the vagina, may help prevent leaking if you have a prolapsed bladder or vagina.

- Nerve stimulation, which sends mild electric current to the nerves around the bladder that help control urination, may be another option.

- Surgery can sometimes improve or cure incontinence if it's caused by a change in the position of the bladder or blockage due to an enlarged prostate.

Even after treatment, some people still leak urine from time to time. There are bladder control products and other solutions, including adult diapers, furniture pads, urine deodorizing pills, and special skin cleansers that may make leaking urine bother you a little less.

Chapter 26

Substance Abuse

Chapter Contents

Section 26.1

Alcohol Use in Older People

This section includes text excerpted from "Facts about Aging and Alcohol," National Institute on Aging (NIA), National Institutes of Health (NIH), August 16, 2017.

Alcohol may act differently in older people than in younger people. Some older people can feel "high" without increasing the amount of alcohol they drink. This "high" can make them more likely to have accidents, including falls and fractures and car crashes.

Drinking too much alcohol over a long time can:

- Lead to some kinds of cancer, liver damage, immune system disorders, and brain damage

- Worsen some health conditions like osteoporosis, diabetes, high blood pressure, stroke, ulcers, memory loss and mood disorders

- Make some medical problems hard for doctors to find and treat—for example, alcohol causes changes in the heart and blood vessels. These changes can dull pain that might be a warning sign of a heart attack.

- Cause some older people to be forgetful and confused—these symptoms could be mistaken for signs of Alzheimer disease.

How Alcohol Affects Safety

Drinking even a small amount of alcohol can lead to dangerous or even deadly situations. Drinking can impair a person's judgment, coordination, and reaction time. This increases the risk of falls, household accidents, and car crashes. Alcohol is a factor in 30 percent of suicides, 40 percent of crashes and burns, 50 percent of drownings and homicides, and 60 percent of falls. People who plan to drive, use machinery, or perform other activities that require attention, skill, or coordination should not drink.

In older adults, too much alcohol can lead to balance problems and falls, which can result in hip or arm fractures and other injuries. Older people have thinner bones than younger people, so their bones break more easily. Studies show that the rate of hip fractures in older adults increases with alcohol use.

Adults of all ages who drink and drive are at higher risk of traffic accidents and related problems than those who do not drink. Drinking slows reaction times and coordination and interferes with eye movement and information processing. People who drink even a moderate amount can have traffic accidents, possibly resulting in injury or death to themselves and others. Even without alcohol, the risk of crashes goes up starting at age 55. Also, older drivers tend to be more seriously hurt in crashes than younger drivers. Alcohol adds to these age-related risks.

In addition, alcohol misuse and abuse can strain relationships with family members, friends, and others. At the extreme, heavy drinking can contribute to domestic violence and child abuse or neglect. Alcohol use is often involved when people become violent, as well as when they are violently attacked. If you feel that alcohol is endangering you or someone else, call 911 or get other help right away.

Section 26.2

Prescription Drug Abuse

This section includes text excerpted from "Misuse of Prescription Drugs," National Institute on Drug Abuse (NIDA), August 2016.

Misuse of prescription drugs means taking a medication in a manner or dose other than prescribed; taking someone else's prescription, even if for a legitimate medical complaint such as pain; or taking a medication to feel euphoria (i.e., to get high). The term nonmedical use of prescription drugs also refers to these categories of misuse. The three classes of medication most commonly misused are:

- opioids—usually prescribed to treat pain

- central nervous system [CNS] depressants (this category includes tranquilizers, sedatives, and hypnotics)—used to treat anxiety and sleep disorders

- stimulants—most often prescribed to treat attention deficit hyperactivity disorder (ADHD)

Prescription drug misuse can have serious medical consequences. Increases in prescription drug misuse over the last 15 years are reflected in increased emergency room visits, overdose deaths associated with prescription drugs and treatment admissions for prescription drug use disorders, the most severe form of which is addiction. Among those who reported past-year nonmedical use of a prescription drug, nearly 12 percent met criteria for prescription drug use disorder. Unintentional overdose deaths involving opioid pain relievers have more than quadrupled since 1999 and have outnumbered those involving heroin and cocaine since 2002.

What Is the Scope of Prescription Drug Misuse?

Misuse of prescription opioids, central nervous system (CNS) depressants, and stimulants is a serious public health problem in the United States. Although most people take prescription medications responsibly, an estimated 54 million people (more than 20 percent of those aged 12 and older) have used such medications for nonmedical reasons at least once in their lifetime. According to results from the 2014 National Survey on Drug Use and Health (NSDUH), an estimated 2.1 million Americans used prescription drugs nonmedically for the first time within the past year, which averages to approximately 5,750 initiates per day. Fifty-four percent were females and about 30 percent were adolescents.

The reasons for the high prevalence of prescription drug misuse vary by age, gender, and other factors, but likely include ease of access. The number of prescriptions for some of these medications has increased dramatically since the early 1990s. Moreover, misinformation about the addictive properties of prescription opioids and the perception that prescription drugs are less harmful than illicit drugs are other possible contributors to the problem.

Although misuse of prescription drugs affects many Americans, certain populations such as youth, older adults, and women may be at particular risk. In addition, while more men than women currently misuse prescription drugs, the rates of misuse and overdose among women are increasing faster than among men.

Older Adults

More than 80 percent of older patients (aged 57 to 85 years) use at least one prescription medication on a daily basis, with more than

50 percent taking more than five medications or supplements daily. This can potentially lead to health issues resulting from unintentionally using a prescription medication in a manner other than how it was prescribed, or from intentional nonmedical use. The high rates of multiple (comorbid) chronic illnesses in older populations, age-related changes in drug metabolism, and the potential for drug interactions makes medication (and other substance) misuse more dangerous in older people than in younger populations. Further, a large percentage of older adults also use over-the-counter medicines and dietary supplements, which (in addition to alcohol) could compound any adverse health consequences resulting from nonmedical use of prescription drugs.

Is It Safe to Use Prescription Drugs in Combination with Other Medications?

The safety of using prescription drugs in combination with other substances depends on a number of factors including the types of medications, dosages, other substance use (e.g., alcohol), and individual patient health factors. Patients should talk with their healthcare provider about whether they can safely use their prescription drugs with other substances, including prescription and over-the-counter (OTC) medications as well as alcohol, tobacco, and illicit drugs. Specifically, drugs that slow down breathing rate, such as opioids, alcohol, antihistamines, prescription central nervous system depressants (including barbiturates and benzodiazepines), or general anesthetics, should not be taken together because these combinations increase the risk of life-threatening respiratory depression. Stimulants should also not be used with other medications unless recommended by a physician. Patients should be aware of the dangers associated with mixing stimulants and OTC cold medicines that contain decongestants, as combining these substances may cause blood pressure to become dangerously high or lead to irregular heart rhythms.

Which Classes of Prescription Drugs Are Commonly Misused?

What Are Opioids?

Opioids are medications that act on opioid receptors in both the spinal cord and brain to reduce the intensity of pain-signal perception. They also affect brain areas that control emotion, which can further diminish the effects of painful stimuli. They have been used for centuries to treat pain, cough, and diarrhea. The most common modern use of opioids is to treat acute pain. However, since the 1990s, they have been increasingly used to treat chronic pain, despite sparse evidence for their effectiveness when used long term. Indeed, some patients experience a worsening of their pain or increased sensitivity to pain as a result of treatment with opioids, a phenomenon known as hyperalgesia. Importantly, in addition to relieving pain, opioids also activate reward regions in the brain causing the euphoria—or high—that underlies the potential for misuse and addiction. Chemically, these medications are very similar to heroin, which was originally synthesized from morphine as a pharmaceutical in the late 19th century. These properties confer an increased risk of addiction and overdose even in patients who take their medication as prescribed.

Prescription opioid medications include hydrocodone (e.g., Vicodin®), oxycodone (e.g., OxyContin®, Percocet®), oxymorphone (e.g., Opana®), morphine (e.g., Kadian®, Avinza®), codeine, fentanyl, and others. Hydrocodone products are the most commonly prescribed in the United States for a variety of indications, including dental- and injury-related pain. Oxycodone and oxymorphone are also prescribed for moderate to severe pain relief. Morphine is often used before and after surgical procedures to alleviate severe pain, and codeine is typically prescribed for milder pain. In addition to their pain-relieving properties, some of these drugs—codeine and diphenoxylate (Lomotil®), for example—are used to relieve coughs and severe diarrhea.

How Do Opioids Affect the Brain and Body?

Opioids act by attaching to and activating opioid receptor proteins, which are found on nerve cells in the brain, spinal cord, gastrointestinal tract, and other organs in the body. When these drugs attach to their receptors, they inhibit the transmission of pain signals. Opioids can also produce drowsiness, mental confusion, nausea, constipation, and respiratory depression, and since these drugs also act on brain regions involved in reward, they can induce euphoria, particularly when they are taken at a higher-than-prescribed dose or administered in other ways than intended. For example, OxyContin® is an oral medication used to treat moderate to severe pain through a slow, steady release of the opioid. Some people who misuse OxyContin® intensify their experience by snorting or injecting it. This is a very dangerous practice, greatly increasing the person's risk for serious medical complications, including overdose.

Understanding Dependence, Addiction, and Tolerance

Dependence occurs as a result of physiological adaptations to chronic exposure to a drug. It is often a part of addiction, but they are not equivalent. Addiction involves other changes to brain circuitry and is distinguished by compulsive drug seeking and use despite negative consequences.

Those who are dependent on a medication will experience unpleasant physical withdrawal symptoms when they abruptly reduce or stop use of the drug. These symptoms can be mild to severe (depending on the drug) and can usually be managed medically or avoided by slowly tapering down the drug dosage.

Tolerance, or the need to take higher doses of a medication to get the same effect, often accompanies dependence. When tolerance occurs, it can be difficult for a physician to evaluate whether a patient is developing a drug problem or has a medical need for higher doses to control his or her symptoms. For this reason, physicians should be vigilant and attentive to their patients' symptoms and level of functioning and should screen for substance misuse when tolerance or dependence is present.

What Are the Possible Consequences of Prescription Opioid Misuse?

When taken as prescribed, patients can often use opioids to manage pain safely and effectively. However, it is possible to develop a substance use disorder when taking opioid medications as prescribed. This risk and the risk for overdose increase when these medications are misused. Even a single large dose of an opioid can cause severe respiratory depression (slowing or stopping of breathing), which can be fatal; taking opioids with alcohol or sedatives increases this risk.

When properly managed, short-term medical use of opioid pain relievers—taken for a few days following oral surgery, for instance—rarely leads to an opioid use disorder or addiction. But regular (e.g., several times a day, for several weeks or more) or longer-term use of opioids can lead to dependence (physical discomfort when not taking the drug), tolerance (diminished effect from the original dose, leading to increasing the amount taken), and, in some cases, addiction (compulsive drug seeking and use). With both dependence and addiction, withdrawal symptoms may occur if drug use is suddenly reduced or stopped. These symptoms may include restlessness, muscle and bone pain, insomnia, diarrhea, vomiting, cold flashes with goose bumps, and involuntary leg movements. Misuse of prescription opioids is also a risk factor for transitioning to heroin use.

How Is Prescription Opioid Misuse Related to Chronic Pain?

Healthcare providers have long wrestled with how best to treat the more than 100 million Americans who suffer from chronic pain. Opioids have been the most common treatment for chronic pain since the late 1990s, but recent research has cast doubt both on their safety and their efficacy in the treatment of chronic pain when it is not related to cancer or palliative care. The potential risks involved with long-term opioid treatment, such as the development of drug tolerance, hyperalgesia, and addiction, present doctors with a dilemma, as there is limited research on alternative treatments for chronic pain. Patients themselves may even be reluctant to take an opioid medication prescribed to them for fear of becoming addicted.

Estimates of the rate of opioid addiction among chronic pain patients vary from about 3 percent up to 26 percent. This variability is the result of differences in treatment duration, insufficient research on long-term outcomes, and disparate study populations and measures used to assess nonmedical use or addiction.

What Are CNS Depressants?

Central nervous system (CNS) depressants, a category that includes tranquilizers, sedatives, and hypnotics, are substances that can slow brain activity. This property makes them useful for treating anxiety and sleep disorders. The following are among the medications commonly prescribed for these purposes:

- Benzodiazepines, such as diazepam (Valium®), clonazepam (Klonopin®), and alprazolam (Xanax®), are sometimes prescribed to treat anxiety, acute stress reactions, and panic attacks. Clonazepam may also be prescribed to treat seizure disorders. The more sedating benzodiazepines, such as triazolam (Halcion®) and estazolam (Prosom®) are prescribed for short-term treatment of sleep disorders. Usually, benzodiazepines are not prescribed for long-term use because of the high risk for developing tolerance, dependence, or addiction.

- Nonbenzodiazepine sleep medications, such as zolpidem (Ambien®), eszopiclone (Lunesta®), and zaleplon (Sonata®), known as z-drugs, have a different chemical structure but act on the same GABA type A receptors in the brain as benzodiazepines. They are thought to have fewer side effects and less risk of dependence than benzodiazepines.

- Barbiturates, such as mephobarbital (Mebaral®), phenobarbital (Luminal®), and pentobarbital sodium (Nembutal®), are used less frequently to reduce anxiety or to help with sleep problems because of their higher risk of overdose compared to benzodiazepines. However, they are still used in surgical procedures and to treat seizure disorders.

What Are the Possible Consequences of CNS Depressant Misuse?

Despite their beneficial therapeutic effects, benzodiazepines and barbiturates have the potential for misuse and should be used only as prescribed. The use of nonbenzodiazepine sleep aids, or z-drugs, is less well-studied, but certain indicators have raised concern about their psychoactive properties as well.

During the first few days of taking a depressant, a person usually feels sleepy and uncoordinated, but as the body becomes accustomed to the effects of the drug and tolerance develops, these side effects begin to disappear. If one uses these drugs long term, he or she may need larger doses to achieve the therapeutic effects. Continued use can also lead to dependence and withdrawal when use is abruptly reduced or stopped. Because all sedatives work by slowing the brain's activity, when an individual stops taking them, there can be a rebound effect, resulting in seizures or other harmful consequences.

Although withdrawal from benzodiazepines can be problematic, it is rarely life threatening, whereas withdrawal from prolonged use of barbiturates can have life-threatening complications. Therefore, someone who is thinking about discontinuing a sedative or who is suffering withdrawal from CNS depressants should speak with a physician or seek immediate medical treatment.

What Are Stimulants?

Stimulants increase alertness, attention, and energy, as well as elevate blood pressure, heart rate, and respiration. Historically, stimulants were used to treat asthma and other respiratory problems, obesity, neurological disorders, and a variety of other ailments. But as their potential for misuse and addiction became apparent, the number of conditions treated with stimulants has decreased. Now, stimulants are prescribed for the treatment of only a few health conditions, including attention deficit hyperactivity disorder (ADHD), narcolepsy, and occasionally treatment-resistant depression.

How Do Stimulants Affect the Brain and Body?

Stimulants, such as dextroamphetamine (Dexedrine®, Adderall®) and methylphenidate (Ritalin®, Concerta®), act in the brain on the family of monoamine neurotransmitter systems, which include norepinephrine and dopamine. Stimulants enhance the effects of these chemicals. An increase in dopamine signaling from nonmedical use of stimulants can induce a feeling of euphoria, and these medications' effects on norepinephrine increase blood pressure and heart rate, constrict blood vessels, increase blood glucose, and open up breathing passages.

What Are the Possible Consequences of Stimulant Misuse?

As with other drugs in the stimulant category, such as cocaine, it is possible for people to become dependent on or addicted to prescription stimulants. Withdrawal symptoms associated with discontinuing stimulant use include fatigue, depression, and disturbed sleep patterns. Repeated misuse of some stimulants (sometimes within a short period) can lead to feelings of hostility or paranoia, or even psychosis. Further, taking high doses of a stimulant may result in dangerously high body temperature and an irregular heartbeat. There is also the potential for cardiovascular failure or seizures.

Cognitive Enhancers

The dramatic increases in stimulant prescriptions over the last 2 decades have led to their greater availability and to increased risk for diversion and nonmedical use. When taken to improve properly diagnosed conditions, these medications can greatly enhance a patient's quality of life. However, because many perceive them to be generally safe and effective, prescription stimulants such as Adderall® and Modafinil® are being misused more frequently.

Stimulants increase wakefulness, motivation, and aspects of cognition, learning, and memory. Some people take these drugs in the absence of medical need in an effort to enhance mental performance. Militaries have long used stimulants to increase performance in the face of fatigue, and the United States Armed Forces allow for their use in limited operational settings. The practice is now reported by some professionals to increase their productivity, by older people to offset declining cognition, and by both high school and college students to improve their academic performance.

Nonmedical use of stimulants for cognitive enhancement poses potential health risks, including addiction, cardiovascular events, and psychosis. The use of pharmaceuticals for cognitive enhancement has also sparked debate over the ethical implications of the practice. Issues of fairness arise if those with access and willingness to take these drugs have a performance edge over others, and implicit coercion takes place if a culture of cognitive enhancement gives the impression that a person must take drugs in order to be competitive.

How Can Prescription Drug Misuse Be Prevented?

- **Clinicians.** More than 80 percent of Americans had contact with a healthcare professional in the past year, placing doctors in a unique position to identify nonmedical use of prescription drugs and take measures to prevent the escalation of a patient's misuse to a substance use disorder. By asking about all drugs, physicians can help their patients recognize that a problem exists, provide or refer them to appropriate treatment, and set recovery goals. Evidence-based screening tools for nonmedical use of prescription drugs can be incorporated into routine medical visits. Doctors should also take note of rapid increases in the amount of medication needed or frequent, unscheduled refill requests. Doctors should be alert to the fact that those misusing prescription drugs may engage in "doctor shopping"—moving from provider to provider—in an effort to obtain multiple prescriptions for their drug(s) of choice.

Prescription drug monitoring programs (PDMPs), state-run electronic databases used to track the prescribing and dispensing of controlled prescription drugs to patients, are also important tools for preventing and identifying prescription drug misuse. While research regarding the impact of these programs is currently mixed, the use of PDMPs in some states has been associated with lower rates of opioid prescribing and overdose, though issues of best practices, ease of use, and interoperability remain to be resolved.

In 2015, the federal government launched an initiative directed toward reducing opioid misuse and overdose, in part by promoting more cautious and responsible prescribing of opioid medications. In line with these efforts, in 2016 the Centers for Disease Control and Prevention (CDC) published its *CDC Guideline for Prescribing Opioids for Chronic Pain* to establish clinical standards for balancing the benefits and risks of chronic opioid treatment.

Preventing or stopping nonmedical use of prescription drugs is an important part of patient care. However, certain patients can benefit from prescription stimulants, sedatives, or opioid pain relievers. Therefore, physicians should balance the legitimate medical needs of patients with the potential risk for misuse and related harms.

- **Patients.** Patients can take steps to ensure that they use prescription medications appropriately by:

    - following the directions as explained on the label or by the pharmacist

    - being aware of potential interactions with other drugs as well as alcohol

    - never stopping or changing a dosing regimen without first discussing it with the doctor

    - never using another person's prescription, and never giving their prescription medications to others

    - storing prescription stimulants, sedatives, and opioids safely

Additionally, patients should properly discard unused or expired medications by following U.S. Food and Drug Administration (FDA) guidelines or visiting U.S. Drug Enforcement Administration (DEA) collection sites. In addition to describing their medical problem, patients should always inform their healthcare professionals about all the prescriptions, over-the-counter medicines, and dietary and herbal supplements they are taking before they obtain any other medications.

- **Pharmacists.** Pharmacists can help patients understand instructions for taking their medications. In addition, by being watchful for prescription falsifications or alterations, pharmacists can serve as the first line of defense in recognizing problematic patterns in prescription drug use. Some pharmacies have developed hotlines to alert other pharmacies in the region when they detect a fraudulent prescription. Along with physicians, pharmacists can use PDMPs to help track opioid-prescribing patterns in patients.

Medication Formulation and Regulation

Manufacturers of prescription drugs continue to work on new formulations of opioid medications, known as abuse-deterrent formulations (ADF), which include technologies designed to prevent people from misusing them by snorting or injection. Approaches currently being used or studied for use include:

- **physical or chemical barriers** that prevent the crushing, grinding, or dissolving of drug products

- **agonist/antagonist combinations** that cause an antagonist (which will counteract the drug effect) to be released if the product is manipulated

- **aversive substances** that are added to create unpleasant sensations if the drug is taken in a way other than directed

- **delivery systems** such as long-acting injections or implants that slowly release the drug over time

- **new molecular entities** or prodrugs that attach a chemical extension to a drug that renders it inactive unless it is taken orally

Several ADF opioids are on the market, and the FDA has also called for the development of ADF stimulants. While ADF opioids have been shown to decrease the illicit value of a drug, in the absence of reduced demand, they can shift use to other formulations. Medication regulation has been shown to be effective in decreasing the prescribing of opioid medications. In 2014, the Drug Enforcement Administration (DEA) moved hydrocodone products from schedule III to the more restrictive schedule II, which resulted in a decrease in hydrocodone prescribing that did not result in any attendant increases in the prescribing of other opioids.

Development of Safer Medications

The development of effective, nonaddicting pain medications is a public health priority. A growing number of older adults and an increasing number of injured military service members add to the urgency of finding new treatments. Researchers are exploring alternative treatment approaches that target other signaling systems in the body such as the endocannabinoid system, which is also involved in pain. More research is also needed to better understand effective chronic pain management, including identifying factors that predispose some patients to substance use disorders and developing measures to prevent the nonmedical use of prescription medications.

How Can Prescription Drug Addiction Be Treated?

Years of research have shown that substance use disorders are brain disorders that can be treated effectively. Treatment must take into account the type of drug used and the needs of the individual. Successful treatment may need to incorporate several components, including detoxification, counseling, and medications, when available. Multiple courses of treatment may be needed for the patient to make a full recovery.

The two main categories of drug addiction treatment are behavioral treatments (such as contingency management and cognitive behavioral therapy) and medications. Behavioral treatments help patients stop drug use by changing unhealthy patterns of thinking and behavior; teaching strategies to manage cravings and avoid cues and situations that could lead to relapse; or, in some cases, providing incentives for abstinence. Behavioral treatments, which may take the form of individual, family, or group counseling, also can help patients improve their personal relationships and their ability to function at work and in the community.

Addiction to prescription opioids can additionally be treated with medications including buprenorphine, methadone, and naltrexone. These drugs can counter the effects of opioids on the brain or relieve withdrawal symptoms and cravings, helping the patient avoid relapse. Medications for the treatment of addiction are administered in combination with psychosocial supports or behavioral treatments, known as medication-assisted treatment (MAT).

Chapter 27

Heat Stroke

Too much heat is not safe for anyone. It is even riskier if you are older or have health problems. It is important to get relief from the heat quickly. If not, you might begin to feel confused or faint. Your heart could become stressed and stop beating.

Being hot for too long can be a problem. It can cause several illnesses, all grouped under the name hyperthermia.

- **Heat syncope** is a sudden dizziness that can happen when you are active in hot weather. If you take a heart medication called a beta blocker or are not used to hot weather, you are even more likely to feel faint. Rest in a cool place, put your legs up, and drink water to make the dizzy feeling go away.

- **Heat cramps** are the painful tightening of muscles in your stomach, arms, or legs. Cramps can result from hard work or exercise. Though your body temperature and pulse usually stay normal during heat cramps, your skin may feel moist and cool. Find a way to cool your body down. Rest in the shade or in a cool building. Drink plenty of fluids, but not those with alcohol or caffeine.

- **Heat edema** is a swelling in your ankles and feet when you get hot. Put your legs up to help reduce swelling. If that doesn't work fairly quickly, check with your doctor.

This chapter includes text excerpted from "Hot Weather Safety for Older Adults," National Institute on Aging (NIA), National Institutes of Health (NIH), July 18, 2017.

- **Heat exhaustion** is a warning that your body can no longer keep itself cool. You might feel thirsty, dizzy, weak, uncoordinated, and nauseated. You may sweat a lot. Your body temperature may stay normal, but your skin may feel cold and clammy. Some people with heat exhaustion have a rapid pulse. Rest in a cool place and get plenty of fluids. If you don't feel better soon, get medical care. Be careful—heat exhaustion can progress to heat stroke.

Heat Stroke—A Medical Emergency

If you have heat stroke, you need to get medical help right away. Older people living in homes or apartments without air conditioning or fans are at most risk. People who become dehydrated or those with chronic diseases or alcoholism are also at most risk. Signs of heat stroke are:

- Fainting (possibly the first sign) or becoming unconscious

- A change in behavior—confusion, agitation, staggering, being grouchy, or acting strangely

- Body temperature over 104°F (40°C)

- Dry, flushed skin and a strong, rapid pulse or a slow, weak pulse

- Not sweating even if it is hot

Who Is at Risk?

Each year, most people who die from hyperthermia are over 50 years old. Health problems that put you at greater risk include:

- Heart or blood vessel problems

- Poorly working sweat glands or changes in your skin caused by normal aging

- Heart, lung, or kidney disease, as well as any illness that makes you feel weak all over or results in a fever

- Conditions treated by drugs, such as diuretics, sedatives, tranquilizers, and some heart and high blood pressure medicines; they may make it harder for your body to cool itself

- Taking several prescription drugs; ask your doctor if any of your medications make you more likely to become overheated.

- Being very overweight or underweight

- Drinking alcoholic beverages

How Can I Lower My Risk?

Things you can do to lower your risk of heat-related illness:

- Drink plenty of liquids, such as water or fruit or vegetable juices. Stay away from drinks containing alcohol or caffeine. If your doctor has told you to limit your liquids, ask what you should do when it is very hot.

- If you live in a home or apartment without fans or air conditioning, try to keep your house as cool as possible. Limit your use of the oven. Keep your shades, blinds, or curtains closed during the hottest part of the day. Open your windows at night.

- If your house is hot, try to spend time during mid-day some place that has air conditioning—for example, go to the shopping mall, movies, library, senior center, or a friend's house.

- If you need help getting to a cool place, ask a friend or relative. Some religious groups, senior centers, and Area Agencies on Aging provide this service. If necessary, take a taxi or call for senior transportation. Don't stand outside in the heat waiting for a bus.

- Dress for the weather. Some people find natural fabrics, such as cotton, to be cooler than synthetic fibers.

- Don't try to exercise or do a lot of activities outdoors when it's hot.

- Avoid crowded places when it's hot outside. Plan trips during nonrush hour times.

Listen to Weather Reports

If the temperature or humidity is going up or an air pollution alert is in effect, you are at increased risk for a heat-related illness. Play it safe by checking the weather report before going outside.

What Should I Remember?

Older people can have a tough time dealing with heat and humidity. The temperature inside or outside does not have to reach 100°F (38°C) to put them at risk for a heat-related illness.

Headache, confusion, dizziness, or nausea could be a sign of a heat-related illness. Go to the doctor or an emergency room to find out if you need treatment.

To keep heat-related illnesses from becoming a dangerous heat stroke, remember to:

- Get out of the sun and into a cool place—air conditioning is best.

- Drink fluids, but avoid alcohol and caffeine. Water and fruit or vegetable juices are good choices.

- Shower, bathe, or sponge off with cool water.

- Lie down and rest in a cool place.

- Visit your doctor or go to an emergency room if you don't cool down quickly.

A Senior Watch

During hot weather, think about making daily visits to older relatives and neighbors. Remind them to drink lots of water or juice, as long as their doctor hasn't recommended otherwise because of a preexisting condition. If there is a heat wave, offer to help them go someplace cool, such as air conditioned malls, libraries, or senior centers.

Part Four

Geriatric Healthcare

Chapter 28

Stay Healthy after 50

Chapter Contents

Section 28.1

Women: Stay Healthy after 50

This section includes text excerpted from "Women: Stay Healthy at 50+," Agency for Healthcare Research and Quality (AHRQ), U.S. Department of Health and Human Services (HHS), April 2014. Reviewed September 2017.

Get the Screenings You Need

Screenings are tests that look for diseases before you have symptoms. Blood pressure checks and mammograms are examples of screenings. You can get some screenings, such as blood pressure readings, in your doctor's office. Others, such as mammograms, need special equipment, so you may need to go to a different office. After a screening test, it's important to ask when you will see the results and who you should talk to about them.

Breast Cancer. Talk with your healthcare team about whether you need a mammogram.

BRCA 1 and 2 **Genes.** If you have a family member with breast, ovarian, or peritoneal cancer, talk with your doctor or nurse about your family history. Women with a strong family history of certain cancers may benefit from genetic counseling and *BRCA* genetic testing.

Cervical Cancer. Get a Pap smear every 3 years or get a combination Pap smear and human papilloma virus (HPV) test every 5 years until age 65. If you are older than 65 or have had a hysterectomy, talk with your doctor or nurse about whether you still need to be screened.

Colon Cancer. If you are 75 or younger, get a screening test for colorectal cancer. Several different tests—for example, a stool test or a colonoscopy—can detect this cancer. Your healthcare team can help you decide which is best for you. If you are between the ages of 76 and 85, talk with your doctor or nurse about whether you should continue to be screened.

Depression. Your emotional health is as important as your physical health. Talk to your healthcare team about being screened for depression, especially if during the last 2 weeks:

• You have felt down, sad, or hopeless.

• You have felt little interest or pleasure in doing things.

Diabetes. Get screened for diabetes (high blood sugar) if you have high blood pressure or if you take medication for high blood pressure. Diabetes can cause problems with your heart, brain, eyes, feet, kidneys, nerves, and other body parts.

Hepatitis C Virus (HCV). Get screened one time for HCV infection if:

• You were born between 1945 and 1965.

• You have ever injected drugs.

• You received a blood transfusion before 1992.

If you currently are an injection drug user, you should be screened regularly.

High Blood Cholesterol. Have your cholesterol checked regularly with a blood test if:

• You use tobacco.

• You are overweight or obese.

• You have a personal history of heart disease or blocked arteries.

• A male relative in your family had a heart attack before age 50 or a female relative, before age 60.

High Blood Pressure. Have your blood pressure checked at least every 2 years.

Human Immunodeficiency Virus (HIV). If you are 65 or younger, get screened for HIV. If you are older than 65, talk to your doctor or nurse about whether you should be screened.

Lung Cancer. Talk to your doctor or nurse about getting screened for lung cancer if you are between the ages of 55 and 80, have a 30 pack-year smoking history, and smoke now or have quit within the past 15 years. (Your pack-year history is the number of packs of cigarettes smoked per day times the number of years you have smoked.)

Know that quitting smoking is the best thing you can do for your health.

Osteoporosis (Bone Thinning). Have a screening test at age 65 to make sure your bones are strong. The most common test is a Dual-energy X-ray absorptiometry (DEXA) scan—a low-dose X-ray of the spine and hip. If you are younger than 65 and at high risk for bone fractures, you should also be screened. Talk with your healthcare team about your risk for bone fractures.

Overweight and Obesity. The best way to learn if you are overweight or obese is to find your body mass index (BMI). A BMI between 18.5 and 25 indicates a normal weight. Persons with a BMI of 30 or higher may be obese. If you are obese, talk to your healthcare team about getting intensive counseling and help with changing your behaviors to lose weight. Overweight and obesity can lead to diabetes and cardiovascular disease.

Get Preventive Medicines If You Need Them

Aspirin. If you are 55 or older, ask your healthcare team if you should take aspirin to prevent strokes. Your healthcare team can help you decide whether taking aspirin to prevent stroke is right for you.

Breast Cancer Drugs. Talk to your doctor about your risks for breast cancer and whether you should take medicines that may reduce those risks. Medications to reduce breast cancer have some potentially serious harms, so think through both the potential benefits and harms.

Vitamin D to Avoid Falls. If you are 65 or older and have a history of falls, mobility problems, or other risks for falling, ask your doctor about taking a vitamin D supplement to help reduce your chances of falling. Exercise and physical therapy may also help.

Immunizations:

- Get a flu shot every year.
- Get shots for tetanus and whooping cough. Get a tetanus booster if it has been more than 10 years since your last shot.
- If you are 60 or older, get a shot to prevent shingles.
- If you are 65 or older, get a pneumonia shot.
- Talk with your healthcare team about whether you need other vaccinations.

Take Steps to Good Health

- Be physically active and make healthy food choices.

- Get to a healthy weight and stay there. Balance the calories you take in from food and drink with the calories you burn off by your activities.

- Be tobacco free.

- If you drink alcohol, have no more than one drink per day. A standard drink is one 12-ounce bottle of beer or wine cooler, one 5-ounce glass of wine, or 1.5 ounces of 80-proof distilled spirits.

You know your body better than anyone else. Always tell your healthcare team about any changes in your health, including your vision and hearing. Ask them about being checked for any condition you are concerned about, not just the ones here. If you are wondering about diseases such as Alzheimer disease or skin cancer, for example, ask about them.

Section 28.2

Men: Stay Healthy after 50

This section includes text excerpted from "Men: Stay Healthy at 50+," Agency for Healthcare Research and Quality (AHRQ), U.S. Department of Health and Human Services (HHS), March 2014. Reviewed September 2017.

Get the Screenings You Need

Screenings are tests that look for diseases before you have symptoms. Blood pressure checks and tests for high blood cholesterol are examples of screenings. You can get some screenings, such as blood pressure readings, in your doctor's office. Others, such as colonoscopy, a test for colon cancer, need special equipment, so you may need to go to a different office. After a screening test, ask when you will see the results and who you should talk to about them.

Abdominal Aortic Aneurysm. If you are between the ages of 65 and 75 and have ever been a smoker, (smoked 100 or more cigarettes in your lifetime), talk to your healthcare team about being screened for abdominal aortic aneurysm (AAA). AAA is a bulging in your abdominal aorta, your largest artery. An AAA may burst, which can cause dangerous bleeding and death.

An ultrasound, a painless procedure in which you lie on a table while a technician slides a medical device over your abdomen, will show whether an aneurysm is present.

Colon Cancer. If you are 75 or younger, get a screening test for colorectal cancer. Several different tests—for example, a stool test or a colonoscopy—can detect this cancer. Your doctor or nurse can help you decide which is best for you. If you are between the ages of 76 and 85, talk to your doctor or nurse about whether you should continue to be screened.

Depression. Your emotional health is as important as your physical health. Talk to your doctor or nurse about being screened for depression especially if during the last 2 weeks:

- You have felt down, sad, or hopeless.

- You have felt little interest or pleasure in doing things.

Diabetes. Get screened for diabetes (high blood sugar) with a blood test if you have high blood pressure or take medication for high blood pressure. Diabetes can cause problems with your heart, brain, eyes, feet, kidneys, nerves, and other body parts.

Hepatitis C Virus (HCV). Get screened one time for HCV infection if:

- You were born between 1945 and 1965.

- You have ever injected drugs.

- You received a blood transfusion before 1992.

If you currently are an injection drug user, you should be screened regularly.

High Blood Cholesterol. Have your blood cholesterol checked regularly with a blood test. High blood cholesterol increases your chance of heart disease, stroke, and poor circulation.

High Blood Pressure. Have your blood pressure checked at least every 2 years. High blood pressure can cause strokes, heart attacks, kidney and eye problems, and heart failure.

Human Immunodeficiency Virus (HIV). If you are 65 or younger, get screened for HIV. If you are older than 65, ask your doctor or nurse if you should be screened.

Lung Cancer. Talk to your doctor or nurse about getting screened for lung cancer if you are between the ages of 55 and 80, have a 30 pack-year smoking history, and smoke now or have quit within the past 15 years. (Your pack-year history is the number of packs of cigarettes smoked per day times the number of years you have smoked.) Know that quitting smoking is the best thing you can do for your health.

Lung cancer can be detected with low-dose computed tomography (LCT). For LCT, you lie on a table while a large machine passes over you to scan your lungs.

Overweight and Obesity. The best way to learn if you are overweight or obese is to find your body mass index (BMI). A BMI between 18.5 and 25 indicates a normal weight. Persons with a BMI of 30 or higher may be obese. If you are obese, talk to your doctor or nurse about getting intensive counseling and help with changing your behaviors to lose weight. Overweight and obesity can lead to diabetes and cardiovascular disease.

Get Preventive Medicines If You Need Them

Aspirin. Your doctor or nurse can help you decide whether taking aspirin to prevent a heart attack is right for you.

Vitamin D to Avoid Falls. If you are 65 or older and have a history of falls, mobility problems, or other risks for falling, ask your doctor about taking a vitamin D supplement to help reduce your chances of falling. Exercise and physical therapy may also help.

Immunizations:

- Get a flu shot every year.

- Get a shot for tetanus, diphtheria, and whooping cough. Get a tetanus booster if it has been more than 10 years since your last shot.

- If you are 60 or older, get a shot to prevent shingles.

- If you are 65 or older, get a pneumonia shot.

- Talk with your healthcare team about whether you need other vaccinations.

403

Take Steps to Good Health

- Be physically active and make healthy food choices.

- Get to a healthy weight and stay there. Balance the calories you take in from food and drink with the calories you burn off by your activities.

- Be tobacco free.

- If you drink alcohol, have no more than two drinks per day if you are 65 or younger. If you are older than 65, have no more than one drink a day. A standard drink is one 12-ounce bottle of beer or wine cooler, one 5-ounce glass of wine, or 1.5 ounces of 80-proof distilled spirits.

You know your body better than anyone else. Always tell your doctor or nurse about any changes in your health, including your vision and hearing. Ask them about being checked for any condition you are concerned about, not just the ones here. If you are wondering about diseases such as Alzheimer disease or skin cancer, for example, ask about them.

Chapter 29

Pain Management

You've probably been in pain at one time or another. Maybe you've had a headache or bruise—pain that doesn't last too long. But, many older people have ongoing pain from health problems like arthritis, cancer, diabetes, or shingles. They may even have many different kinds of pain. Pain can be your body's way of warning you that something is wrong. Always tell the doctor where you hurt and exactly how it feels.

Acute Pain and Chronic Pain

There are two kinds of pain. Acute pain begins suddenly, lasts for a short time, and goes away as your body heals. You might feel acute pain after surgery or if you have a broken bone, infected tooth, or kidney stone.

Pain that lasts for several months or years is called chronic (or persistent) pain. This pain often affects older people. Examples include rheumatoid arthritis (RA) and sciatica. In some cases, chronic pain follows after acute pain from an injury or other health issue has gone away, like postherpetic neuralgia after shingles.

Living with any type of pain can be very hard. It can cause many other problems. For instance, pain can:

- Get in the way of your daily activities

- Disturb your sleep and eating habits

This chapter includes text excerpted from "Pain: You Can Get Help," National Institute on Aging (NIA), National Institutes of Health (NIH), July 18, 2017.

- Make it difficult to continue working

- Cause depression or anxiety

Describing Pain

Many people have a hard time describing pain. Think about these questions when you explain how the pain feels:

- Where does it hurt?

- When did it start? Does the pain come and go?

- What does it feel like? Is the pain sharp, dull, or burning? Would you use some other word to describe it?

- Do you have other symptoms?

- When do you feel the pain? In the morning? In the evening? After eating?

- Is there anything you do that makes the pain feel better or worse? For example, does using a heating pad or ice pack help? Does changing your position from lying down to sitting up make it better? Have you tried any over-the-counter medications for it?

Your doctor or nurse may ask you to rate your pain on a scale of 0 to 10, with 0 being no pain and 10 being the worst pain you can imagine. Or, your doctor may ask if the pain is mild, moderate, or severe. Some doctors or nurses have pictures of faces that show different expressions of pain. You point to the face that shows how you feel.

Attitudes about Pain

Everyone reacts to pain differently. Many older people have been told not to talk about their aches and pains. Some people feel they should be brave and not complain when they hurt. Other people are quick to report pain and ask for help.

Worrying about pain is a common problem. This worry can make you afraid to stay active, and it can separate you from your friends and family. Working with your doctor, you can find ways to continue to take part in physical and social activities despite being in pain.

Some people put off going to the doctor because they think pain is just part of aging and nothing can help. This is not true! It is important to see a doctor if you have a new pain. Finding a way to manage your pain is often easier if it is addressed early.

Treating Pain

Treating, or managing, chronic pain is important. The good news is that there are ways to care for pain. Some treatments involve medications, and some do not. Your doctor may make a treatment plan that is specific for your needs.

Most treatment plans do not just focus on reducing pain. They also include ways to support daily function while living with pain. Pain doesn't always go away overnight. Talk with your doctor about how long it may take before you feel better. Often, you have to stick with a treatment plan before you get relief. It's important to stay on a schedule. Sometimes this is called "staying ahead" or "keeping on top" of your pain. As your pain lessens, you can likely become more active and will see your mood lift and sleep improve.

Medicines to Treat Pain

Your doctor may prescribe one or more of the following pain medications:

- **Acetaminophen** may help all types of pain, especially mild to moderate pain. Acetaminophen is found in over-the-counter and prescription medicines. People who drink a lot of alcohol or who have liver disease should not take acetaminophen. Be sure to talk with your doctor about whether it is safe for you to take and what would be the right dose.

- **Nonsteroidal anti-inflammatory drugs (NSAIDs)** include medications like aspirin, naproxen, and ibuprofen. Some types of NSAIDs can cause side effects, like internal bleeding, which make them unsafe for many older adults. For instance, you may not be able to take ibuprofen if you have high blood pressure or had a stroke. Talk to your doctor before taking NSAIDs to see if they are safe for you.

- **Narcotics** (also called opioids) are used for severe pain and require a doctor's prescription. They may be habit-forming. Examples of narcotics are codeine, morphine, and oxycodone.

- **Other medications** are sometimes used to treat pain. These include antidepressants, anticonvulsive medicines, local pain-killers like nerve blocks or patches, and ointments and creams.

As people age, they are at risk for developing more serious side effects from medication. It's important to take exactly the amount of pain medicine your doctor prescribes.

Mixing any pain medication with alcohol or other drugs, such as tranquilizers, can be dangerous. Make sure your doctor knows all the medicines you take, including over-the-counter drugs and herbal supplements, as well as the amount of alcohol you drink.

Remember: If you think the medicine is not working, don't change it on your own. Talk to your doctor or nurse. You might say, "I've been taking the medication as you directed, but it still hurts too much to play with my grandchildren. Is there anything else I can try?"

Pain Specialist

Some doctors receive extra training in pain management. If you find that your regular doctor can't help you, ask him or her for the name of a pain medicine specialist. You also can ask for suggestions from friends and family, a nearby hospital, or your local medical society.

What Other Treatments Help with Pain?

In addition to drugs, there are a variety of complementary and alternative approaches that may provide relief. Talk to your doctor about these treatments. It may take both medicine and other treatments to feel better.

- **Acupuncture** uses hair-thin needles to stimulate specific points on the body to relieve pain.

- **Biofeedback** helps you learn to control your heart rate, blood pressure, and muscle tension. This may help reduce your pain and stress level.

- **Cognitive behavioral therapy** is a form of short-term counseling that may help reduce your reaction to pain.

- **Distraction** can help you cope with pain by learning new skills that may take your mind off your discomfort.

- **Electrical nerve stimulation** uses electrical impulses in order to relieve pain.

- **Guided imagery** uses directed thoughts to create mental pictures that may help you relax, manage anxiety, sleep better, and have less pain.

- **Hypnosis** uses focused attention to help manage pain.

- **Massage therapy** can release tension in tight muscles.

- **Physical therapy** uses a variety of techniques to help manage everyday activities with less pain and teaches you ways to improve flexibility and strength.

Helping Yourself

There are things you can do yourself that might help you feel better. Try to:

- Keep a healthy weight. Putting on extra pounds can slow healing and make some pain worse. Keeping a healthy weight might help with knee pain, or pain in the back, hips, or feet.

- Be active. Try to keep moving. Pain might make you inactive, which can lead to a cycle of more pain and loss of function. Mild activity can help.

- Get enough sleep. It will improve healing and your mood.

- Avoid tobacco, caffeine, and alcohol. They can get in the way of your treatment and increase your pain.

- Join a pain support group. Sometimes, it can help to talk to other people about how they deal with pain. You can share your ideas and thoughts while learning from others.

- Participate in activities you enjoy. Taking part in activities that you find relaxing, like listening to music or doing art, might help take your mind off of some of the pain.

Pain Management for Conditions

Cancer Pain

Some people with cancer are more afraid of the pain than of the cancer. But, most pain from cancer or cancer treatments can be controlled. As with all pain, it's best to start managing cancer pain early. It might take a while to find the best approach. Talk with your doctor so the pain management plan can be corrected to work for you.

One special concern in managing cancer pain is "breakthrough pain." This is a pain that comes on quickly and can take you by surprise. It can be very upsetting. After one attack, many people worry it will happen again. This is another reason why it is so important to talk with your doctor about having a pain management plan in place.

Alzheimer Disease and Pain

People who have Alzheimer disease may not be able to tell you when they're in pain. When you're caring for someone with Alzheimer disease, watch for clues. A person's face may show signs of being in pain or feeling ill. You may also notice sudden changes in behavior such as increased yelling, striking out, or spending more time in bed. It's important to find out if there is something wrong. If you're not sure what to do, call the doctor for help.

Pain at the End of Life

Not everyone who is dying is in pain. But if a person has pain at the end of life, there are ways to help. Experts often believe it's best to focus on making the person comfortable, without worrying about possible addiction or drug dependence.

Speak to a palliative care or pain management specialist if you are concerned about pain for yourself or a loved one. These specialists are trained to manage pain and other symptoms for people with serious illnesses.

Caring for Someone in Pain

It's hard to see a loved one hurting. Caring for a person in pain can leave you feeling tired and discouraged. To keep from feeling overwhelmed, you might consider asking other family members and friends for help. Or, some community service organizations might offer short-term, or respite, care. The Eldercare Locator might help you find a local group that offers this service.

Chapter 30

Medicines: Use Them Wisely

As you get older you may be faced with more health conditions that you need to treat on a regular basis. It is important to be aware that more use of medicines and normal body changes caused by aging can increase the chance of unwanted or maybe even harmful drug interactions. The more you know about your medicines and the more you talk with your healthcare professionals, the easier it is to avoid problems with medicines.

As you get older, body changes can affect the way medicines are absorbed and used. For example, changes in the digestive system can affect how fast medicines enter the bloodstream. Changes in body weight can influence the amount of medicine you need to take and how long it stays in your body. The circulatory system may slow down, which can affect how fast drugs get to the liver and kidneys. The liver and kidneys also may work more slowly, affecting the way a drug breaks down and is removed from the body.

Drug Interactions

Because of these body changes, there is also a bigger risk of drug interactions among older adults. Therefore, it's important to know about drug interactions.

This chapter includes text excerpted from "As You Age: You and Your Medicines," U.S. Food and Drug Administration (FDA), June 23, 2015.

411

- **Drug-drug interactions** happen when two or more medicines react with each other to cause unwanted effects. This kind of interaction can also cause one medicine to not work as well or even make one medicine stronger than it should be. For example, you should not take aspirin if you are taking a prescription blood thinner, such as warfarin, unless your healthcare professional tells you to.

- **Drug-condition interactions** happen when a medical condition you already have makes certain drugs potentially harmful. For example, if you have high blood pressure or asthma, you could have an unwanted reaction if you take a nasal decongestant.

- **Drug-food interactions** result from drugs reacting with foods or drinks. In some cases, food in the digestive tract can affect how a drug is absorbed. Some medicines also may affect the way nutrients are absorbed or used in the body.

- **Drug-alcohol interactions** can happen when the medicine you take reacts with an alcoholic drink. For instance, mixing alcohol with some medicines may cause you to feel tired and slow your reactions.

It is important to know that many medicines do not mix well with alcohol. As you grow older, your body may react differently to alcohol, as well as to the mix of alcohol and medicines. Keep in mind that some problems you might think are medicine-related, such as loss of coordination, memory loss, or irritability, could be the result of a mix between your medicine and alcohol.

What Are Side Effects?

Side effects are unplanned symptoms or feelings you have when taking a medicine. Most side effects are not serious and go away on their own; others can be more bothersome and even serious. To help prevent possible problems with medicines, seniors must know about the medicine they take and how it makes them feel. Keep track of side effects to help your doctor know how your body is responding to a medicine. New symptoms or mood changes may not be a result of getting older, but could be from the medicine you're taking or another factor, such as a change in diet or routine. If you have an unwanted side effect, call your doctor right away.

Talk to Your Healthcare Professionals

It is important to go to all your medical appointments and to talk to your team of healthcare professionals (doctors, pharmacists, nurses, or physician assistants) about your medical conditions, the medicines you take, and any health concerns you have. It may help to make a list of comments, questions, or concerns before your visit or call to a healthcare professional. Also, think about having a close friend or relative come to your appointment with you if you are unsure about talking to your healthcare professional or would like someone to help you understand and remember answers to your questions. Here are some other things to keep in mind:

- **All medicines count.** Tell your team of healthcare professionals about all the medicines you take, including prescription and over-the-counter (OTC) medicines, such as pain relievers, antacids, cold medicines, and laxatives. Don't forget to include eye drops, dietary supplements, vitamins, herbals, and topical medicines, such as creams and ointments.

- **Keep in touch with your doctors.** If you regularly take a prescription medicine, ask your doctor to check how well it is working. Check to see whether you still need to take it and, if so, whether there is anything you can do to cut back. Don't stop taking the medicine on your own without first talking with your doctor.

- **Medical history.** Tell your healthcare professional about your medical history. The doctor will want to know whether you have any food, medicine, or other allergies. He or she also will want to know about other conditions you have or had and how you are being treated or were treated for them by other doctors. It is helpful to keep a written list of your health conditions that you can easily share with your doctors. Your primary care doctor should also know about any specialist doctors you may see on a regular basis.

- **Eating habits.** Mention your eating habits. If you follow or have recently changed to a special diet (a very low-fat diet, for instance, or a high-calcium diet), talk to your doctor about this. Tell your doctor about how much coffee, tea, or alcohol you drink each day and whether you smoke. These things may make a difference in the way your medicine works.

- **Recognizing and remembering to take your medicines.**
  Let your healthcare professional know whether you have trouble telling your medicines apart. The doctor can help you find better ways to recognize your medicines. Also tell your doctor if you have problems remembering when to take your medicines or how much to take. Your doctor may have some ideas to help, such as a calendar or pill box.

- **Swallowing tablets.** If you have trouble swallowing tablets, ask your doctor, nurse, or pharmacist for ideas. Maybe there is a liquid medicine you could use or maybe you can crush your tablets. Do not break, crush, or chew tablets without first asking your healthcare professional.

- **Your lifestyle.** If you want to make your medicine schedule more simple, talk about it with your doctor. He or she may have another medicine or other ideas. For example, if taking medicine four times a day is a problem for you, maybe the doctor can give you a medicine you only need to take once or twice a day.

- **Put it in writing.** Ask your healthcare professional to write out a complete medicine schedule, with directions on exactly when and how to take your medicines. Find out from your primary care doctor how your medicine schedule should be changed if you see more than one doctor.

- **Keep a record of your medicines.** List all prescription and OTC medicines, dietary supplements, vitamins, and herbals you take.

Your Pharmacist Can Help, Too

One of the most important services a pharmacist can offer is to talk to you about your medicines. A pharmacist can help you understand how and when to take your medicines, what side effects you might expect, or what interactions may occur. A pharmacist can answer your questions privately in the pharmacy or over the telephone. Here are some other ways your pharmacist can help:

- Many pharmacists keep track of medicines on their computer. If you buy your medicines at one store and tell your pharmacist all the OTC and prescription medicines or dietary supplements you take, your pharmacist can help make sure your medicines don't interact harmfully with one another.

- Ask your pharmacist to place your prescription medicines in easy-to-open containers if you have a hard time taking off child-proof caps and do not have young children living in or visiting your home. Remember to keep all medicines out of the sight and reach of children.

- Your pharmacist may be able to print labels on prescription medicine containers in larger type, if reading the medicine label is hard for you.

- Your pharmacist may be able to give you written information to help you learn more about your medicines. This information may be available in large type or in a language other than English.

What to Ask Your Doctor or Pharmacist

- What is the name of the medicine and what is it supposed to do? Is there a less expensive alternative?

- How and when do I take the medicine and for how long?

- Should it be taken with water, food, or with a special medicine, or at the same time as other medicines?

- What do I do if I miss or forget a dose?

- Should it be taken before, during, or after meals?

- What is the proper dose? For example, does "four times a day" mean you have to take it in the middle of the night?

- What does your doctor mean by "as needed"?

- Are there any other special instructions to follow?

- What foods, drinks, other medicines, dietary supplements, or activities should I avoid while taking this medicine?

- Will any tests or monitoring be required while I am taking this medicine? Do I need to report back to the doctor?

- What are the possible side effects and what do I do if they occur?

- When should I expect the medicine to start working, and how will I know if it is working?

- Will this new prescription work safely with the other prescription and OTC medicines or dietary supplements I am taking?

- Do you have a patient profile form for me to fill out? Does it include space for my OTC drugs and any dietary supplements?

- Is there written information about my medicine? Ask the pharmacist to review the most important information with you. (Ask if it's available in large print or in a language other than English if you need it.)

- What is the most important thing I should know about this medicine? Ask the pharmacist any questions that may not have been answered by your doctor.

- Can I get a refill? If so, when?

- How and where should I store this medicine?

Cutting Medicine Costs

Medicines are an important part of treating an illness because they often allow people to remain active and independent. But medicine can be expensive. Here are some ideas to help lower costs:

- **Tell your doctor if you are worried about the cost of your medicine.** Your doctor may not know how much your prescription costs, but may be able to tell you about another less expensive medicine, such as a generic drug or OTC product.

- **Ask for a senior citizen's discount.**

- **Shop around.** Look at prices at different stores or pharmacies. Lower medicine prices may not be a bargain if you need other services, such as home delivery, patient medicine profiles, or pharmacist consultation, or if you cannot get a senior citizen discount.

- **Ask for medicine samples.** If your doctor gives you a prescription for a new medicine, ask your doctor for samples you can try before filling the prescription.

- **Buy bulk.** If you need to take medicine for a long period of time and your medicine does not expire quickly, you may be able to buy a larger amount of the medicine for less money.

- **Try mail order.** Mail-order pharmacies can provide medications at lower prices. However, it is a good idea to talk with your doctor before using such a service. Make sure to find a backup pharmacy in case there is a problem with the mail service.

- **Buy OTC medicines when they are on sale.** Check the expiration dates and use them before they expire. If you need help choosing an OTC medicine, ask the pharmacist for help.

If you decide to buy medicines on the Internet, check the website for the Verified Internet Pharmacy Practice Sites (VIPPS) program seal of approval to make sure the site is properly licensed and has been successfully reviewed and inspected by the National Association of Boards of Pharmacy (NABP).

Chapter 31

Leaving the Hospital

Returning home from a hospital stay can result in unexpected challenges for many seniors. Finding themselves back at home after a hospital stay, many older adults struggle to manage their medications and make follow-up doctor's appointments as well as obtain the physical assistance and inhome support they may require, at least on a temporary basis. As a result, many older adults do not successfully make the transition home well and end up returning to the hospital. In fact, one in five Medicare patients are readmitted to a hospital within 30 days after discharge. Studies have shown that nearly half of the readmissions are linked to social problems and lack of access to community resources problems.

You can help ensure that you or your loved one makes a successful transition home from the hospital if you start planning for your hospital visit before you are admitted for a planned procedure or for unexpected visits to start planning for discharge the day of admission. Planning goes a long way to help patients address the questions that arise during the discharge process and make a safe and smooth return home.

This chapter is meant to help stimulate thinking about the answers to these and other questions. It is intended for older adults and their family and friends who will help them transition successfully from a hospital back home.

This chapter includes text excerpted from "Hospital to Home Plan for a Smooth Transition," Eldercare Locator, U.S. Administration on Aging (AOA), August 19, 2017.

Prehospital

If you have a planned admission, and you know that you will be staying in the hospital for at least one night for an elective (non-emergency) surgery, tests or special procedures, planning takes several steps.

What do you need to do before you are admitted? What do you need to bring?

You will likely get a packet of preadmission papers. Ask for this packet if the hospital does not offer it. The packet will have basic information about:

- Tests you need before admission

- Where to go on the day of admission and what time to arrive

- Hospital policies, such as visiting hours

- Information about payment

Hospital Kit

Leading up to your hospital admission, you should create a kit to take to the hospital. Here are some items to include:

- Insurance information and identification card

- List of your doctors, with contact information

- Emergency contact numbers

- Test reports, lab results and copies of recent X-rays

- Names and dosages of all your medications. Besides prescription drugs, be sure to include vitamins, herbals, laxatives, and other over-the-counter products. You can use a "Medication Management Form" to assist you.

- List of any allergies

- Healthcare Proxy and Advance Directives. You should prepare these papers whether or not you are going to the hospital, but if you have not done this, the hospital can give you information.

- Other items to bring: Eyeglasses, dentures, hearing aids, and toiletries.

- DO NOT bring jewelry, money, or other valuable items

Posthospital

Hospital stays are often very short. As soon as a doctor says you are "medically stable," the hospital will want to discharge you. Depending on the condition, patients often transition from the hospital to home or to a short-term rehabilitation program in a nursing home. This chapter focuses on important considerations when you are heading home from the hospital or a rehab program. Make sure you or your family caregiver talks to a discharge planner, someone at the hospital who helps plan a smooth transition home. There are a lot of details to work out and the sooner you start the better. Here are some important issues to keep in mind:

Your Home

Make sure to order all the needed equipment and supplies. A member of your hospital team can help you with this task. If you are eligible for home care agency services, find out what the agency provides and what you must get on your own. Here are some good questions to ask:

- Will I need a hospital bed, shower chair, commode, oxygen supply, or other equipment? If so, where do I get these items?

- What supplies do I need? This may be diapers, disposable gloves, and skin care items. Where do I get these?

- Will my insurance pay for the equipment and supplies?

Additionally, your home should be comfortable and safe, and a good place for care. Ask the hospital team if you need to do anything special to get ready. This might be to:

- Make room for a hospital bed or other large equipment

- Move out items that can cause falls, such as area rugs and electric cords (a good idea in any event)

- Create a comfortable space for a family member or friend who might be staying with you for a few days

- Find a place for important information, such as a bulletin board, notebook or a drawer

Healthcare Tasks

You and/or a caregiver will likely do certain tasks as part of your care. What will you be able to do by yourself? What will you need help with? It is important that you and/or your caregiver know how to do these tasks safely and properly. You and any caregivers you might have should try to learn as much as possible while you are still in the hospital. You can do this by watching hospital staff as they do these tasks and asking them to watch as you try these tasks yourself.

Sometimes, hospital staff will not teach these tasks until the day you leave the hospital. This may not be a good time to learn if you feel rushed or overwhelmed. Learn what you can and ask who to call if you have questions at home. You might be told to call someone from the hospital, a home care nurse or other healthcare professional.

If you are a caregiver, speak up if you are afraid of doing certain tasks (such as wound care) or cannot help with personal hygiene (like bathing or changing adult diapers). The hospital team needs to know what tasks you can and cannot do so they can help you plan for any needed help.

Medication Management

It is important to be taking the right medications, at the right time and in the right amount. Here are some questions to ask that can help you do this job well:

- What new medications will I take? How long will I take them?
- Should these medications be taken with meals? At certain times each day?
- Do they have any side effects?
- Can new medications be taken with those I was taking prior to being admitted?
- Are any new medications listed in the "Medication Management Form," along with other prescriptions, over-the-counter medications, vitamins and herbal supplements?
- Do I get these medications from my pharmacy or the hospital?
- Will my insurance pay for these medications? If not, are there generic alternatives?

Know Who to Call and What to Do

You may have a lot of questions during the first few days at home. Make sure you have phone numbers for people on the hospital team, as well as any home care agency involved with your care and a listing of community services you may need.

Make sure you know what to do for your care. This includes knowing:

- Are there any symptoms that you must report right away, such as fever, intense pain, or shortness of breath? If you notice these symptoms, who do you call and what should you do?

- Are there limits or restrictions on what your can do? For example, you might not be able to drive, take a bath, lift heavy things or walk up or down stairs.

- Is it safe to be alone? How often should I ask a family member or friend to check in?

Chapter 32

Complementary
and Integrative Health for
Older Adults

Many older adults are turning to complementary and integrative health approaches, often as a reflection of a healthy self-empowered approach to well-being. Natural products often sold as dietary supplements are frequently used by many older people for various reasons despite safety concerns or a lack of evidence to support their use. Although there is a widespread public perception that the botanical and traditional agents included in dietary supplements can be viewed as safe, these products can contain pharmacologically active compounds and have the associated dangers.

Mind and body practices, including relaxation techniques and meditative exercise forms such as yoga, tai chi, and qi gong are being widely used by older Americans, both for fitness and relaxation, and because of perceived health benefits. A number of systematic reviews point to the potential benefit of mind and body approaches for symptom management, particularly for pain. However, research on these mind and body approaches is still hampered by methodological issues, including a lack of consensus on appropriate controls and lack of intervention

This chapter includes text excerpted from "Complementary and Integrative Health for Older Adults," National Center for Complementary and Integrative Health (NCCIH), April 2015.

425

standardization. While much of the clinical data is inconclusive, these approaches may help older adults maintain motivation to incorporate physical exercise into their regular activities.

Osteoarthritis (OA)

Mind and Body Practices for Osteoarthritis

In 2012, the American College of Rheumatology (ACR) issued recommendations for using pharmacologic and nonpharmacologic approaches for Osteoarthritis (OA) of the hand, hip, and knee:

- The guidelines conditionally recommend tai chi, along with other nondrug approaches such as manual and thermal therapies, self-management programs, and walking aids, for managing knee OA.

- Acupuncture is also conditionally recommended for those who have chronic moderate-to-severe knee pain and are candidates for total knee replacement but are unwilling or unable to undergo surgical repair.

Acupuncture for Osteoarthritis

Studies of acupuncture for OA have focused primarily on OA of the knee. There is also evidence that acupuncture may help to improve pain and function in other joints such as the hip. There are few complications associated with acupuncture, but adverse effects such as minor bruising or bleeding can occur; infections can result from the use of nonsterile needles or poor technique from an inexperienced practitioner.

Massage for Osteoarthritis

Massage therapy appears to have few risks if it is used appropriately and provided by a trained massage professional.

Tai Chi for Osteoarthritis

A few studies of tai chi for OA have been promising for managing symptoms of OA of the knee. Tai chi is considered to be a safe practice.

Natural Products for Osteoarthritis

Glucosamine, Chondroitin Sulfate, or the Combination: Glucosamine and chondroitin sulfate—taken separately or together—are marketed for supporting joint health. They have also been widely used for treating OA. The preponderance of evidence indicates little or no meaningful effect on pain or function.

Safety

Glucosamine and chondroitin appear to be relatively safe and well tolerated when used in suggested doses over a 2-year period. In a few specific situations, however, possible side effects or drug interactions should be considered:

- No serious side effects have been reported in large, well-conducted studies of people taking glucosamine, chondroitin, or both for up to 3 years. However, glucosamine or chondroitin may interact with warfarin.

- Although studies conducted by the U.S. Food and Drug Administration (FDA) show that high doses of glucosamine hydrochloride taken by mouth in rats may promote cartilage regeneration and repair, this dose was also found to cause severe kidney problems in the rats—a serious side effect of the treatment.

Cognitive Decline and Alzheimer Disease

Natural Products for Cognitive Decline and Alzheimer Disease

Although a few trials of natural products for the prevention of cognitive decline or dementia have shown some modest effects, direct evidence is lacking. The evidence base on efficacy of natural products for cognitive function and dementia, including Alzheimer disease, consists of many randomized controlled trials, particularly on omega-3 fatty acids and ginkgo biloba supplementation.

- Omega-3 fatty acid supplements usually do not have negative side effects. When side effects do occur, they typically consist of minor gastrointestinal symptoms. Omega-3 supplements may extend bleeding time. People who take anticoagulants or nonsteroidal anti-inflammatory drugs, should use caution.

- Side effects of ginkgo supplements may include headache, nausea, gastrointestinal upset, diarrhea, dizziness, or allergic skin reactions. More severe allergic reactions have occasionally been reported. There are some data to suggest that ginkgo can increase bleeding risk.

Sleep Disorders

Mind and Body Practices for Sleep Disorders

Relaxation Techniques

Relaxation techniques include progressive relaxation, guided imagery, biofeedback, self-hypnosis, and deep breathing exercises. The goal is similar in all: to consciously produce the body's natural relaxation response, characterized by slower breathing, lower blood pressure, and a feeling of calm and well-being. Relaxation techniques are also used to induce sleep, reduce pain, and calm emotions.

Evidence suggests that using relaxation techniques before bedtime can be helpful components of a successful strategy to improve sleep habits. Other components include maintaining a consistent sleep schedule; avoiding caffeine, alcohol, heavy meals, and strenuous exercise too close to bedtime; and sleeping in a quiet, cool, dark room.

Safety

- Relaxation techniques are generally considered safe. There have been rare case reports of worsening of symptoms in people with epilepsy or certain psychiatric conditions, or with a history of abuse or trauma.

- Relaxation techniques are generally used as components of a treatment plan, and not as the only approach for potentially serious health conditions.

Other Mind and Body Practices for Sleep Disorders

Other mind and body practices which have been studied for their effects on insomnia and other sleep disorders include mindfulness-based stress reduction, yoga, massage therapy, and acupuncture.

- Meditation is considered to be safe for healthy people. There have been rare reports that meditation could cause or worsen symptoms in people who have certain psychiatric problems, but this question has not been fully researched. People with physical limitations may not be able to participate in certain meditative practices involving physical movement. Individuals with existing mental or physical health conditions should speak with their healthcare providers prior to starting a meditative practice and make their meditation instructor aware of their condition.

- Overall, clinical data suggest yoga as taught and practiced in certain research studies under the guidance of skilled teacher has a low rate of minor side effects. However, injuries from yoga, some of them serious, have been reported in the popular press. People with health conditions should work with an experienced teacher who can help modify or avoid some yoga poses to prevent side effects.

- Massage therapy appears to have few risks when performed by a trained practitioner. However, massage therapists should take some precautions with certain health conditions. In some cases, pregnant women should avoid massage therapy. Forceful and deep tissue massage should be avoided by people with conditions such as bleeding disorders or low blood platelet counts, and by people taking anticoagulants. Massage should not be done in any potentially weak area of the skin, such as wounds. Deep or intense pressure should not be used over an area where the patient has a tumor or cancer, unless approved by the patient's healthcare provider.

- Acupuncture is generally considered safe when performed by an experienced practitioner using sterile needles. Reports of serious adverse events related to acupuncture are rare, but include infections and punctured organs.

Natural Products for Sleep Disorders

Melatonin

Melatonin is a hormone known to shift circadian rhythms. Research suggest that melatonin may be useful in treating several sleep disorders, such as jet lag, delayed sleep phase disorder, and sleep problems related to shift work.

- Melatonin supplements appear to be relatively safe for short-term use, although modest adverse effects on mood were seen with melatonin use in elderly people (most of whom had dementia) in one study. The long-term safety of melatonin supplements has not been established.

- Melatonin can have additive effects with alcohol and other sedating medications, and older people should be cautioned about its use.

Menopausal Symptoms

Mind and Body Practices for Menopausal Symptoms

Overall, evidence suggests that some mind and body approaches, such as yoga, tai chi, and meditation-based programs may provide some benefit in reducing common menopausal symptoms.

- Meditation is considered to be safe for healthy people. There have been rare reports that meditation could cause or worsen symptoms in people who have certain psychiatric problems, but this question has not been fully researched. People with physical limitations may not be able to participate in certain meditative practices involving physical movement. Individuals with existing mental or physical health conditions should speak with their healthcare providers prior to starting a meditative practice and make their meditation instructor aware of their condition.

- Overall, clinical trial data suggest yoga as taught and practiced in these research studies under the guidance of skilled teacher has a low rate of minor side effects. However, injuries from yoga, some of them serious, have been reported in the popular press. People with health conditions should work with an experienced teacher who can help modify or avoid some yoga poses to prevent side effects.

- Tai chi is considered to be a safe practice.

- There are few complications associated with acupuncture, but adverse effects such as minor bruising or bleeding can occur; infections can result from the use of nonsterile needles or poor technique from an inexperienced practitioner.

Natural Products for Menopausal Symptoms

Many natural products have been studied for their effects on menopausal symptoms, but there is little evidence that they are useful. While some herbs and botanicals are often found in over-the-counter formulas and combinations, many of these combination products have not been studied. Further, because natural products used for menopausal symptoms can have side effects and can interact with other botanicals or supplements or with medications.

Black Cohosh (Actaea Racemosa, Cimicifuga Racemosa)

- United States Pharmacopeia (USP) experts suggest that women should discontinue use of black cohosh and consult a healthcare practitioner if they have a liver disorder or develop symptoms of liver trouble, such as abdominal pain, dark urine, or jaundice.

- There have been several case reports of hepatitis, as well as liver failure, in women who were taking black cohosh. It is not known if black cohosh was responsible for these problems. Although these cases are very rare and the evidence is not definitive, there is concern about the possible effects of black cohosh on the liver.

Benign Prostatic Hyperplasia (BPH)

Natural Products for Benign Prostatic Hyperplasia (BPH)

Although several small studies have suggested modest benefit of saw palmetto for treating symptoms of BPH, a large study evaluating high doses of saw palmetto and a Cochrane review found that saw palmetto was not more effective than placebo for treatment of urinary symptoms related to BPH. Saw palmetto appears to be well tolerated by most users. It may cause mild side effects, including stomach discomfort.

Age-Related Macular Degeneration

Natural Products for Age-Related Macular Degeneration

There is some evidence that natural products such as antioxidant vitamins and minerals may delay the development of advanced age-related macular degeneration (AMD) in people who are at high risk for the disease. However, other studies of vitamin E and beta carotene supplementation did not show benefit in preventing the onset of AMD.

Safety

- Although generally regarded as safe, vitamin supplements may have harmful effects, and clear evidence of benefit is needed before they can be recommended.

- Omega-3s appear to be safe for most adults at low-to-moderate doses. The FDA has concluded that omega-3 dietary supplements from fish are "generally recognized as safe." Fish oil supplements may cause minor gastrointestinal upsets, including diarrhea, heartburn, indigestion, and abdominal bloating.

- Side effects of ginkgo supplements may include headache, nausea, gastrointestinal upset, diarrhea, dizziness, or allergic skin reactions. More severe allergic reactions have occasionally been reported. There are some data to suggest that ginkgo can increase bleeding risk.

Herpes Zoster (Shingles)

Mind and Body Practices for Herpes Zoster

There have only been a few studies on the effects of tai chi on cell-mediated immunity to varicella zoster virus following vaccination, but the results of these studies have shown some benefit. Other interventions such as acupuncture, cupping, neural therapy, and intravenous vitamin C (ascorbic acid) have been studied for their effects on duration of neuropathic pain and postherpetic neuralgia due to herpes zoster, but these studies have been small.

Chapter 33

Online Health Information: Is It Reliable?

Many older adults share a common concern: "How can I trust the health information I get on the Internet?". There are thousands of medical websites. Some provide reliable health information. Some do not. Some of the medical news is current. Some of it is not. Choosing which websites to trust is an important part of using the Internet.

How Do I Find Reliable Health Information Online?

As a rule, health websites sponsored by Federal Government agencies are good sources of information. You can reach all Federal websites by visiting www.usa.gov. Large professional organizations and well-known medical schools may also be good sources of health information.

How Do I Navigate Health Websites?

The home page is like a lobby to other areas of the website; however, it may not be the first page you see. The first page you see depends on the link you click to get to the website, for example, from a search engine.

This chapter includes text excerpted from "Online Health Information: Is It Reliable?" National Institute on Aging (NIA), National Institutes of Health (NIH), August 16, 2017.

Even if you don't start on the homepage, you can still use the website menu. Usually, you can find the menu at the top of a page or along the left side. No matter where you start, you should be able to spot the name of the sponsor or owner of the site right away.

Where Can I Find Reliable Health Information Online?

Sometimes, it's hard to know where to begin to look for trustworthy health information. The National Institutes of Health (NIH) website, www.nih.gov, is a good place to start for reliable health information. Here are a few other helpful websites hosted by NIH:

- National Institute on Aging (NIA) (www.nia.nih.gov) has a variety of resources about health and aging, including information about Alzheimer disease.

- MedlinePlus (www.medlineplus.gov), a website from the National Library of Medicine (NLM), has dependable information about more than 700 health-related topics.

- National Heart, Lung, and Blood Institute (NHLBI) (www.nhlbi.nih.gov) has information about managing heart disease and other topics.

- National Institute on Deafness and Other Communication Disorders (NIDCD) (www.nidcd.nih.gov) has information about hearing loss and deafness.

- National Institute of Dental and Craniofacial Research (NIDCR) (www.nidcr.nih.gov) offers, for example, tips on taking care of dentures.

Questions to Ask before Trusting a Website

As you search online, you are likely to find websites for many health agencies and organizations that are not well-known. By answering the following questions you should be able to find more information about these websites. A lot of these details might be found under the heading "About Us."

1. **Who sponsors/hosts the website? Is that information easy to find?**

   Websites cost money. Is the source of funding (sponsor) clear? Sometimes the website address is helpful. For example:

- **.gov** identifies a U.S. government agency

- **.edu** identifies an educational institution, like a school, college, or university

- **.org** usually identifies nonprofit organizations (such as professional groups; scientific, medical, or research societies; advocacy groups)

- **.com** identifies commercial websites (such as businesses, pharmaceutical companies, and sometimes hospitals)

2. **Is it clear how you can reach the sponsor?**

   Trustworthy websites will have contact information for you to use to reach the site's sponsor or authors. An email address, toll-free phone number, and/or mailing address might be listed at the bottom of every page or on a separate "About Us" or "Contact Us" page.

3. **Who wrote the information?**

   Authors and contributors are often but not always identified. For example, most government sites have many authors and contributors and, rather than list the names of the people, they will often credit a department. A contributor's connection to the website, and any financial interest he or she has in the information on the website, should be clear.

   Be careful about testimonials. Personal stories may be helpful and comforting, but not everyone experiences health problems the same way. Also, there is a big difference between a website developed by a single person interested in a topic and a website developed using strong scientific evidence (that is, information gathered from research). No information should replace seeing a doctor or other health professional.

4. **Who reviews the information? Does the website have editors?**

   Read the "About Us" page to see if experts check the information before putting it online. Find out if the list includes actual experts in the field. Dependable websites tell you where the health information came from and how it has been reviewed.

5. **When was the information written?**

   Look for websites that stay current on their health information. You don't want to make decisions about your care based

435

on out-of-date information. Often the bottom of the page will have a date. Pages on the same site may be updated at different times. Some may be updated more often than others. Older information isn't useless. Many websites provide older articles as historical background.

6. **Is your privacy protected? Does the website clearly state a privacy policy?**

Take time to read the website's privacy policy, which can usually be found at the bottom of the page or on a separate page titled "About Us," "Privacy Policy," or "Our Policies." If the website says something like, "We share information with companies that can provide you with products," that's a sign your information isn't private.

BE CAREFUL about sharing your Social Security number. Find out why your number is needed, how it will be used, and what will happen if you do not share your number. Some websites, like for your health insurance, might need your Social Security number to process claims.

7. **Are your privacy rights, as a consumer, protected when making an online purchase?**

If you are asked for personal information, be sure to find out how the information will be used. Contact the website sponsor by phone or mail, or use the "Contact Us" feature on the website. Be careful when buying things online. Websites without security may not protect your credit card or bank account information. Look for information saying that a website has a "secure server" before buying anything online. Secure websites that collect personal information have an "s" after "http" in the start of their website address (https://) and often require that you create a username and password.

8. **Does the website offer quick and easy solutions to your health problems? Are miracle cures promised?**

Be careful of websites or companies that claim any one remedy will cure a lot of different illnesses. Question dramatic writing or amazing cures. Make sure you can find other websites with the same information. Even if the website links to a trustworthy source, it doesn't mean that the site has the other organization's endorsement or support—any website can link to another without permission.

Trust Yourself and Talk to Your Doctor

Use common sense and good judgment when looking at health information online. There are websites on nearly every health topic, and many have no rules overseeing the quality of the information provided. Take a deep breath and think a bit before acting on any health information you find online. Don't count on any one website and check your sources. And, remember to talk with your doctor about what you learn online before making any changes in your healthcare.

A Quick Checklist

You can use the following checklist to help make sure that the health information you are reading online can be trusted. You might want to keep this checklist by your computer.

1. Is the sponsor/owner of the website a Federal agency, medical school, or large professional or nonprofit organization, or is it related to one of these?

2. If not sponsored by a Federal agency, medical school, or large professional or nonprofit organization, does the website reference one of these trustworthy sources for its health information?

3. Is the mission or goal of the sponsor clear?

4. Can you see who works for the agency or organization and who authored the information? Is there a way to contact the sponsor of the website?

5. When was the information written or webpage last updated?

6. Is your privacy protected?

7. Does the website offer unbelievable solutions to your health problem(s)? Are quick, miracle cures promised?

Chapter 34

Assistive Technology

Chapter Contents

Section 34.1

Assistive Technology: Overview

This section includes text excerpted from "Assistive Technology," Eldercare Locator, U.S. Administration on Aging (AOA), October 15, 2015.

Assistive technology (AT) is any service or tool that helps older adults or persons with disabilities perform activities that might otherwise be difficult or impossible.

For older adults, such technology may be a walker to improve mobility or an amplification device to make sounds easier to hear. It could also include a magnifying glass for someone who has poor vision or a scooter that makes it possible for someone to travel over distances that are too far to walk. In short, AT is anything that aids continued participation in daily activities.

AT allows many people to live independently without long-term nursing or home healthcare. For some, it is critical to the ability to perform simple activities of daily living, such as bathing.

Choosing AT

Older adults should carefully evaluate their needs before purchasing AT. Using AT may change the mix of services that they require or affect the way that those services are provided. Needs assessment and planning are very important.

Usually, a needs assessment is most effective when done by a team working with the older adult in a place where the AT will be used. For example, someone who has trouble communicating or hearing might consult his or her doctor, an audiology specialist, a speech-language therapist, and family and friends. Together, they can identify precise challenges and help select the most effective devices available at the lowest cost. A professional member of the team, such as the audiology specialist, can also arrange for any training needed to use the equipment.

When considering AT, it is useful to consider high-tech and low-tech solutions. Older adults should also think about how their needs might change over time. High-tech devices tend to be more expensive but may address many different needs. Low-tech equipment is usually less expensive but also less adaptable.

Paying for AT

Right now, not all private insurance plans or public programs will pay for all types of AT under any circumstances. However, Medicare Part B will cover up to 80 percent of the cost, if the items are durable medical equipment—devices that are "primarily and customarily used to serve a medical purpose, and generally are not useful to a person in the absence of illness or injury." Contact Medicare to determine whether a particular type of AT is covered.

Depending on where you live, the state-run Medicaid program may pay for some AT. Keep in mind that when Medicaid covers part of the cost, the benefits do not usually provide the total amount needed to buy an expensive piece of equipment, such as a power wheelchair.

Older adults who are eligible for veteran benefits may be eligible for assistance from the U.S. Department of Veterans Affairs (VA), which has a model structure in place to pay for the large volume of equipment that it buys. The VA also invests in training people to use assistive devices.

Subsidy programs provide some types of AT at a reduced cost or for free. Many businesses and nonprofit groups offer discounts, grants, or rebates to get consumers to try a specific product. Older adults should be cautious about participating in subsidy programs run by businesses with commercial interests in the product or service because of the potential for fraud.

Section 34.2

Assistive Devices for People with Hearing, Voice, Speech, or Language Disorders

This section includes text excerpted from "Assistive Devices for People with Hearing, Voice, Speech, or Language Disorders," National Institute on Deafness and Other Communication Disorders (NIDCD), March 6, 2017.

What Are Assistive Devices?

The terms *assistive device or assistive technology* can refer to any device that helps a person with hearing loss or a voice, speech, or language disorder to communicate. These terms often refer to devices that help a person to hear and understand what is being said more clearly or to express thoughts more easily. With the development of digital and wireless technologies, more and more devices are becoming available to help people with hearing, voice, speech, and language disorders communicate more meaningfully and participate more fully in their daily lives.

What Types of Assistive Devices Are Available?

Health professionals use a variety of names to describe assistive devices:

- **Assistive listening devices (ALDs)** help amplify the sounds you want to hear, especially where there's a lot of background noise. ALDs can be used with a hearing aid or cochlear implant to help a wearer hear certain sounds better.

- **Augmentative and alternative communication (AAC)** devices help people with communication disorders to express themselves. These devices can range from a simple picture board to a computer program that synthesizes speech from text.

- **Alerting devices** connect to a doorbell, telephone, or alarm that emits a loud sound or blinking light to let someone with hearing loss know that an event is taking place.

What Types of Assistive Listening Devices (ALDs) Are Available?

Several types of ALDs are available to improve sound transmission for people with hearing loss. Some are designed for large facilities such as classrooms, theaters, places of worship, and airports. Other types are intended for personal use in small settings and for one-on-one conversations. All can be used with or without hearing aids or a cochlear implant. ALD systems for large facilities include hearing loop systems, frequency-modulated (FM) systems, and infrared systems.

Hearing loop (or induction loop) systems use electromagnetic energy to transmit sound. A hearing loop system involves four parts:

- A sound source, such as a public address system, microphone, or home TV or telephone

- An amplifier

- A thin loop of wire that encircles a room or branches out beneath carpeting

- A receiver worn in the ears or as a headset

Amplified sound travels through the loop and creates an electro-magnetic field that is picked up directly by a hearing loop receiver or a telecoil, a miniature wireless receiver that is built into many hearing aids and cochlear implants. To pick up the signal, a listener must be wearing the receiver and be within or near the loop. Because the sound is picked up directly by the receiver, the sound is much clearer, without as much of the competing background noise associated with many listening environments. Some loop systems are portable, making it possible for people with hearing loss to improve their listening environments, as needed, as they proceed with their daily activities. A hearing loop can be connected to a public address system, a television, or any other audio source. For those who don't have hearing aids with embedded telecoils, portable loop receivers are also available.

FM systems use radio signals to transmit amplified sounds. They are often used in classrooms, where the instructor wears a small microphone connected to a transmitter and the student wears the receiver, which is tuned to a specific frequency, or channel. People who have a telecoil inside their hearing aid or cochlear implant may also wear a wire around the neck (called a neckloop) or behind their aid or implant (called a silhouette inductor) to convert the signal into magnetic signals

443

that can be picked up directly by the telecoil. FM systems can transmit signals up to 300 feet and are able to be used in many public places. However, because radio signals are able to penetrate walls, listeners in one room may need to listen to a different channel than those in another room to avoid receiving mixed signals. Personal FM systems operate in the same way as larger scale systems and can be used to help people with hearing loss to follow one-on-one conversations.

Infrared systems use infrared light to transmit sound. A transmitter converts sound into a light signal and beams it to a receiver that is worn by a listener. The receiver decodes the infrared signal back to sound. As with FM systems, people whose hearing aids or cochlear implants have a telecoil may also wear a neckloop or silhouette inductor to convert the infrared signal into a magnetic signal, which can be picked up through their telecoil. Unlike induction loop or FM systems, the infrared signal cannot pass through walls, making it particularly useful in courtrooms, where confidential information is often discussed, and in buildings where competing signals can be a problem, such as classrooms or movie theaters. However, infrared systems cannot be used in environments with too many competing light sources, such as outdoors or in strongly lit rooms.

Personal amplifiers are useful in places in which the above systems are unavailable or when watching TV, being outdoors, or traveling in a car. About the size of a cell phone, these devices increase sound levels and reduce background noise for a listener. Some have directional microphones that can be angled toward a speaker or other source of sound. As with other ALDs, the amplified sound can be picked up by a receiver that the listener is wearing, either as a headset or as earbuds.

What Types of Augmentative and Alternative Communication (AAC) Devices Are Available for Communicating Face-To-Face?

The simplest AAC device is a picture board or touch screen that uses pictures or symbols of typical items and activities that make up a person's daily life. For example, a person might touch the image of a glass to ask for a drink. Many picture boards can be customized and expanded based on a person's age, education, occupation, and interests.

Keyboards, touch screens, and sometimes a person's limited speech may be used to communicate desired words. Some devices employ a text display. The display panel typically faces outward so that two people can exchange information while facing each other. Spelling and word prediction software can make it faster and easier to enter information.

Speech-generating devices go one step further by translating words or pictures into speech. Some models allow users to choose from several different voices, such as male or female, child or adult, and even some regional accents. Some devices employ a vocabulary of prerecorded words while others have an unlimited vocabulary, synthesizing speech as words are typed in. Software programs that convert personal computers into speaking devices are also available.

What Augmentative and Alternative Communication Devices Are Available for Communicating by Telephone?

For many years, people with hearing loss have used text telephone or telecommunications devices, called TTY or TDD machines, to communicate by phone. This same technology also benefits people with speech difficulties. A TTY machine consists of a typewriter keyboard that displays typed conversations onto a readout panel or printed on paper. Callers will either type messages to each other over the system or, if a call recipient does not have a TTY machine, use the national toll-free telecommunications relay service at 711 to communicate. Through the relay service, a communications assistant serves as a bridge between two callers, reading typed messages aloud to the person with hearing while transcribing what's spoken into type for the person with hearing loss.

With today's new electronic communication devices, however, TTY machines have almost become a thing of the past. People can place phone calls through the telecommunications relay service using almost any device with a keypad, including a laptop, personal digital assistant, and cell phone. Text messaging has also become a popular method of communication, skipping the relay service altogether.

Another system uses voice recognition software and an extensive library of video clips depicting American Sign Language to translate a signer's words into text or computer-generated speech in real time. It is also able to translate spoken words back into sign language or text.

Finally, for people with mild to moderate hearing loss, captioned telephones allow you to carry on a spoken conversation, while providing a transcript of the other person's words on a readout panel or computer screen as back-up.

What Types of Alerting Devices Are Available?

Alerting or alarm devices use sound, light, vibrations, or a combination of these techniques to let someone know when a particular event is occurring. Clocks and wake-up alarm systems allow a person to choose to wake up to flashing lights, horns, or a gentle shaking.

Visual alert signalers monitor a variety of household devices and other sounds, such as doorbells and telephones. When the phone rings, the visual alert signaler will be activated and will vibrate or flash a light to let people know. In addition, remote receivers placed around the house can alert a person from any room. Portable vibrating pagers can let parents and caretakers know when a baby is crying. Some baby monitoring devices analyze a baby's cry and light up a picture to indicate if the baby sounds hungry, bored, or sleepy.

Chapter 35

Personal Safety

Chapter Contents

Section 35.1

Elder Abuse and Its Impact

This section includes text excerpted from "Elder Abuse,"
National Institute on Aging (NIA), National Institutes of
Health (NIH), July 18, 2017.

Abuse can happen in many places, including the older person's home, a family member's house, an assisted living facility, or a nursing home.

Types of Abuse

There are many types of abuse:

- **Physical abuse** happens when someone causes bodily harm by hitting, pushing, or slapping.

- **Emotional abuse,** sometimes called psychological abuse, can include a caregiver saying hurtful words, yelling, threatening, or repeatedly ignoring the older person. Keeping that person from seeing close friends and relatives is another form of emotional abuse.

- **Neglect** occurs when the caregiver does not try to respond to the older person's needs.

- **Abandonment** is leaving a senior alone without planning for his or her care.

- **Sexual abuse** involves a caregiver forcing an older adult to watch or be part of sexual acts.

Money Matters

Financial abuse happens when money or belongings are stolen. It can include forging checks, taking someone else's retirement and Social Security benefits, or using another person's credit cards and bank accounts. It also includes changing names on a will, bank account, life insurance policy, or title to a house without permission from the older person. Financial abuse is becoming a widespread and hard-to-detect issue. Even someone you've never met can steal your financial information using the telephone or email. Be careful about sharing any financial information over the phone or online—you don't know who will use it.

Healthcare fraud can be committed by doctors, hospital staff, and other healthcare workers. It includes overcharging, billing twice for the same service, falsifying Medicaid or Medicare claims, or charging for care that wasn't provided. Older adults and caregivers should keep an eye out for this type of fraud.

Who Is Being Abused?

Most victims of abuse are women, but some are men. Likely targets are older people who have no family or friends nearby and people with disabilities, memory problems, or dementia.

Abuse can happen to any older person, but often affects those who depend on others for help with activities of everyday life—including bathing, dressing, and taking medicine. People who are frail may appear to be easy victims.

What Are Signs of Abuse?

You may see signs of abuse or neglect when you visit an older person at home or in an eldercare facility. You may notice the person:

- Has trouble sleeping
- Seems depressed or confused
- Loses weight for no reason
- Displays signs of trauma, like rocking back and forth
- Acts agitated or violent
- Becomes withdrawn
- Stops taking part in activities he or she enjoys
- Has unexplained bruises, burns, or scars
- Looks messy, with unwashed hair or dirty clothes
- Develops bed sores or other preventable conditions

If you see signs of abuse, try talking with the older person to find out what's going on. For instance, the abuse may be from another resident and not from someone who works at the nursing home or assisted living facility. Most importantly, get help.

What Is the Long-Term Effect of Abuse?

Most physical wounds heal in time. But, any type of mistreatment can leave the abused person feeling fearful and depressed. Sometimes, the victim thinks the abuse is his or her fault. Protective services agencies can suggest support groups and counseling that can help the abused person heal the emotional wounds.

Who Can Help?

Elder abuse will not stop on its own. Someone else needs to step in and help. Many older people are too ashamed to report mistreatment. Or, they're afraid if they make a report it will get back to the abuser and make the situation worse.

If you think someone you know is being abused—physically, emotionally, or financially—talk with him or her when the two of you are alone. You could say you think something is wrong and you're worried. Offer to take him or her to get help, for instance, at a local adult protective services agency.

Many local, state, and national social service agencies can help with emotional, legal, and financial problems.

The Administration for Community Living (ACL) has a National Center on Elder Abuse (NCEA) where you can learn about how to report abuse, where to get help, and state laws that deal with abuse and neglect. Call the Eldercare Locator weekdays at 1-800-677-1116.

Most states require that doctors and lawyers report elder mistreatment. Family and friends can also report it. Do not wait. Help is available.

If you think someone is in urgent danger, call 911 or your local police to get help right away.

Section 35.2

Preventing Falls

This section includes text excerpted from "Bone Basics—Falls and Fractures," National Institute of Arthritis and Musculoskeletal and Skin Diseases (NIAMS), November 2014. Reviewed September 2017.

Falls are serious at any age, but especially for older people who are more likely to break a bone when they fall.

If you have a disease called osteoporosis, you are more likely to break a bone if you fall. Osteoporosis is called the "silent disease" because bones become weak with no symptoms. You may not know that you have it until a strain, bump, or fall causes a bone to break.

Falls are especially dangerous for people with osteoporosis. If you break a bone, you might need a long time to recover. Learning how to prevent falls can help you avoid broken bones and the problems they can cause.

Why Do People Fall?

Some of the reasons people fall are:

- Tripping or slipping due to loss of footing or traction
- Slow reflexes, which make it hard to keep your balance or move out of the way of a hazard
- Balance problems
- Reduced muscle strength
- Poor vision
- Illness
- Taking medicines
- Drinking alcohol

Illness and some medicines can make you feel dizzy, confused, or slow. Medicines that may increase the risk of falls are:

- Blood pressure pills

- Heart medicines
- Diuretics (water pills)
- Muscle relaxants
- Sleeping pills

Drinking alcohol can lead to a fall because it can:

- Slow your reflexes
- Cause you to feel dizzy or sleepy
- Alter your balance
- Cause you to take risks that can lead to falls

How Can I Prevent Falling?

At any age, people can make changes to lower their risk of falling. Some tips to help prevent falls outdoors are:

- Use a cane or walker
- Wear rubber-soled shoes so you don't slip
- Walk on grass when sidewalks are slick
- Put salt or kitty litter on icy sidewalks

Some ways to help prevent falls indoors are:

- Keep rooms free of clutter, especially on floors
- Use plastic or carpet runners
- Wear low-heeled shoes
- Do not walk in socks, stockings, or slippers
- Be sure rugs have skid-proof backs or are tacked to the floor
- Be sure stairs are well lit and have rails on both sides
- Put grab bars on bathroom walls near tub, shower, and toilet
- Use a nonskid bath mat in the shower or tub
- Keep a flashlight next to your bed
- Use a sturdy stepstool with a handrail and wide steps
- Add more lights in rooms

- Buy a cordless phone so that you don't have to rush to the phone when it rings and so that you can call for help if you fall

You can also do exercises to improve your balance. While holding the back of a chair, sink, or counter:

- Stand on one leg at a time for a minute and then slowly increase the time. Try to balance with your eyes closed or without holding on.
- Stand on your toes for a count of 10, and then rock back on your heels for a count of 10.
- Make a big circle to the left with your hips, and then to the right. Do not move your shoulders or feet. Repeat five times.

How Can I Prevent Broken Bones If I Fall?

Sometimes you cannot prevent a fall. If you do fall, you can try to prevent breaking a bone. Try to fall forwards or backwards (on your buttocks), because if you fall to the side you may break your hip. You can also use your hands or grab things around you to break a fall. Some people wear extra clothes to pad their hips or use special hip pads.

How Can I Keep My Bones Healthy?

Some ways to protect your bones are:

- Get enough calcium and vitamin D each day.
- Walk, climb stairs, lift weights, or dance each day.
- Talk with your doctor about having a bone mineral density (BMD) test.
- Talk with your doctor about taking medicine to make your bones stronger.

Table 35.1. Recommended Calcium and Vitamin D Intakes

Life-Stage Group	Calcium mg/day	Vitamin D (IU/day)
51- to 70-year-old males	1,000	600
51- to 70-year-old females	1,200	600
>70 years old	1,200	800

Definitions: mg = milligrams; IU = International Units

Section 35.3

Heating in the Winter

This section includes text excerpted from "Winter Warmth and Safety: Home Energy Tips for Older Adults," Eldercare Locator, U.S. Administration on Aging (AOA), August 19, 2017.

Everyone appreciates a warm, comfortable home during the cold winter months. Yet with escalating energy costs, many older Americans will find it a challenge to keep up with home heating bills this winter. With a little planning and preparation, you can reduce the amount you owe and still stay warm during the winter. The Eldercare Locator and the U.S. Environmental Protection Agency (EPA) offer some economical ways to stay warm and safe at home.

Find out about Financial Energy Assistance Programs

- Many states, counties and cities provide programs that assist older adults with winter heating costs. Your local Area Agency on Aging is a good source of information about available community programs and eligibility requirements. To identify the Area Agency on Aging serving your community, contact the Eldercare Locator at 800-677-1116 or www.eldercare.gov.

- **Ask about the Low-Income Home Energy Assistance Program (LIHEAP)**—the federally funded program that helps eligible low-income homeowners and renters meet home heating needs. The name of this program and eligibility requirements may vary across states. Be mindful that there is an application deadline for assistance, except for emergency situations. Depending on where you live, LIHEAP may offer one or more of the following types of help:

  - Heating funds (i.e., fuel subsidies) to increase the affordability of home energy;

  - Low-cost residential weatherization and other home repairs to safely increase the efficiency of a household's use of home energy, thus lowering energy bills and making homes more comfortable; and

- Energy crisis intervention to address weather-related and fuel supply shortages and other household energy-related emergencies, such as utility shutoffs.

- Get information about the **Weatherization Assistance Program (WAP)**. Most state and local governments receive federal funds to help low-income families permanently reduce their energy bills by making their homes more energy efficient. WAP assistance is free and preference is given to people over age 60 and households with children or people with disabilities. You must apply to determine eligibility.

Be Aware of Help Provided by Utility Companies

- Check with your gas, water and electricity suppliers to see if they offer a monthly budget plan to help spread out energy costs throughout the year. Often they have special heating assistance funds, as well as "no cut off" guidelines to avoid termination of service for older adults, people with disabilities and ill customers who may have difficulty paying their bills.

- Utility companies are also a great source for energy conservation information. They might be able to refer you to an expert to inspect your home for ways to make it more energy efficient, or provide a list of contractors to tune up your furnace so that it operates at peak efficiency.

Look for Ways to Cut down on Winter Energy Use

- The ENERGY STAR Program, run by the EPA offers tips to help make your home more energy efficient (888-782-7937 or www. energystar.gov). ENERGY STAR is a widely recognized and trusted label that identifies and promotes energy-efficient products, including major appliances, office equipment, lighting, home electronics and more. These products can help you save about one third on energy bills without sacrificing features, style or comfort.

- Simple, inexpensive energy-saving things you can do yourself:

  - Have a friend or relative seal air leaks. Weather strip and insulate the attic hatch or door to prevent warm air from leaking out of the house. Replace your screens with storm windows to provide an extra barrier to the cold outside air.

• Use a programmable thermostat that can automatically adjust the temperature of your home when you are asleep or away. To maximize savings without sacrificing comfort, program the thermostat to lower the heat by 8 degrees Fahrenheit or more when away and asleep.

• Dirt and neglect are the number one causes of heating system failure, so be sure to schedule a fall checkup of your heating equipment with a licensed contractor to make sure your system is operating at peak performance. Also, check your system's air filter every month and when it is dirty, change it. At a minimum change it every three months.

• While a log fire in your fireplace is attractive, it does not efficiently heat your home. Your chimney creates a draft that removes the combustion byproducts from a fire. That same draft also pulls air from your home up the chimney—air that you have paid to heat with your heating system. So be sure to close your fireplace damper when not in use, and consider the use of a fireplace "balloon" to make it even tighter. Fireplace balloons and other "chimney plugs" will save energy. But you must remember to remove them before lighting a fire in the fireplace.

Ensure Your Health and Safety

In addition to addressing the need to stay warm during winter, consider safety as well. For example:

• Avoid the risk of home fires. Do not use your stove or oven to heat your home. Keep batteries and battery-powered flashlights available. When needed, use flashlights instead of candles. Check to make sure that electrical cords on space heaters are not damaged and do not pose a tripping hazard.

• Make sure that smoke and carbon monoxide detectors are installed and working properly. It is recommended that you replace the batteries at least once a year. As a reminder, pick a holiday or your birthday and replace the batteries each year on that day.

• Insulate water pipes to avoid freezing and bursting. When freezing temperatures are expected, leave water taps slightly open so they drip continuously. Drain and turn off outside water spouts.

- Have a fire extinguisher ready to use. Fire extinguishers should be inspected at least once a year to assure they will operate effectively and safely when needed. Consult your telephone directory or local fire department for fire extinguisher service.

Have a Back-Up Plan

Before you need them, consider alternative arrangements should extreme weather conditions require emergency action.

- Identify temporary living arrangements in case you are unable to stay in your own home and have a plan for getting there.

- Keep in touch with family and friends. Ask someone to check on you daily—especially if you live alone.

- Plan for your medical needs. Have extra medications on hand or identify a pharmacy that will deliver them to you.

- If you or a loved one in your home has medical equipment, be sure you know how it will need to be maintained or moved in an emergency.

- Share emergency contact information with everyone who would need it.

Indoor Pollutants and Carbon Monoxide Information

In winter, most people spend a majority of their time indoors. It is important to remember that pollutants are not only outdoors, but they can be indoors too. Be aware of possible indoor pollutants in your home and take steps to reduce your exposure.

- Avoid smoking and second hand smoke. Fix water leaks promptly and eliminate mold. Clean up pet dander, dust, pollens and other fine particles as these can cause health problems and trigger an asthma attack.

- Carbon monoxide (CO) poisoning is the most common cause of poisoning death in the United States.

- There are approximately 500 deaths and 15,000 visits to the emergency room that occur annually due to unintentional CO poisoning.

457

- You can prevent CO poisoning by installing a CO monitor to alert you if there is a dangerous level of carbon monoxide in your home.

- Install a CO and smoke detector in your home. Make sure that your detectors are working properly.

- The batteries should be replaced at least once a year. Choose a holiday or your birthday to replace the batteries each year.

Section 35.4

Stay Safe in Cold Weather!

This section includes text excerpted from "Cold Weather Safety for Older Adults," National Institute on Aging (NIA), National Institutes of Health (NIH), June 29, 2017.

If you are like most people, you feel cold every now and then during the winter. What you may not know is that just being really cold can make you very sick. Older adults can lose body heat fast— faster than when they were young. Changes in your body that come with aging can make it harder for you to be aware of getting cold. A big chill can turn into a dangerous problem before an older person even knows what's happening. Doctors call this serious problem hypothermia.

What Is Hypothermia?

Hypothermia is what happens when your body temperature gets very low. For an older person, a body temperature colder than 95°F can cause many health problems, such as a heart attack, kidney problems, liver damage, or worse.

Being outside in the cold, or even being in a very cold house, can lead to hypothermia. Try to stay away from cold places, and pay attention to how cold it is where you are. You can take steps to lower your chance of getting hypothermia.

Keep Warm Inside

Living in a cold house, apartment, or other building can cause hypothermia. In fact, hypothermia can happen to someone in a nursing home or group facility if the rooms are not kept warm enough. If someone you know is in a group facility, pay attention to the inside temperature and to whether that person is dressed warmly enough.

People who are sick may have special problems keeping warm. Do not let it get too cold inside and dress warmly. Even if you keep your temperature between 60 and 65 degrees Fahrenheit, your home or apartment may not be warm enough to keep you safe. This is a special problem if you live alone because there is no one else to feel the chilliness of the house or notice if you are having symptoms of hypothermia.

Here are some tips for keeping warm while you're inside:

- Set your heat at 68°F or higher. To save on heating bills, close off rooms you are not using. Close the vents and shut the doors in these rooms, and keep the basement door closed. Place a rolled towel in front of all doors to keep out drafts.

- Make sure your house isn't losing heat through windows. Keep your blinds and curtains closed. If you have gaps around the windows, try using weather stripping or caulk to keep the cold air out.

- Dress warmly on cold days even if you are staying in the house. Throw a blanket over your legs. Wear socks and slippers.

- When you go to sleep, wear long underwear under your pajamas, and use extra covers. Wear a cap or hat.

- Make sure you eat enough food to keep up your weight. If you don't eat well, you might have less fat under your skin. Body fat helps you to stay warm.

- Drink alcohol moderately, if at all. Alcoholic drinks can make you lose body heat.

- Ask family or friends to check on you during cold weather. If a power outage leaves you without heat, try to stay with a relative or friend.

You may be tempted to warm your room with a space heater. But, some space heaters are fire hazards, and others can cause carbon monoxide poisoning.

Bundle up on Windy, Cold Days

A heavy wind can quickly lower your body temperature. Check the weather forecast for windy and cold days. On those days, try to stay inside or in a warm place. If you have to go out, wear warm clothes, and don't stay out in the cold and wind for a long time.

Here are some other tips:

- Dress for the weather if you have to go out on chilly, cold, or damp days.

- Wear loose layers of clothing. The air between the layers helps to keep you warm.

- Put on a hat and scarf. You lose a lot of body heat when your head and neck are uncovered.

- Wear a waterproof coat or jacket if it's snowy.

Illness, Medicines, and Cold Weather

Some illnesses may make it harder for your body to stay warm. Diabetes, thyroid problems, Parkinson disease, memory loss, and arthritis are problems that can make it harder for older adults to stay warm. Talk with your doctor about your health problems and how to prevent hypothermia.

Taking some medicines and not being active also can affect body heat. These include medicines you get from your doctor and those you buy over-the-counter. Ask your doctor if the medicines you take may affect body heat. Always talk with your doctor before you stop taking any medication.

Here are some topics to talk about with your doctor to stay safe in cold weather:

- Ask your doctor about signs of hypothermia.

- Talk to your doctor about any health problems and medicines that can make hypothermia a special problem for you. Your doctor can help you find ways to prevent hypothermia.

- Ask about safe ways to stay active even when it's cold outside.

What Are the Warning Signs of Hypothermia?

Sometimes it is hard to tell if a person has hypothermia. Look for clues. Is the house very cold? Is the person not dressed for cold weather? Is the person speaking slower than normal and having trouble keeping his or her balance?

Watch for the signs of hypothermia in yourself, too. You might become confused if your body temperature gets very low. Talk to your family and friends about the warning signs so they can look out for you.

Early signs of hypothermia:

- Cold feet and hands

- Puffy or swollen face

- Pale skin

- Shivering (in some cases the person with hypothermia does not shiver)

- Slower than normal speech or slurring words

- Acting sleepy

- Being angry or confused

Later signs of hypothermia:

- Moving slowly, trouble walking, or being clumsy

- Stiff and jerky arm or leg movements

- Slow heartbeat

- Slow, shallow breathing

- Blacking out or losing consciousness

Call 911 right away if you think someone has warning signs of hypothermia.

What to do after you call 911:

- Try to move the person to a warmer place.

- Wrap the person in a warm blanket, towels, or coats—whatever is handy. Even your own body warmth will help. Lie close, but be gentle.

- Give the person something warm to drink, but avoid drinks with alcohol or caffeine, such as regular coffee.

- Do not rub the person's legs or arms.

- Do not try to warm the person in a bath.

- Do not use a heating pad.

Hypothermia and the Emergency Room

The only way to tell for sure that someone has hypothermia is to use a special thermometer that can read very low body temperatures. Most hospitals have these thermometers. In the emergency room, doctors will warm the person's body from inside out. For example, they may give the person warm fluids directly by using an intravenous (IV). Recovery depends on how long the person was exposed to the cold and his or her general health.

Is There Help for My Heating Bills?

If you are having a hard time paying your heating bills, there are some resources that might help. Contact the National Energy Assistance Referral service at 1-866-674-6327 (toll-free; TTY, 1-866-367-6228) or email energyassistance@ncat.org to get information about the Low Income Home Energy Assistance Program.

If your home doesn't have enough insulation, contact your state or local energy agency or the local power or gas company. They may be able to give you information about weatherizing your home. This can help keep heating bills down. These agencies and companies may also have special programs for people who have a limited income and qualify for help paying the heating bill. Your local Area Agency on Aging, senior center, or social service agency may have information on these programs.

Chapter 36

Caregiver Stress

What Is a Caregiver?

A caregiver is anyone who provides care for another person in need, such as a child, an aging parent, a husband or wife, a relative, friend, or neighbor. A caregiver also may be a paid professional who provides care in the home or at a place that is not the person's home.

People who are not paid to give care are called informal caregivers or family caregivers. This chapter focuses on family caregivers who provide care on a regular basis for a loved one with an injury, an illness such as dementia, or a disability. The family caregiver often has to manage the person's daily life. This can include helping with daily tasks like bathing, eating, or taking medicine. It can also include arranging activities and making health and financial decisions.

Who Are Caregivers?

Most Americans will be informal caregivers at some point during their lives. A 2012 survey found that 36 percent of Americans provided unpaid care to another adult with an illness or disability in the past year. That percentage is expected to go up as the proportion of people in the United States who are elderly increases. Also, changes in healthcare mean family caregivers now provide more home-based

This chapter includes text excerpted from "Caregiver Stress," Office on Women's Health (OWH), U.S. Department of Health and Human Services (HHS), January 25, 2015.

medical care. Nearly half of family caregivers in the survey said they give injections or manage medicines daily.

Also, most caregivers are women. And nearly three in five family caregivers have paid jobs in addition to their caregiving.

What Is Caregiver Stress?

Caregiver stress is due to the emotional and physical strain of caregiving. Caregivers report much higher levels of stress than people who are not caregivers. Many caregivers are providing help or are "on call" almost all day. Sometimes, this means there is little time for work or other family members or friends. Some caregivers may feel overwhelmed by the amount of care their aging, sick or disabled family member needs.

Although caregiving can be very challenging, it also has its rewards. It feels good to be able to care for a loved one. Spending time together can give new meaning to your relationship.

Remember that you need to take care of yourself to be able to care for your loved one.

Who Gets Caregiver Stress?

Anyone can get caregiver stress, but more women caregivers say they have stress and other health problems than men caregivers. And some women have a higher risk for health problems from caregiver stress, including those who:

- **Care for a loved one who needs constant medical care and supervision.** Caregivers of people with Alzheimer disease or dementia are more likely to have health problems and to be depressed than caregivers of people with conditions that do not require constant care.

- **Care for a spouse.** Women who are caregivers of spouses are more likely to have high blood pressure, diabetes, and high cholesterol and are twice as likely to have heart disease as women who provide care for others, such as parents or children.

Women caregivers also may be less likely to get regular screenings, and they may not get enough sleep or regular physical activity.

What Are the Signs and Symptoms of Caregiver Stress?

Caregiver stress can take many forms. For instance, you may feel frustrated and angry one minute and helpless the next. You may make mistakes when giving medicines. Or you may turn to unhealthy behaviors like smoking or drinking too much alcohol.

Other signs and symptoms include:

- Feeling overwhelmed
- Feeling alone, isolated, or deserted by others
- Sleeping too much or too little
- Gaining or losing a lot of weight
- Feeling tired most of the time
- Losing interest in activities you used to enjoy
- Becoming easily irritated or angered
- Feeling worried or sad often
- Having headaches or body aches often

Talk to your doctor about your symptoms and ways to relieve stress. Also, let others give you a break. Reach out to family, friends, or a local resource.

How Does Caregiver Stress Affect My Health?

Some stress can be good for you, as it helps you cope and respond to a change or challenge. But long-term stress of any kind, including caregiver stress, can lead to serious health problems.

Some of the ways stress affects caregivers include:

- **Depression and anxiety.** Women who are caregivers are more likely than men to develop symptoms of anxiety and depression. Anxiety and depression also raise your risk for other health problems, such as heart disease and stroke.

- **Weak immune system.** Stressed caregivers may have weaker immune systems than noncaregivers and spend more days sick with the cold or flu. A weak immune system can also make vaccines such as flu shots less effective. Also, it may take longer to recover from surgery.

- **Obesity.** Stress causes weight gain in more women than men. Obesity raises your risk for other health problems, including heart disease, stroke, and diabetes.

- **Higher risk for chronic diseases.** High levels of stress, especially when combined with depression, can raise your risk for

465

health problems, such as heart disease, cancer, diabetes, or arthritis.

- **Problems with short-term memory or paying attention.** Caregivers of spouses with Alzheimer disease are at higher risk for problems with short-term memory and focusing.

Caregivers also report symptoms of stress more often than people who are not caregivers.

What Can I Do to Prevent or Relieve Caregiver Stress?

Taking steps to relieve caregiver stress helps prevent health problems. Also, taking care of yourself helps you take better care of your loved one and enjoy the rewards of caregiving.

Here are some tips to help you prevent or manage caregiver stress:

- **Learn ways to better help your loved one.** Some hospitals offer classes that can teach you how to care for someone with an injury or illness. To find these classes, ask your doctor or call your local Area Agency on Aging.

- **Find caregiving resources in your community to help you.** Many communities have adult daycare services or respite services to give primary caregivers a break from their caregiving duties.

- **Ask for and accept help.** Make a list of ways others can help you. Let helpers choose what they would like to do. For instance, someone might sit with the person you care for while you do an errand. Someone else might pick up groceries for you.

- **Join a support group for caregivers.** You can find a general caregiver support group or a group with caregivers who care for someone with the same illness or disability as your loved one. You can share stories, pick up caregiving tips, and get support from others who face the same challenges as you do.

- **Get organized.** Make to-do lists, and set a daily routine.

- **Take time for yourself.** Stay in touch with family and friends, and do things you enjoy with your loved ones.

- **Take care of your health.** Find time to be physically active on most days of the week, choose healthy foods, and get enough sleep.

- **See your doctor for regular checkups.** Make sure to tell your doctor or nurse you are a caregiver. Also, tell her about any symptoms of depression or sickness you may have.

If you work outside the home and are feeling overwhelmed, consider taking a break from your job. Under the federal Family and Medical Leave Act, eligible employees can take up to 12 weeks of unpaid leave per year to care for relatives. Ask your human resources office about your options.

What Caregiving Services Can I Find in My Community?

Caregiving services include:

- Meal delivery
- Home healthcare services, such as nursing or physical therapy
- Nonmedical home care services, such as housekeeping, cooking, or companionship
- Making changes to your home, such as installing ramps or modified bathtubs
- Legal and financial counseling
- Respite care, which is substitute caregiving (someone comes to your home, or you may take your loved one to an adult day care center or day hospital)

The National Eldercare Locator, a service of the U.S. Administration on Aging (AOA), can help you find caregiving services in your area. You also can contact your local Area Agency on Aging.

How Can I Pay for Home Healthcare and Other Caregiving Services?

Medicare, Medicaid, and private insurance companies will cover some costs of home healthcare. Other costs you will have to pay for yourself.

- If the person who needs care has insurance, check with the person's insurance provider to find out what's included in the plan.
- If the person who needs care has Medicare, find out what home health services are covered.
- If the person who needs care has Medicaid, coverage of home health services vary between states. Check with your state's Medicaid program to learn what the benefits are.

Part Five

Senior Living Options and End-of-Life Care

Chapter 37

Deciding What Living Solution Is Best

Chapter Contents

Section 37.1

Having the Conversation

This section includes text excerpted from "Let's Talk
Starting the Conversation about Health, Legal, Financial and
End-of-Life Issues," Eldercare Locator, U.S. Administration on
Aging (AOA), August 17, 2017.

A national survey by The Conversation Project found that 9 in 10
Americans want to discuss their loved ones' and their own end-of-life
care, but approximately 3 in 10 Americans have actually had these
types of conversations. For older adults, families and close friends
these conversations may be tough to initiate, but they are valuable and
necessary for all involved. This section is meant to help you prepare
for these conversations, offer helpful tips for starting a discussion and
provide a range of topics for your consideration.

Why Is It Important to Have the Conversation with Loved Ones?

Initiating conversations about health, legal, financial and end-of-life
issues may be difficult for you and your loved ones, but having these
conversations will ensure that a plan is created that accurately reflects
your wishes and prepares and engages those who you love. A conversation can provide a shared understanding of what matters most to you
and guide your loved ones if and when they need to make decisions on
your behalf. Planning in advance will save time, energy and money,
allowing everyone to think about what they want for the future.

Preparing for the Conversation

Prior to talking openly with loved ones, it may be useful to gather
your thoughts. Remember:

- Get yourself ready. Think about the conversation.

- It might be useful to write a letter—to yourself, your family or a
friend.

- Consider having a practice conversation with a friend.

- These conversations may reveal that you and your loved ones disagree on some things. **That's okay.** It's important to simply know this, and to continue talking about it now—not during a crisis situation.

Thinking about basic aspects of the conversation may also be helpful. Here are some areas to consider:

- Select a time to talk. Holidays, family get-togethers and other special occasions are all times when family and friends gather together, presenting an opportunity to include many of your loved ones in these conversations.

- Determine the location for the conversation to take place. A location you and your loved ones are comfortable with such as your home, on a walk or at a park.

- Decide who should be involved in the conversation.

- Make a list of the topics that are most important for you to discuss.

Starting the Conversation

To ease everyone in, certain conversation starters can be used, such as sharing a story of someone else's experiences or using a letter or video as a starting point. Here are some additional ways you can break the ice:

- "I need your help with something."

- "I was thinking about what happened to _____ and it made me realize..."

- "I just answered some questions about how I want the end of my life to be. I want you to see my answers and I'm wondering what your answers would be."

- Ask for help with planning the future.

Conversation Reminders:

- Be patient. Some people may need a little more time to think.

- You don't have to steer the conversation; just let it happen.

- Don't judge.

- Nothing is set in stone. You and your loved ones can always change your minds.

- Every attempt at a conversation is valuable.

- This is the first of many conversations—you do not have to cover everything right now.

What to Talk About

There may be a variety of topics you want to address in these conversations. Here is some guidance on possible health, legal, financial and end-of-life considerations. This list doesn't cover everything you may need to think about or discuss, but it offers a good place to start.

Health

Awareness of any health conditions and the location of useful health information will help avoid any confusion or mistakes later on. Some of the useful health documents include:

- List of your doctors and pharmacy contact information

- Medical Records

- Medicare and/or Medicaid Number and Identification Card

- Insurance Policies

- Living Will

- Durable Power of Attorney for healthcare

- List of medications you are taking, dosage and cost

Legal

There are various legal and medical documents where your advance planning wishes can be recorded to ensure they will be honored when needed. Here are some of the steps to consider in advance care planning:

- Appoint a Durable Power of Attorney for property matters, and fully discuss finances and plans with them.

- Determine if a Trust arrangement is useful.

- Create a Will.

- Choose an agent under a Health Care Power of Attorney and fully discuss healthcare expectations and wishes with them and other important people.

- Create a Health Care Advance Directive and note if it only includes a Health Care Power of Attorney or a Living Will, or if it is comprehensive and includes both.

- Talk with your physicians about your wishes and provide them with a copy of the Health Care Advance Directive.

- Place legal, personal and financial papers in an easily found location and share that location with the agent and essential loved ones.

- Identify where legal help can be provided for any planning questions.

After completing the legal tools, it is important to make these tools available. For financial planning tools, such as a durable power of attorney, an agent should have access to an original copy and any legal advice should be followed. For a healthcare advance directive, a copy should be provided to the doctor to place in the medical record. The agent should also have a copy, and should be aware of how to obtain the original document. It is important to continue to review documents and make sure they reflect any changes in circumstances or thinking.

Creating legal documents is only part of what is needed. Just as important, is talking with family and loved ones about what the documents mean and how you want decisions made, if you are unable to make decisions for yourself. The conversation about your wishes is just as important, maybe more important, than the actual legal documents.

Financial

When having legal, health or end-of-life conversations with loved ones, you should also determine and record where critical financials items will be stored to prevent future confusion. Documents should include:

- Birth Certificate

- Credit Cards

- Social Security Card

- Passwords to Online Accounts

- Life Insurance Policy
- List of Assets and Debts
- Long-Term Care Insurance
- List of Household Bills
- Mortgage or Rental Documents and Bills
- Federal and State Tax Returns
- Bank Contact or Financial Planner Contact Information
- Utility Bills
- Car Insurance/Title
- Power of Attorney
- Bank Records

End-of-Life Issues

Here are some considerations when discussing end-of-life care:

- When you think about the last phase of your life, what's most important to you? How would you like this phase to be handled?
- Any particular health concerns.
- Who do you want (or not want) to be involved in your care? Who would you like to make decisions on your behalf if you're not able to? (This person is your healthcare proxy).
- Would you prefer to be actively involved in decisions about your care? Or would you rather have your doctors do what they think is best?
- Who will make decisions on financial and healthcare matters? (They do not have to be the same person).
- Are there any disagreements or family tensions that you're concerned about?
- Acceptable and/or unacceptable medical treatment/care.
- Any important milestones to meet if possible.
- Acceptable and/or unacceptable places to receive care (home, nursing facility, hospital).
- When would it be okay to shift from a focus on curative care to a focus on comfort care alone?

- What affairs should be in order and discussed with loved ones (personal finances, property, relationships)?

Keep the Conversation Going

Every conversation you have will empower you and your loved ones to truly understand each other's wishes. After the first conversation, it is important to write down what was discussed and to continue talking with family and friends when necessary. A way to ensure wishes reflect any changes in thinking following a life change is by **reviewing plans when any of the "5 Ds" occur:**

- Every new *Decade* of life

- After the *Death* of a loved one

- After a *Divorce*

- After any significant *Diagnosis*

- After any significant *Decline* in functioning

Section 37.2

Warning Signs That a Loved One Needs Help

This section includes text excerpted from "10 Warning Signs Your Older Family Member May Need Help," Eldercare Locator, U.S. Administration on Aging (AOA), October 15, 2015.

Changes in physical and cognitive abilities that may occur with age can be difficult to detect—for older adults and their family members, friends, and caregivers. To help in determining when an older adult may need assistance in the home, the Eldercare Locator has compiled this list of 10 warning signs. Any one of the following behaviors may indicate the need to take action. It is also important to inform the older adult's physician of these changes.

1. Changing eating habits, resulting in weight loss, appetite loss, or missed meals.

2. Neglecting personal hygiene, including clothing, body odor, oral health, nails, and skin.

3. Neglecting the home, with a noticeable change in tidiness and/ or sanitation.

4. Exhibiting inappropriate behavior, such as being unusually loud, quiet, paranoid, or agitated, or making phone calls at unusual hours.

5. Changing relationship patterns, causing friends and neighbors to express concern.

6. Showing physical injuries, such as burns, which may have resulted from general weakness, forgetfulness, or misuse of alcohol or medication.

7. Decreasing or stopping participation in activities that were once enjoyable, such as a bridge or book club, dining with friends, or attending religious services.

8. Exhibiting forgetfulness, resulting in unopened mail, newspaper piles, unfilled prescriptions, or missed appointments.

9. Mishandling finances, such as not paying bills or paying them more than once and losing or hiding money.

10. Making unusual purchases, such as more than one subscription to the same magazine, entering an unusually large number of contests, or increasing purchases from television advertisements.

Chapter 38

Housing Options for Seniors

One of the most important decisions older adults make is their choice of housing. Their future contentment, comfort and even safety may depend on careful consideration of all the housing options available to them. Fortunately, an array of housing options and living arrangements can meet the needs of those who are aging. Understanding what the options are and the needs they fill is the first step in making a wise choice.

Many will want to stay in a cherished home for as long as possible—but will make some changes to make it safer and more comfortable. Others will seek a group setting, where companionship and planned activities fill the day or where inhome support services may be easier to obtain.

Housing appropriate for one older adult may be completely unacceptable for another. An older person who needs assistance may require a different type of housing than one who can live independently. What's most important is matching, as closely as possible, housing and living arrangements with an older adult's needs and desires.

If you are beginning to think about your options, or need to make a decision in the near future, this chapter can help you. It can increase your understanding of your housing choices—and help you make informed housing decisions. This chapter provides an overview of the many housing options now available. It also discusses key benefits

---

This chapter includes text excerpted from "Housing Options for Older Adults," Eldercare Locator, U.S. Administration on Aging (AOA), August 29, 2017.

and challenges to consider for each housing option and describes the primary legal considerations relevant for each option.

It helps to know beforehand that the terms for housing options for older adults can be very confusing. In some cases, no standard "vocabulary" clearly distinguishes one housing type from another.

An example is the term "assisted living." There is not a standard definition for this term. In some states, where assisted living is not licensed or regulated, the term may be used very loosely. Facilities in these states may not provide the services usually associated with assisted living. In other states, the term is used to describe a specific type of housing option. Those investigating various housing options should make sure they have confirmed all the features and services offered by a provider.

For those considering the housing options covered in this chapter, it is important that they ask themselves these general questions:

- What kind of lifestyle do I want? What will my living conditions be like?

- How important is my choice of location? How close would I like to be to family and friends, doctors, pharmacies, other medical facilities, shopping, senior centers, religious facilities, and other amenities?

- Does my current health status require that I look for features that will help me move about more comfortably?

- How much will the housing option cost?

- What, if any, inhome support services will I receive for my money?

- Am I eligible for any publiclyfunded or subsidized services, such as Medicare or Medicaid?

- What inhome support services are available now, and in the future, to meet my health and social needs?

- Have I involved family members and friends in my decision-making, as appropriate?

- What role will others have in making these decisions?

- Would it be advisable for me to talk with an attorney so that I understand my rights and any legal concerns?

Whatever the housing decision, the best choice is the one that ensures that the older adult's health, social and financial needs are met, and that the older adult's legal rights are protected.

Owning a Home

This housing option needs no explanation. The types of housing available for purchase include single family homes, condominiums, cooperatives and manufactured or mobile homes. When in their own homes, many older adults live independently. Depending on the locality, homeowners may be able to obtain inhome support services and community services to support their continued independence.

Many older adults want to stay in the homes where they have lived for many years. For others, downsizing to a smaller home is an alternative. Active adult communities and retirement communities are increasingly an option. While remaining in one's own home may be highly desirable for older adults, the wisdom of choosing that option depends on making certain that their health, social and financial needs are met.

Benefits: The most significant benefit for many is staying close to family, friends and neighbors. Older adults may relish the comfort and familiarity of their social networks, as well as their neighborhood and community. They may want to continue to attend the same religious services and shop in their favorite local stores. Often older adults are very committed to continuing long-term relationships with physicians in their community. They enjoy the privacy of their home. Those who plan to stay in their home may have made certain that essential health and social services are available, either in their home or community.

Some older adults want a life filled with planned activities that they share with others in their age range. They may pull up stakes and find new companions and many amenities in active adult and retirement communities. These communities offer a variety of housing options for purchase.

And for homeowners, protecting the home as a financial asset can be very important. They may be counting on it as a future financial resource.

Challenges: The challenges to being a homeowner include the responsibility for the home's physical maintenance and upkeep. It may need modifications to make it possible to live in comfortably and safely. For those who have difficulty driving or walking, visiting friends or attending social events may no longer be possible. And homeowners may face a significant financial burden if they have a fixed or limited income.

Personal Considerations—Questions to Ask about Home Ownership

- Is remaining at home a short-term or a long-term plan?

- If I remain at home, how will my social, health and financial needs be met?

- Do I have equity in my home? If so, what are ways to obtain a loan and use it?

- Is house sharing an option to consider?

- Am I eligible for any home repair programs that are completed by volunteers?

- Are there programs available to help me pay for the costs of home repairs, home modifications, home heating expenses, weatherization, utility bills and other expenses of maintaining a home

- Would modifying my home permit me to continue living there? If so, how do I find a qualified remodeler? Is the remodeler I am considering a Certified Aging-in-Place Specialist? Are there volunteers from my local Area Agency on Aging who can help me?

- What universally design products and features should I consider to make my home safer and more comfortable?

- Am I eligible for any property tax relief programs in my state?

- Am I eligible for any inhome support services through federal, state or local programs, such as Medicare or Medicaid?

- Can I use my long-term care insurance policy to pay for in-home support services?

Primary Legal Issues to Understand about Home Ownership

- The uses for reverse mortgage loans. These loans can be used to pay for expenses, such as medical and long-term care needs, and home repairs and modifications.

- The impact that a reverse mortgage loan or the income from house sharing may have on eligibility for public benefits.

- The effect of receiving Medicaid services on the transfer of the title of the home after the homeowner dies.

- The use of a life estate to allow the homeowner to remain in the home if the sale or transfer of the property is being considered.

- The importance of having a will, if a homeowner's wishes are to be followed regarding the person or entity to receive the home after the homeowner's death.

Renting a Home

Renting a home may be an attractive choice. Many housing options are available as rentals, and some offer special services and amenities. Rental options include singlefamily houses, apartments, mobile homes in parks, retirement communities, and apartment complexes specifically designed for adults over 55 years of age. Most rental units are private, although it is possible to pay rent to share a home, or to rent a single room in a home. Rental housing may be publicly or privately-owned, operated or managed.

Benefits: Renters may take advantage of the availability of a range of housing choices. Those who rent are also free of many of the financial and physical responsibilities of being a homeowner. When owners sell their homes prior to renting, they may use the equity to help pay some of their expenses. Some renters may be eligible for either public housing or subsidized housing such as Section 8.

Challenges: Challenges include less independence for tenants, restrictions on pet ownership, and the need to rely on others to make necessary repairs and modifications. Landlords may end their tenants' leases before residents want to move. In some communities, suitable or affordable rental units may not be available.

Personal Considerations—Questions to Ask about Rental Housing

- If I anticipate the need to make physical changes to the unit to make it more accessible, who is responsible for the cost of the modifications?
- Are pets allowed and if not, would it be possible to have a pet if I pay a pet deposit? If a pet deposit policy is in place, is it refundable if there's no damage when I move out?
- Can the landlord object or ask me to move if I receive inhome support services?
- Am I eligible for any inhome support services through federal, state or local programs?
- Can I use my longterm care insurance policy to pay for inhome support services?
- Am I eligible for any state or federal rent subsidy programs?
- Am I eligible for any state rent rebate programs?

Primary Legal Issues to Understand about Renting

- The rights and responsibilities of renters under state landlord/tenant laws and under the federal Fair Housing Act.

- The landlord's duties and obligations under state landlord/tenant laws and under the federal Fair Housing Act.

- The frequency with which the landlord can raise the rent.

- The options if the new amount is unaffordable.

- The question of whether or not a landlord can ask to see medical records before renting a unit.

Living in a Group Setting

Group living arrangements are another housing option very important to many older adults. Group settings provide housing, a range of in-home support services and some social activities. Both the housing and in-home support services are designed to meet the individual needs of those who require help with "activities of daily living" or "instrumental activities of daily living." However, group housing does not offer the level of medical care provided in nursing homes.

- **Activities of Daily Living are activities relating to personal care:**

  - Bathing or showering

  - Dressing

  - Eating

  - Getting in or out of bed or chairs

- **Using the toilet Instrumental Activities of Daily Living are activities related to independent living:**

  - Using the telephone

  - Doing light or heavy housework

  - Preparing meals

  - Shopping for groceries or personal items

  - Managing money

It is very important to determine whether a particular type of group housing is the right match for an individual.

The following are some of the terms used for group housing for older adults. They may refer to very similar group settings—the only difference may be what they are called and how they are licensed in a state.

Board and Care Homes

Board and care homes are private and in residential settings. A board and care home is often a converted or adapted single-family home. This type of home provides the following services: a basic room, which may be shared with another person; meals; help with instrumental activities of daily living; the arrangements for or provision of transportation to medical and other appointments; reminders to take medications; and daily contact with staff. Services such as meals, supervision and transportation are usually handled by the home's owner or manager.

Adult Foster Care Homes

An adult foster care home provides room, board and in-home support services in a family setting. Generally, an adult foster care home provides more in-home support services than a board and care home. These homes may meet the needs of adults who require periodic or regular assistance with activities of daily living. Some adult foster care homes may offer more complex care if the staff has experience and is trained to provide it. In some cases, visiting nurses provide the necessary assistance.

Adult Care Facilities

- Adult care facilities provide room, board and in-home support services to six or more adults who are not related to the operator. Services for residents may be similar to a board and care home or an adult foster care home. Adult care facilities generally have more residents. They are therefore less likely to resemble family life. Adult care facilities may also be called congregate housing.

- These facilities are available for older adults who are no longer able or willing to live completely independently. Generally, residents live in a private apartment and are capable of getting to the communal dining area independently. They usually receive help with grocery shopping, meal preparation and housework.

Residential Care Facilities

A residential care facility is a group residence that provides each resident with, at a minimum, assistance with bathing, dressing, and help with medications on a 24-hour-a-day basis. The facility may also provide medical services under certain circumstances.

Assisted Living Facilities

This term is probably the most confusing. In some states, the term "assisted living" or "assisted living facility" includes all types of group settings that provide some level of in-home support services. In other states, assisted living facilities are specifically licensed and regulated by state law. In these states, assisted living facilities must provide the services and features the state requires.

Assisted living facilities are a housing option for those who need a wide range of in-home support services to help them with activities of daily living. However, residents in these facilities do not require the level of continuous nursing care that a nursing home offers.

People who live in newer assisted living facilities usually have their own private apartment. Private apartments generally are self-contained, with their own bedroom, bathroom, small kitchen and living area. Alternatively, individual living spaces, consisting of a private or semiprivate sleeping area and a shared bathroom, may resemble a dormitory or hotel. There are usually common areas for socializing with other residents.

Continuing Care Retirement Communities (CCRC)

A continuing care retirement community provides a comprehensive, lifetime range of services, to include housing, residential services and nursing care. A person moving into a CCRC is required to sign a contract with the provider which contains information on the services that are available and the costs of those services. All housing is usually part of one campus setting.

- In these housing communities, residents live in the type of housing appropriate for their needs and desires. They can move from one level of care to another, while remaining in the CCRC. For example, a resident could start out living independently in a private individual home or apartment. If daily care becomes necessary, the resident could then move into an assisted living facility. The CCRC's nursing home cares for those who require higher levels of care. CCRC contracts usually require that residents use the CCRC nursing home if the resident needs nursing care. CCRCs generally require a large payment, called an entry fee, before new residents move in. CCRCs also charge a monthly fee.

- These general descriptions of the various group settings portray some of the basic differences between them. Many of these options are available throughout the country. It is not a good idea to rely on advertisements to learn about these various group housing options. It is best to get the most objective information available. What is most important when considering group settings is this: focus not on what it's called but on the type of housing units that are available, the types of services that are provided and the monthly costs.

- **Benefits:** Group housing options offer a wide range of inhome support services, a variety of housing types and the choice of location of facilities. They also give residents opportunities for socializing with others.

- **Challenges:** Group settings may limit privacy. Residents who need more care or supervision may need to obtain additional services or relocate. Some older adults may not be able to afford certain group settings.

Personal Considerations—Questions to Ask about Group Housing

- What is the basic monthly rate and what inhome support services are included in that rate? How many hours of service are included?

- Can I save hours that I do not use during a day or week for a later time when I do need them?

- Is there an entrance fee? Is it refundable?

- Is there a waiting list?

- Am I eligible for any inhome support services through federal, state or local programs?

- Can I use my longterm care insurance policy to pay for inhome support services?

- Can I purchase additional services? If so, what types of services and how many hours a day or week are they available? What would those additional costs be and how would I be billed

- What happens if my needs change or increase?

- Will I be asked to sign an admissions agreement or a contract before I move in? Are there resources available to help me understand the contract?

- Are my utilities included?

- How will I be assigned a room? Can I bring my own furnishings?

- Can I have a pet?

- Will the facility honor my special food and dietary preferences?

- Can I have guests in my unit?

- What is the provider's background and experience? Is the provider financially sound?

- What are the professional qualifications for staff and how many people does each staff person serve?

- What are the training requirements for the facility administrator and for the staff?

- Is the facility close to shopping, senior centers, religious facilities, medical facilities and other amenities that are important to me?

- Do rooms have a telephone and television? How is billing for those handled?

- Does the facility have safety features? Does it have a disaster relief plan?

- What happens if the facility asks me to leave? Have I received a copy of the facility's statement of resident rights?

- Is there a resident council? Can I participate in facility management and decision making?

Primary Legal Issues to Understand about Group Housing

- The terms and conditions of the admissions agreement.

- The terms and conditions of a CCRC contract.

- The standards for quality of care and services, and who is responsible for enforcing and monitoring those standards.

- The rights of those who are abused or neglected.

- A negotiated risk agreement, if asked to sign one.

- The transfer or discharge process and the rights of residents in the process.

- The facility policy for residents who temporarily leave the facility.

- The eviction process and the rights of residents in the process.

Living in a Nursing Home

A nursing home, also known as a long-term care facility, is typically the last option for people who can no longer be cared for at home or in a community-based facility, and who need 24-hour nursing supervision.

Chapter 39

Growing Old at Home

You may share the often-heard wish—"I want to stay in my own home!" The good news is that with the right help you might be able to do just that. Staying in your own home as you get older is called "aging in place." This chapter contains suggestions to help you find the help you need to continue to live independently.

Planning Ahead to Stay in Your Home

Planning ahead is hard because you never know how your needs might change. The first step is to think about the kinds of help you might want in the near future. Maybe you live alone, so there is no one living in your home who is available to help you. Maybe you don't need help right now, but you live with a spouse or family member who does. Everyone has a different situation.

One way to begin planning is to look at any illnesses, like diabetes or emphysema, that you or your spouse might have. Talk with your doctor about how these health problems could make it hard for someone to get around or take care of him- or herself in the future. If you're a caregiver for an older adult, learn how you can get them the support they need to stay in their own home.

This chapter includes text excerpted from "Aging in Place: Growing Old at Home," National Institute on Aging (NIA), National Institutes of Health (NIH), August 16, 2017.

What Support Can Help Me Stay at Home?

You can get almost any type of help you want in your home—often for a cost. You can get more information on many of the services listed here from your local Area Agency on Aging, local and State offices on aging or social services, tribal organization, or nearby senior center.

Personal care. Is bathing, washing your hair, or dressing getting harder to do? Maybe a relative or friend could help. Or, you could hire a trained aide for a short time each day.

Household chores. Do you need help with chores like housecleaning, yard work, grocery shopping, or laundry? Some grocery stores and drug stores will take your order over the phone and bring the items to your home. There are cleaning and yard services you can hire, or maybe someone you know has a housekeeper or gardener to suggest. Some housekeepers will help with laundry. Some drycleaners will pick up and deliver your clothes.

Meals. Worried that you might not be eating nutritious meals or tired of eating alone? Sometimes you could share cooking with a friend or have a potluck dinner with a group of friends. Find out if meals are served at a nearby senior center or house of worship. Eating out may give you a chance to visit with others. Is it hard for you to get out? Ask someone to bring you a healthy meal a few times a week. Meal delivery programs bring hot meals into your home; some of these programs are free or low-cost.

Money management. Do you worry about paying bills late or not at all? Are health insurance forms confusing? Maybe you can get help with these tasks. Ask a trusted relative to lend a hand. Volunteers, financial counselors, or geriatric care managers can also help. Just make sure you get the referral from a trustworthy source, like your local Area Agency on Aging. If you use a computer, you could pay your bills online. Check with your bank about this option. Some people have regular bills, like utilities and rent or mortgage, paid automatically from their checking account.

Be careful to avoid money scams. Never give your Social Security number, bank or credit card numbers, or other sensitive information to someone on the phone (unless you placed the call) or in response to an email. Always check all bills, including utility bills, for charges you do not recognize.

Even though you might not need it now, think about giving someone you trust permission to discuss your bills with creditors or your Social Security or Medicare benefits with those agencies.

Healthcare. Do you forget to take your medicine? There are devices available to remind you when it is time for your next dose. Special pill boxes allow you or someone else to set out your pills for an entire week. Have you just gotten out of the hospital and still need nursing care at home for a short time? The hospital discharge planner can help you make arrangements, and Medicare might pay for a home health aide to come to your home.

If you can't remember what the doctor told you to do, try to have someone go to your doctor visits with you. Ask them to write down everything you are supposed to do or, if you are by yourself, ask the doctor to put all recommendations in writing.

Aging in Place: Common Concerns

If staying in your home is important to you, you may still have concerns about safety, getting around, or other activities of daily life. Find suggestions below to help you think about some of these worries.

Getting around—at home and in town. Are you having trouble walking? Perhaps a walker would help. If you need more, think about getting an electric chair or scooter. These are sometimes covered by Medicare. Do you need someone to go with you to the doctor or shopping? Volunteer escort services may be available. If you are no longer driving a car, find out if there are free or low-cost public transportation and taxis in your area. Maybe a relative, friend, or neighbor would take you along when they go on errands or do yours for you.

Activities and friends. Are you bored staying at home? Your local senior center offers a variety of activities. You might see friends there and meet new people too. Is it hard for you to leave your home? Maybe you would enjoy visits from someone. Volunteers are sometimes available to stop by or call once a week. They can just keep you company, or you can talk about any problems you are having. Call your local Area Agency on Aging to see if they are available near you.

Safety. Are you worried about crime in your neighborhood, physical abuse, or losing money as a result of a scam? Talk to the staff at your local Area Agency on Aging. If you live alone, are you afraid of becoming sick with no one around to help? You might want to get an emergency alert system. You just push a special button that you wear, and emergency medical personnel are called. There is typically a monthly fee for this service.

Housing. Would a few changes make your home easier and safer to live in? Think about things like a ramp at the front door, grab bars in the tub or shower, nonskid floors, more comfortable handles on doors or faucets, and better insulation. Sound expensive? You might be able to get help paying for these changes. Check with your local Area Agency on Aging, State housing finance agency, welfare department, community development groups, or the Federal Government.

Help during the day. Do you need care but live with someone who can't stay with you during the day? For example, maybe they work. Adult day care outside the home is sometimes available for older people who need help caring for themselves. The day care center can pick you up and bring you home. If your caretaker needs to get away overnight, there are places that provide temporary respite care.

Where Can I Look for Help Staying at Home?

Here are some resources to start with:

People you know. Family, friends, and neighbors are the biggest source of help for many older people. Talk with those close to you about the best way to get what you need. If you are physically able, think about trading services with a friend or neighbor. One could do the grocery shopping, and the other could cook dinner, for example.

Community and local government resources. Learn about the services in your community. Healthcare providers and social workers may have suggestions. The local Area Agency on Aging, local and State offices on aging or social services, and your tribal organization may have lists of services. If you belong to a religious group, talk with the clergy, or check with its local office about any senior services they offer.

Geriatric care managers. These specially trained professionals can help find resources to make your daily life easier. They will work with you to form a long-term care plan and find the services you need. Geriatric care managers can be helpful when family members live far apart.

Federal Government sources. The Federal Government offers many resources for seniors. Longtermcare.gov, from the Administration for Community Living, is a good place to start.

How Much Will It Cost to Get Help at Home?

An important part of planning is thinking about how you are going to pay for the help you need. Some things you want may cost a lot. Others may be free. Some might be covered by Medicare or other health insurance. Some may not. Check with your insurance provider(s). It's possible that paying for a few services out of pocket could cost less than moving into an independent living, assisted living, or long-term care facility. And you will have your wish of still living on your own. Resources like Benefits.gov and BenefitsCheckUp can help you find out about possible benefits you might qualify for.

Are you eligible for benefits from the U.S. Department of Veterans Affairs (VA)? The VA sometimes provides medical care in your home. In some areas, they offer homemaker/ home health aide services, adult day healthcare, and hospice.

Be Prepared for a Medical Emergency

If you were to suddenly become sick and unable to speak for yourself, you probably would want someone who knows you well to decide on your medical care. To make sure this happens, think about giving someone you trust permission to discuss your healthcare with your doctor and make necessary decisions. Talk with your doctor about whether you should get a medical alert ID bracelet or necklace.

Chapter 40

Home Improvement Assistance

Home improvements, modifications, and repairs can help older adults maintain their independence and prevent accidents. Work can range from simple changes, like replacing doorknobs with pull handles, to major structural projects such as installing a wheelchair ramp.

Changes can improve the accessibility, adaptability, and/or universal design of a home. Improving accessibility involves things like widening doorways and lowering countertop and light switch heights for someone who uses a wheelchair. Changes that do not require home redesign, such as installing grab bars in bathrooms, are adaptability features. Universal design is usually built in when a home is constructed. It includes features that are sturdy and reliable, easy for all people to use, and flexible enough to be adapted for special needs.

Evaluating Your Needs

Before any changes are made to the home, evaluate your current and future needs room by room. Once you have explored all areas, make a list of potential problems and solutions.

This chapter includes text excerpted from "Home Improvement Assistance," Eldercare Locator, U.S. Administration on Aging (AOA), July 10, 2017.

Financial Assistance

Minor improvements and repairs can cost between $150 and $2,000. Many home remodeling contractors offer reduced rates or sliding-scale fees based on income and ability to pay. Public and private financing options may also be available. Sources of support include the following.

- Modification and repair funds provided by the Older Americans Act are distributed by Area Agencies on Aging (AAA).

- Rebuilding Together, Inc., a national volunteer organization, is able to assist some low-income seniors through its local affiliates.

- Local energy and social service departments can assist through the U.S. Department of Energy's Low-Income Home Energy Assistance Program (LIHEAP) and Weatherization Assistance Program (WAP).

- Many cities and towns make grant funds available through their local departments of community development.

- Lenders may offer home equity conversion mortgages or reverse mortgages that allow homeowners to utilize home equity to pay for improvements.

Hiring a Contractor

For some repairs and improvements, you may choose to hire a professional contractor without a public assistance program. In that case, keep these important tips in mind.

- Make sure the contractor is licensed, bonded, and insured for the specific type of work.

- Check with your local Better Business Bureau and Chamber of Commerce to see whether any complaints against the contractor are on file.

- Talk with family and friends to get recommendations based on their experiences. Contractors with good reputations can usually be counted on to do a good job again.

- Ask for a written agreement that specifies the exact tasks and timeline.

- Your agreement should outline the total estimated cost and require only a small down payment. The terms should require balance payment when the job is completed.

- Consider asking a trusted friend or family member to help you review the contract and/or monitor work throughout the project.

Chapter 41

Independence and Mobility

Have you ever thought about what would happen if the transportation you use is no longer an option? How would you continue to maintain your independence so that you could continue with your daily routines? Who would you turn to for assistance? People often look to friends or relatives to assist with transportation—this may be a good option for you, but it is not always the most convenient for you or for them.

Thinking ahead to alternative transportation options can give you peace of mind should your current means of getting around in your community change in the future. This chapter will assist you to learn about various alternative transportation options and some things to consider to help you make confident decisions about which option would be best for you.

Keep in mind that not all types of transportation are available in every community. Several aging organizations can assist you in learning about the options in your community, such as your local Area Agency on Aging (AAA), Aging and Disability Resource Center (ADRC), and Indian Tribal Organization. Contact the Eldercare Locator at 800-677-1116 or www.eldercare.gov to identify these resources in your area.

This chapter contains text excerpted from the following sources: Text in this chapter begins with excerpts from "Choices for Mobility Independence," Eldercare Locator, U.S. Administration on Aging (AOA), November 28, 2007. Reviewed September 2017; Text under the heading "Older Drivers" is excerpted from "Older Drivers," National Institute on Aging (NIA), National Institutes of Health (NIH), August 7, 2017.

Transportation Options

Depending upon your destination and physical needs, transportation choices in your area might include buses, vans, taxis, or even volunteer drivers from human service organizations. Listed below are descriptions of transportation resources and services for you to think about and explore as you look ahead:

- **Volunteer Driver Programs:** Local faith-based and nonprofit organizations frequently have a network of volunteers who offer flexible transportation for shopping, doctors' appointments, recreation, and other activities. One-way, round-trip, and multi-stop rides are usually available; reservations are needed. These programs are provided free, on a donation basis, through membership dues, or for a minimal cost.

- **Paratransit Service:** Public transit, aging organizations, and private agencies provide door-to-door or curb-to-curb transportation using mini-buses or small vans (vehicles for less than 25 passengers). Paratransit service often requires users to make advanced reservations but still offers a degree of flexibility and personalization in scheduling. Curb-to-curb service provides for passenger pickup and delivery at the curb or roadside; door-to-door service offers a higher level of assistance by picking up passengers at the door of their homes and delivering them to the doors of their destinations. Paratransit and van services offer reduced fares for older adults and persons with disabilities, and some providers may operate on a donation basis.

- **Door-through-Door (Escort) Service:** Agencies provide drivers or escorts who offer personal, hands-on assistance by helping passengers through the doors of their residences and destinations, as needed. This type of service includes several levels of assistance from opening doors and providing verbal guidance, to physical support. Persons with severe physical or mental disabilities typically use this service. Contact your local aging organizations to find out if this service is available in your area.

- **Public Transit/Fixed Route Service:** Public transit agencies provide bus and rail services along established routes with set schedules on a nonreservation basis—also referred to as "public transportation" or "mass transit." Reduced rate fares and additional transportation services are available for older adults and persons with disabilities. Information about routes, schedules, fares, and special services are available through your public transit agency.

- **Travel Training:** Public transit agencies and local aging organizations provide free, hands-on instruction to help older adults and persons with disabilities learn to travel safely and independently within public transit systems. Topics discussed include the best routes to take to reach various destinations, hours of service, the cost of the trip (including available discounts), and how to pay for services (such as fare cards or tokens). Demonstrations on how to ride public buses and trains also are provided.

- **Taxi Service:** Passengers activate this service by calling a dispatcher to request a ride between locations of their choice. Trips usually can be scheduled in advance or on the spot. Some taxis are wheelchair accessible and meet ADA standards; inquire with your local taxi providers. Fares are charged on a per-mile or per-minute basis on top of a base charge for each trip, and may be payable through a transportation voucher program.

- **Transportation Vouchers Programs:** Area Agencies on Aging (AAA), Aging and Disability Resource Centers (ADRC), and other social service organizations often provide fare assistance programs that enable qualified persons (usually economically disadvantaged older adults or persons with disabilities) to purchase vouchers for transportation services at a reduced rate. The vouchers are then used to pay for services from a participating transportation provider that can include public transportation, volunteer programs, or taxis and other private companies. Applications for these programs are required. Participants are responsible for reserving and securing the services they need.

In addition to the services described above, some communities have mobility managers who can guide you through the transportation resources and services that are available. Mobility managers know the community-wide transportation service network and understand how it operates. Their main focus is to assist consumers in choosing the best options to meet their individual travel needs. Contact your local aging organization or public transit agency to determine if a mobility manager is available in your area.

Key Considerations

Depending upon your lifestyle, one or more transportation options can keep you connected to all of your activities. Evaluate what your transportation needs are now or might be in the future—including necessary as well as social activities. When investigating transportation options, there are a few things to consider in order to make a confident decision about which options are best for you. Consider the following questions based on type of transportation provider:

Eligibility

- What, if any, requirements are there to qualify for the service?
- Is any evaluation needed prior to using the service?
- Are rides provided for wheelchair users or other persons with disabilities?
- If needed, can a family member serve as an escort?

Affordability

- What is the cost of the service?
- Are discounts available?
- How are costs calculated?
- Is there a membership fee?
- Is my income a factor for using this service?
- Can an account be setup in advance with the service?
- Will my insurance pay for rides by this service provider?

Accessibility

- What is the service area?
- What times does the service operate?
- Are door-through-door, door-to-door, or curb-to-curb services provided?
- Is a reservation needed, and how far in advance?
- Are rides provided in the evenings, on weekends, or on holidays?
- Are rides provided to social as well as medical or shopping appointments?

- Will driver provide assistance with packages and other carry-ons?

- Are vehicles wheelchair accessible?

- If other passengers will be riding at the same time, what is the maximum length of time of the ride while others are being picked up or dropped off?

Older Drivers

Have you been worried about your driving? Have your family or friends expressed concern? Changes in your health may affect your driving skills over time. Don't risk hurting yourself or others. Talk with your doctor about any concerns you have about your health and driving.

Stiff Joints and Muscles

As you age, your joints may get stiff, and your muscles may weaken. Arthritis, which is common among older adults, might affect your ability to drive. These changes can make it harder to turn your head to look back, turn the steering wheel quickly, or brake safely.

Safe driving tips:

- See your doctor if pain, stiffness, or arthritis seem to get in the way of your driving.

- If possible, drive a car with automatic transmission, power steering, power brakes, and large mirrors.

- Be physically active or exercise to keep and even improve your strength and flexibility.

- Think about getting hand controls for both the gas and brake pedals if you have leg problems.

Trouble Seeing

Your eyesight can change as you get older. It might be harder to see people, things, and movement outside your direct line of sight. It may take longer to read street or traffic signs or even recognize familiar places. At night, you may have trouble seeing things clearly. Glare from oncoming headlights or street lights can be a problem. Depending on the time of the day, the sun might be blinding.

Eye diseases, such as glaucoma, cataracts, and macular degeneration, as well as some medicines, can also cause vision problems.
Safe driving tips:

• If you are 65 or older, see your eye doctor at least every 1 to 2 years. Ask if there are ways to improve your eyesight.

• If you need glasses or contact lenses to see far away while driving, make sure your prescription is up-to-date and correct. Always wear them when you are driving.

• Cut back on or stop driving at night if you have trouble seeing in the dark. Try to avoid driving during sunrise and sunset, when the sun can be directly in your line of vision.

Trouble Hearing

As you get older, your hearing can change, making it harder to notice horns, sirens, or even noises coming from your own car. Hearing loss can be a problem because these sounds warn you when you may need to pull over or get out of the way.
Safe driving tips:

• Have your hearing checked at least every 3 years after age 50.

• Discuss concerns you have about hearing with your doctor. There may be things that can help.

• Try to keep the inside of the car as quiet as possible while driving.

Dementia and Driving

In the early stages of Alzheimer disease or other types of dementia, some people are able to keep driving. But, as memory and decision-making skills get worse, they need to stop.

People with dementia often do not know they are having driving problems. Family and friends need to monitor the person's driving ability and take action as soon as they observe a potential problem, such as forgetting how to find familiar places like the grocery store or even their home. Work with the doctor to let the person know it's no longer safe to keep driving.

Slower Reaction Time and Reflexes

As you get older, your reflexes might get slower, and you might not react as quickly as you could in the past. You might find that you have a shorter attention span, making it harder to do two things at once. Stiff joints or weak muscles also can make it harder to move quickly. Loss of feeling or tingling in your fingers and feet can make it difficult to steer or use the foot pedals. Parkinson disease or limitations following a stroke can make it no longer safe to drive.

Safe driving tips:

- Leave more space between you and the car in front of you.

- Start braking early when you need to stop.

- Avoid heavy traffic areas or rush-hour driving when you can.

- If you must drive on a fast-moving highway, drive in the right-hand lane. Traffic moves more slowly there, giving you more time to make safe driving decisions.

Medications Can Affect Driving

Do you take any medicines that make you feel drowsy, lightheaded, or less alert than usual? Do medicines you take have a warning about driving? Many medications have side effects that can make driving unsafe. Pay attention to how these drugs may affect your driving.

Safe driving tips:

- Read medicine labels carefully. Look for any warnings.

- Make a list of all of your medicines, and talk with your doctor or pharmacist about how they can affect your driving.

- Don't drive if you feel lightheaded or drowsy.

Be a Safe Driver

Maybe you already know that driving at night, on the highway, or in bad weather is a problem for you. Some older drivers also have problems when yielding the right of way, turning (especially making left turns), changing lanes, passing, and using expressway ramps.

Safe driving tips:

- Have your driving skills checked by a driving rehabilitation specialist, occupational therapist, or other trained professional.

- Take a defensive driving course. Some car insurance companies may lower your bill when you pass this type of class. Organizations like AARP, American Automobile Association (AAA), or your car insurance company can help you find a class near you.

- When in doubt, don't go out. Bad weather like rain, ice, or snow can make it hard for anyone to drive. Try to wait until the weather is better, or use buses, taxis, or other transportation services.

- Avoid areas where driving can be a problem. For example, choose a route that avoids highways or other high-speed road-ways. Or, find a way to go that requires few or no left turns.

- Ask your doctor if any of your health problems or medications might make it unsafe for you to drive. Together, you can make a plan to help you keep driving and decide when it is no longer safe to drive.

Is It Time to Give Up Driving?

We all age differently. For this reason, there is no way to set one age when everyone should stop driving. So, how do you know if you should stop? To help decide, ask yourself:

- Do other drivers often honk at me?

- Have I had some accidents, even if they were only "fender benders"?

- Do I get lost, even on roads I know?

- Do cars or people walking seem to appear out of nowhere?

- Do I get distracted while driving?

- Have family, friends, or my doctor said they're worried about my driving?

- Am I driving less these days because I'm not as sure about my driving as I used to be?

- Do I have trouble staying in my lane?

- Do I have trouble moving my foot between the gas and the brake pedals, or do I sometimes confuse the two?

- Have I been pulled over by a police officer about my driving?

If you answered "yes" to any of these questions, it may be time to talk with your doctor about driving or have a driving assessment.

How Will You Get Around?

Are you worried you won't be able to do the things you want and need to do if you stop driving? Many people have this concern, but there may be more ways to get around than you think. For example, some areas provide free or low-cost bus or taxi services for older people. Some communities offer a carpool service or scheduled trips to the grocery store, mall, or doctor's office. Religious and civic groups sometimes have volunteers who will drive you where you want to go.

Your local Area Agency on Aging can help you find services in your area. Call 1-800-677-1116, or go to www.eldercare.gov to find your nearest Area Agency on Aging.

You can also think about using a car service. Sound pricey? Don't forget—it costs a lot to own a car. If you don't have to make car payments or pay for insurance, maintenance, gas, oil, or other car expenses, then you may be able to afford to take taxis or other public transportation. You can also buy gas for friends or family members who give you rides.

More Safe Driving Tips

Before you leave home:

- Plan to drive on streets you know.

- Only drive to places that are easy to get to and close to home.

- Avoid risky spots like ramps and left turns.

- Add extra time for travel if you must drive when conditions are poor.

- Limit how much you drive at night.

- Don't drive when you are stressed or tired.

While you are driving:

- Always wear your seat-belt and make sure your passengers wear their seat belts, too.

- Wear your glasses and/or hearing aid, if you use them.

- Stay off your cell phone.

- Avoid distractions such as eating, listening to the radio, or chatting.

- Use your window defrosters to keep both the front and back windows clear.

Chapter 42

Long-Term Care

What Is Long-Term Care?

Long-term care involves a variety of services designed to meet a person's health or personal care needs during a short or long period of time. These services help people live as independently and safely as possible when they can no longer perform everyday activities on their own.

Long-term care is provided in different places by different caregivers, depending on a person's needs. Most long-term care is provided at home by unpaid family members and friends. It can also be given in a facility such as a nursing home or in the community, for example, in an adult day care center.

The most common type of long-term care is personal care—help with everyday activities, also called "activities of daily living." These activities include bathing, dressing, grooming, using the toilet, eating, and moving around—for example, getting out of bed and into a chair.

Long-term care also includes community services such as meals, adult day care, and transportation services. These services may be provided free or for a fee.

People often need long-term care when they have a serious, ongoing health condition or disability. The need for long-term care can arise

This chapter includes text excerpted from "Long-Term Care—What Is Long-Term Care?" National Institute on Aging (NIA), National Institutes of Health (NIH), August 16, 2017.

suddenly, such as after a heart attack or stroke. Most often, however, it develops gradually, as people get older and frailer or as an illness or disability gets worse.

Who Will Need Long-Term Care?

It is difficult to predict how much or what type of long-term care a person might need. Several things increase the risk of needing long-term care.

- **Age.** The risk generally increases as people get older.
- **Gender.** Women are at higher risk than men, primarily because they often live longer.
- **Marital status.** Single people are more likely than married people to need care from a paid provider.
- **Lifestyle.** Poor diet and exercise habits can increase a person's risk.
- **Health and family history.** These factors also affect risk.

Home-Based Long-Term Care Services

Home-based long-term care includes health, personal, and support services to help people stay at home and live as independently as possible. Most long-term care is provided either in the home of the person receiving services or at a family member's home. In-home services may be short term—for someone who is recovering from an operation, for example—or long term, for people who need ongoing help.

Most home-based services involve personal care, such as help with bathing, dressing, and taking medications, and supervision to make sure a person is safe. Unpaid family members, partners, friends, and neighbors provide most of this type of care.

Home-based long-term care services can also be provided by paid caregivers, including caregivers found informally, and healthcare professionals such as nurses, home healthcare aides, therapists, and homemakers, who are hired through home healthcare agencies. These services include: home healthcare, homemaker services, friendly visitor/companion services, and emergency response systems.

Home Healthcare

Home healthcare involves part-time medical services ordered by a physician for a specific condition. These services may include nursing care to help a person recover from surgery, an accident, or illness. Home healthcare may also include physical, occupational, or speech therapy and temporary home health aide services. These services are provided by home healthcare agencies approved by Medicare, a government insurance program for people over age 65.

Homemaker Services

Home health agencies offer personal care and homemaker services that can be purchased without a physician's order. Personal care includes help with bathing and dressing. Homemaker services include help with meal preparation and household chores. Agencies do not have to be approved by Medicare to provide these kinds of services.

Friendly Visitor / Companion Services

Friendly visitor/companion services are usually staffed by volunteers who regularly pay short visits (less than 2 hours) to someone who is frail or living alone. You can also purchase these services from home health agencies.

Transportation Services

Transportation services help people get to and from medical appointments, shopping centers, and other places in the community. Some senior housing complexes and community groups offer transportation services. Many public transit agencies have services for people with disabilities. Some services are free. Others charge a fee.

Emergency Response Systems

Emergency response systems automatically respond to medical and other emergencies via electronic monitors. The user wears a necklace or bracelet with a button to push in an emergency. Pushing the button summons emergency help to the home. This type of service is especially useful for people who live alone or are at risk of falling. A monthly fee is charged.

Chapter 43

Choosing a Nursing Home or Other Long-Term Care

Chapter Contents

Section 43.1

How to Decide

This section includes text excerpted from "Your Guide to Choosing a
Nursing Home or Other Long-Term Services & Supports," Centers
for Medicare and Medicaid Services (CMS), May 2017.

People go to nursing homes for different reasons, including if they're
sick, hurt, had surgery and need to get better, or have chronic care
needs or disabilities that require on-going nursing care.

Before You Get Started

You may have other long-term care options, like community services, home care, or assisted living, depending on your needs and
resources. Before choosing a nursing home, you can check to see if one
of these other options is available to you, or if they might help after a
nursing home stay.

If You Have Medicare

Medicare covers short-term nursing home stays following hospitalization, but generally doesn't cover long-term care or stays in a nursing
home. Medicare coverage of home- and community-based long-term
care services is very limited.

If You Have Medicaid

Medicaid may cover long-term nursing home stays, and home- and
community-based services. Home- and community-based services provide opportunities for people with Medicaid to get services in their own
home or community, rather than in a specialized facility. These programs serve a variety of groups, including people with mental illnesses,
intellectual or developmental disabilities, and/or physical disabilities.

What Is Nursing Home Care?

Medicare Part A (Hospital Insurance) may cover care in a certified
skilled nursing facility (SNF) if it's medically necessary for you to have

skilled nursing care (like changing sterile dressings). However, most nursing home care is custodial care, like help with bathing or dressing. Medicare doesn't cover custodial care if that's the only care you need.

Your Care Plan

Once you've selected a nursing home and are a resident, the nursing home staff will get your health information and review your health condition to prepare your care plan. You (if you're able), your family (with your permission), or someone acting on your behalf has the right to take part in planning your care with the nursing home staff. **The basic care plan includes:**

- A health assessment (a review of your health condition) that begins on the day you're admitted, and must be completed within 14 days of admission.

- A health assessment at least every 90 days after your first review, and possibly more often if your medical status changes.

- Ongoing, regular assessments of your condition to see if your health status has changed, with adjustments to your care plan as needed.

Nursing homes are required to submit this information to the federal government. Your health assessment information is used to make sure you get quality care, to determine nursing home payment, and as part of state inspections.

Depending on your needs, your care plan may include:

- What kind of personal or healthcare services you need.
- What type of staff should give you these services
- How often you need the services.
- What kind of equipment or supplies you need (like a wheelchair or feeding tube).

Depending on your needs, your care plan may include:

- What kind of diet you need (if you need a special one) and your food preferences.
- How your care plan will help you reach your goals.
- Information on whether you plan on returning to the community and, if so, a plan to help you meet that goal.

Your Resident Rights and Protections

As a resident in a Medicare- and/or Medicaid-certified nursing home, you have certain rights and protections under federal and state law to make sure you get the care and services you need. You have the right to be informed, make your own decisions, and have your personal information kept private.

The nursing home must tell you about these rights and explain them to you in writing in a language you understand. They must also explain in writing how you should act and what you're responsible for while you're in the nursing home. This must be done before or at the time you're admitted, as well as during your stay. You must acknowledge in writing that you got this information.

Here is a brief list of some of your rights.

You have the right to:

- Be free from discrimination.

- Be free from abuse and neglect.

- Exercise your rights as a U.S. citizen.

- Have your representative notified.

- Get proper medical care.

- Be treated with respect.

- Be free from restraints.

- Have protections against involuntary transfer or discharge.

- Participate in activities.

- Spend time with visitors.

- Form or participate in resident groups.

- Manage your money.

- Get information on services and fees.

- Get proper privacy, property, and living arrangements.

- Make complaints.

How Do I Choose a Nursing Home?

Follow these 4 steps to find the nursing home that best meets your needs:

Step 1: Find nursing homes in your area.

Step 2: Compare the quality of the nursing homes you're considering.

Step 3: Visit the nursing homes you're interested in, or have someone visit for you.

Step 4: Choose the nursing home that best meets your needs.

Step 1: Find Nursing Homes in Your Area

There are many ways you can learn about nursing homes in your area:

- Ask people you trust, like your family, friends, or neighbors, if they've had personal experience with nursing homes. They may be able to recommend a nursing home to you.

- Ask your doctor if he or she provides care at any local nursing homes. If so, ask your doctor which nursing homes he or she visits, so you can continue to get care from him or her while you're in the nursing home.

- Contact your local senior and community activity center.

- If you're in the hospital, ask your social worker about discharge planning as early in your hospital stay as possible. The hospital's staff should be able to help you find a nursing home that meets your needs and help with your transfer when you're ready to be discharged.

Step 2: Compare the Quality of the Nursing Homes You're Considering

Medicare's Nursing Home Compare

Visit Medicare.gov/nursinghomecompare to get information on the quality of every Medicare- and Medicaid-certified nursing home in the country. Consider the information you find on Nursing Home Compare carefully. Use it, along with the other information you gather, to help guide your decision.

Step 3: Visit the Nursing Homes You're Interested In, or Have Someone You Trust Visit for You

After you consider what's important to you in a nursing home, visit the nursing homes. It's best to visit the nursing homes that interest you before you make a final decision on which one meets your needs.

A visit gives you the chance to see the residents, staff, and the nursing home setting. It also allows you to ask questions of the nursing home staff and talk with residents and their family members.

If you can't visit the nursing home yourself, you may want to get a family member or friend to visit for you. You can also call for information, however, a visit can help you see the quality of care and life of the actual residents.

Important things to know when visiting nursing homes

- Before you go, call and make an appointment to meet with someone on the staff. You're also encouraged to visit the nursing homes at other times without an appointment.

- Don't be afraid to ask questions.

- Ask the staff to explain anything you see and hear that you don't understand. For example, if you hear a person calling out, it may be because they're confused, not because they're being hurt or neglected.

- Ask who to call if you have further questions, and write down their name and phone number.

- If a resident or a resident's family wishes, you may talk to them about the care offered at the facility and their experience.

- Don't go into resident rooms or care areas without asking the resident and nursing home staff first. Always knock first and ask a resident before entering their room.

- Residents have a right to privacy and can refuse to allow you to come into their rooms.

- After your visit, write down any questions you still have about the nursing home or how the nursing home will meet your needs.

Here are some general things to consider when you visit a nursing home:

- Does the nursing home allow you to participate in social, recreational, religious, or cultural activities that are important to you?

- Is transportation provided to community activities?

- Does the nursing home offer private spaces for when you have visitors?

- Who are the doctors who will care for you? Can you still see your personal doctors? If your personal doctors don't visit the nursing home, who will help you arrange transportation if you choose to continue to see them?

- What does the quality of care and staffing information on Nursing Home Compare at Medicare.gov/nursinghomecompare show about how well this nursing home cares for its residents?

- Will the same nursing home staff take care of you day to day or do they change?

- How many residents is a Certified Nursing Assistant (CNA) assigned to work with during each shift (day and night) and during meals?

- What type of therapy is available at this facility? Are therapy staff available?

- What types of meals does the nursing home serve? (**Note:** Ask the nursing home if you can see a menu.)

- Can you get food and drinks you like at any time? What if you don't like the food that's served?

- Does the nursing home make sure residents get preventive care to help keep them healthy? Are specialists like eye doctors, ear doctors, dentists, and podiatrists (foot doctors) available to see residents on a regular basis? Does the facility help make arrangements to see these specialists? (**Note:** Nursing homes must either provide treatment, or help you make appointments and provide transportation for you to see specialists.)

- Does the nursing home have a screening program for vaccinations, like flu (influenza) and pneumonia? (**Note:** Nursing homes are required to provide flu shots each year, but you have the right to refuse if you don't want the shot, have already been immunized during the immunization period, or if the shots are medically contraindicated.)

- How will you get access to oral care in the nursing home?

- How will you get access to mental healthcare in the nursing home?

- What is the nursing home's policy for the use of antipsychotic medication in dementia patients?

Step 4: Choose the Nursing Home That Meets Your Needs

When you have all the information that's important to you about the nursing homes you're considering, talk with people who understand your personal and healthcare needs. This can include your family, friends, doctor, clergy, spiritual advisor, hospital discharge planner, or social worker.

What If More than One Nursing Home Meets My Needs?

If you find more than one nursing home you like with a bed available, use the information you got to compare them. Trust your senses. If you don't like what you saw on a visit (for example, if the facility wasn't clean or you weren't comfortable talking with the nursing home staff), you may want to choose another nursing home. If you felt that the residents were treated well, the facility was clean, and the staff was helpful, you might feel better about choosing that nursing home.

What If I'm Helping Someone Make a Decision?

If you're helping someone, keep the person you're helping involved in the decision making process as much as possible. People who are involved from the beginning are better prepared when they move into a nursing home. If the person you're helping isn't alert or able to communicate well, keep his or her values and preferences in mind.

What If I Don't like a Nursing Home I Visit?

If you visit a nursing home that you don't like, look at other options, if available. Your happiness and the quality of your care is important.

What If I'm in the Hospital and Don't like the Nursing Home That Has an Available Bed?

If you're in a hospital and decide not to go to a certain nursing home that has an available bed, talk to the hospital discharge planner or your doctor. They may be able to help you find a more suitable nursing home or arrange for other care, like short-term home care, until a bed is available at another nursing home you choose. However, you may be responsible for paying the bill for any additional days you stay in the hospital.

What If I Don't like a Nursing Home I'm Currently In?

If you don't like the nursing home you're currently living in, you can move to another facility with an available bed. Moving can be difficult, but an extra move may be better for you than choosing to stay at a facility that isn't right for you.

The nursing home you leave may require that you let them know ahead of time that you're planning to leave. Talk to the nursing home staff about their rules for leaving. If you don't follow the rules for leaving, you may have to pay extra fees.

I've Chosen a Nursing Home. What Should I Do Next?

Make Arrangements to Be Admitted

After you choose a nursing home, you'll need to make arrangements to be admitted. When you contact the nursing home office, it's helpful to have this information ready:

Information for the nursing home office staff

Insurance information: Provide information about any health coverage and long-term care insurance you have that pays for nursing home care, healthcare, or both. This includes the name of the insurance company and the policy number.

Note: If Medicare or Medicaid will cover your nursing home care, the nursing home can't require you to pay a cash deposit. They may ask that you pay your Medicare coinsurance and other charges you would normally have to pay. The nursing home can't require you to pay more than the rates allowed by Medicare or Medicaid for covered services. There may be charges for items or services that Medicare or Medicaid don't cover, but the nursing home can't require that you accept services that Medicare or Medicaid don't cover as a condition of your continued stay.

It's best to pay charges once they're billed to you, not in advance. You may have to pay a cash deposit before you're admitted to a nursing home if your care won't be covered by either Medicare or Medicaid, and the nursing home isn't limited to the rates allowed by Medicare or Medicaid.

Information for the nursing home medical staff

- **Information on your medical history:** Your doctor may give the staff some of this information. This includes a list of any current or past health problems, any past surgeries or treatments, any shots you've had, and allergies you have to food or medicine.

- **Information on your current health status:** Your doctor should give the staff this information, including a list of your current health problems, recent diagnostic test results, and information about any activities of daily living that might be difficult for you to do by yourself.

- **A list of your current medicines:** Include the dose, how often you take it, when you take it, and why you take it.

- **A list of all your healthcare providers:** Include names, addresses, and phone numbers.

- **A list of family members to call in case of an emergency:** Include names, addresses, and phone numbers.

Other important information to have ready
Healthcare advance directives

You may be asked if you have a healthcare advance directive, which is a written legal document that says how you want medical decisions to be made if you become unable to make decisions for yourself. There are 2 common types of healthcare advance directives:

1. **A living will:** A living will is a written legal document that shows what type of treatments you want or don't want in case you can't speak for yourself, like whether you want life support. Usually, this document only comes into effect if you're unconscious.

2. **A durable power of attorney for healthcare:** A durable power of attorney for healthcare is a legal document that names someone else to make healthcare decisions for you. This is helpful if you become unable to make your own decisions.

If you don't have a healthcare advance directive and need help preparing one, or you need more information, talk to a social worker, discharge planner, your doctor, or the nursing home staff.

Personal needs accounts

You may want to open an account managed by the nursing home, although the nursing home may not require this. You can deposit money into the account for personal use. Check with the nursing home to see how they manage these accounts. You may only have access to the account at certain times.

Information the nursing home must give you

Once you choose a nursing home, they must give you (orally and in writing), and prominently display, information about how to apply for and use Medicare and Medicaid benefits. They must also give you information on how to get refunds for previous payments you may have made that are covered by these benefits.

Section 43.2

Ask about Physical Activities

This section includes text excerpted from "Choosing a Retirement Community," *Go4Life*, National Institutes of Health (NIH), July 28, 2017.

As you visit potential retirement communities, consider their physical activity offerings. If you're already active, you know you want to stay that way. If you're not, then take this great opportunity to become physically active. Here are 10 questions to ask to make sure you can be active in your retirement community.

1. Is there a pool or fitness center?

2. Are there other physical activity features, like walking trails, tennis courts, or a pool?

3. Are there exercise classes or a personal trainer? Is the trainer certified to work with older adults and those with a variety of health issues?

4. What does it cost, if anything, to use the fitness facilities and classes?

5. If your living space is small, does the community provide a place where you can securely store a bike?

6. If the community doesn't have fitness or physical activity facilities, is there a nearby Y, senior center, or gym that you can use?

7. Are the stairs well lit and easily accessible? Do they have sturdy handrails?

8. Does the community have well-lit, well-maintained sidewalks so you can walk safely during the evening as well as the day?

9. Are there parks nearby?

10. Does the community offer physically active social events, like dances, bowling outings, and sports activities?

Section 43.3

Assisted Living

This section includes text excerpted from "Assisted Living," Eldercare Locator, U.S. Administration on Aging (AOA), April 13, 2012. Reviewed September 2017.

Assisted living facilities offer a housing alternative for older adults who may need help with dressing, bathing, eating, and toileting, but do not require the intensive medical and nursing care provided in nursing homes.

Assisted living facilities may be part of a retirement community, nursing home, senior housing complex, or may stand-alone. Licensing requirements for assisted living facilities vary by state and can be known by as many as 26 different names including: residential care, board and care, congregate care, and personal care.

What Services Are Provided?

Residents of assisted living facilities usually have their own units or apartment. In addition to having a support staff and providing meals, most assisted living facilities also offer at least some of the following services:

- Healthcare management and monitoring

- Help with activities of daily living such as bathing, dressing, and eating

- Housekeeping and laundry

- Medication reminders and/or help with medications

- Recreational activities

- Security
- Transportation

How to Choose a Facility?

The following suggestions can help you get started in your search for a safe, comfortable, and appropriate assisted living facility:

- Think ahead. What will the resident's future needs be and how will the facility meet those needs?
- Is the facility close to family and friends? Are there any shopping centers or other businesses nearby (within walking distance)?
- Do admission and retention policies exclude people with severe cognitive impairments or severe physical disabilities?
- Does the facility provide a written statement of the philosophy of care?
- Visit each facility more than once, sometimes unannounced.
- Visit at meal times, sample the food, and observe the quality of mealtime and the service.
- Observe interactions among residents and staff.
- Check to see if the facility offers social, recreational, and spiritual activities.
- Talk to residents.
- Learn what types of training staff receive and how frequently they receive training.
- Review state licensing reports.

The following steps should also be considered:

- Contact your state's long-term care ombudsman to see if any complaints have recently been filed against the assisted living facility you are interested in. In many states, the ombudsman checks on conditions at assisted living units as well as nursing homes.
- Contact the local Better Business Bureau to see if that agency has received any complaints about the assisted living facility.
- If the assisted living facility is connected to a nursing home, ask for information about it, too.

What Is the Cost for Assisted Living?

Although assisted living costs less than nursing home care, it is still fairly expensive. Depending on the kind of assisted living facility and type of services an older person chooses, the price costs can range from less than $25,000 a year to more than $50,000 a year. Because there can be extra fees for additional services, it is very important for older persons to find out what is included in the basic rate and how much other services will cost.

Primarily, older persons or their families pay the cost of assisted living. Some health and long-term care insurance policies may cover some of the costs associated with assisted living. In addition, some residences have their own financial assistance programs.

The federal Medicare program does not cover the costs of assisted living facilities or the care they provide. In some states, Medicaid may pay for the service component of assisted living.

Chapter 44

End-of-Life Care

Chapter Contents

Section 44.1

Hospice

This section contains text excerpted from the following sources:
Text under the heading "What Is End-of-Life Care?" is excerpted
from "End of Life—What Is End-of-Life Care?" National Institute on
Aging (NIA), National Institutes of Health (NIH), August 16, 2017;
Text under the heading "Hospice" is excerpted from "End of Life—
What Are Palliative Care and Hospice Care?" National Institute on
Aging (NIA), National Institutes of Health (NIH), August 16, 2017.

What Is End-of-Life Care?

At the end of life, each story is different. Death comes suddenly,
or a person lingers, gradually fading. For some older people, the body
weakens while the mind stays alert. Others remain physically strong,
but cognitive losses take a huge toll. Although everyone dies, each loss
is personally felt by those close to the one who has died.

End-of-life care is the term used to describe the support and medical care given during the time surrounding death. Such care does not
happen only in the moments before breathing ceases and the heart
stops beating. Older people often live with one or more chronic illnesses
and need a lot of care for days, weeks, and even months before death.

When a doctor says something like, "I'm afraid the news is not good.
There are no other treatments for us to try. I'm sorry," it may close
the door to the possibility of a cure, but it does not end the need for
medical support. Nor does it end the involvement of family and friends.

There are many ways to provide care for an older person who is
dying. Such care often involves a team. Being a caregiver for someone
at the end of life can be physically and emotionally exhausting. In the
end, accept that there may be no perfect death, just the best you can
do for the one you love. And, the pain of losing someone close to you
may be softened a little because, when you were needed, you did what
you could.

The chapter provides information for caregivers and include suggestions from healthcare providers with expertise in helping individuals
and families through this difficult time. Read about what you or a
loved one might expect near the end of life, including:

Hospice

Hospice can be provided in any setting—home, nursing home, assisted living facility, or inpatient hospital. At some point, it may not be possible to cure a serious illness, or a patient may choose not to undergo certain treatments. Hospice is designed for this situation. The patient beginning hospice care understands that his or her illness is not responding to medical attempts to cure it or to slow the disease's progress.

Hospice provides comprehensive comfort care as well as support for the family, but, in hospice, attempts to cure the person's illness are stopped. Hospice is provided for a person with a terminal illness whose doctor believes he or she has 6 months or less to live if the illness runs its natural course. Hospice is an approach to care, so it is not tied to a specific place. It can be offered in two types of settings—at home or in a facility such as a nursing home, hospital, or even in a separate hospice center.

Hospice care brings together a team of people with special skills— among them nurses, doctors, social workers, spiritual advisors, and trained volunteers. Everyone works together with the person who is dying, the caregiver, and/or the family to provide the medical, emotional, and spiritual support needed.

A member of the hospice team visits regularly, and someone is always available by phone—24 hours a day, 7 days a week. Hospice may be covered by Medicare and other insurance companies; check to see if insurance will cover your particular situation.

It is important to remember that stopping treatment aimed at curing an illness does not mean discontinuing all treatment. A good example is an older person with cancer. If the doctor determines that the cancer is not responding to chemotherapy and the patient chooses to enter into hospice care, then the chemotherapy will stop. Other medical care may continue as long as it is helpful. For example, if the person has high blood pressure, he or she will still get medicine for that.

Although hospice provides a lot of support, the day-to-day care of a person dying at home is provided by family and friends. The hospice team coaches family members on how to care for the dying person and even provides respite care when caregivers need a break. Respite care can be for as short as a few hours or for as long as several weeks.

Families of people who received care through a hospice program are more satisfied with end-of-life care than are those of people who did not have hospice services. Also, hospice recipients are more likely to have their pain controlled and less likely to undergo tests or be given medicines they don't need, compared with people who don't use hospice care.

What Does the Hospice 6-Month Requirement Mean?

Some people misinterpret their doctors' suggestion to consider hospice. They think it means death is very near. But, that's not always the case. Sometimes, people don't begin hospice care soon enough to take full advantage of the help it offers. Perhaps they wait too long to begin hospice; they are too close to death. Or, some people are not eligible for hospice care soon enough to receive its full benefit.

In the United States, people enrolled in Medicare can receive hospice care if their healthcare provider thinks they have less than 6 months to live should the disease take its usual course. Doctors have a hard time predicting how long an older, sick person will live. Health often declines slowly, and some people might need a lot of help with daily living for more than 6 months before they die.

Talk to the doctor if you think a hospice program might be helpful. If he or she agrees, but thinks it is too soon for Medicare to cover the services, then you can investigate how to pay for the services that are needed.

What happens if someone under hospice care lives longer than 6 months? If the doctor continues to certify that that person is still close to dying, Medicare can continue to pay for hospice services. It is also possible to leave hospice care for a while and then later return if the healthcare provider still believes that the patient has less than 6 months to live.

Section 44.2

Palliative Care

This section includes text excerpted from "End of Life—What
Are Palliative Care and Hospice Care?" National Institute on
Aging (NIA), National Institutes of Health (NIH), August 16, 2017.

Doctors can provide treatment to seriously ill patients in the hopes of a cure for as long as possible. These patients may also receive medical care for their symptoms, or palliative care, along with curative treatment.

A palliative care consultation team is a multidisciplinary team that works with the patient, family, and the patient's other doctors to provide medical, social, emotional, and practical support. The team is made of palliative care specialist doctors and nurses, and includes others such as social workers, nutritionists, and chaplains.

Palliative care can be provided in hospitals, nursing homes, outpatient palliative care clinics and certain other specialized clinics, or at home. Medicare, Medicaid, and insurance policies may cover palliative care. Veterans may be eligible for palliative care through the Department of Veterans Affairs (VA). Private health insurance might pay for some services. Health insurance providers can answer questions about what they will cover. Check to see if insurance will cover your particular situation.

In palliative care, you do not have to give up treatment that might cure a serious illness. Palliative care can be provided along with curative treatment and may begin at the time of diagnosis. Over time, if the doctor or the palliative care team believes ongoing treatment is no longer helping, there are two possibilities. Palliative care could transition to hospice care if the doctor believes the person is likely to die within 6 months. Or, the palliative care team could continue to help with increasing emphasis on comfort care.

Who Can Benefit from Palliative Care?

Palliative care is a resource for anyone living with a serious illness, such as heart failure, chronic obstructive pulmonary disease, cancer, dementia, Parkinson disease, and many others. Palliative care can be helpful at any stage of illness and is best provided from the point of diagnosis.

In addition to improving quality of life and helping with symptoms, palliative care can help patients understand their choices for medical treatment. The organized services available through palliative care may be helpful to any older person having a lot of general discomfort and disability very late in life. Palliative care can be provided along with curative treatment and does not depend on prognosis.

Section 44.3

Understanding Healthcare Decisions at the End of Life

This section includes text excerpted from "Understanding Healthcare Decisions at the End of Life," National Institute on Aging (NIA), National Institutes of Health (NIH), August 16, 2017.

It can be overwhelming to be asked to make healthcare decisions for someone who is dying and is no longer able to make his or her own decisions. It is even more difficult if you do not have written or verbal guidance. How do you decide what type of care is right for someone? Even when you have written documents, some decisions still might not be clear since the documents may not address every situation you could face.

Two approaches might be useful. One is to put yourself in the place of the person who is dying and try to choose as he or she would. This is called substituted judgment. Some experts believe that decisions should be based on substituted judgment whenever possible.

Another approach, known as best interests, is to decide what would be best for the dying person. This is sometimes combined with substituted judgment.

If you are making decisions for someone at the end of life and are trying to use one of these approaches, it may be helpful to think about the following questions:

- Has the dying person ever talked about what he or she would want at the end of life?

- Has he or she expressed an opinion about how someone else was being treated?

- What were his or her values in life? What gave meaning to life? Maybe it was being close to family—watching them grow and making memories together. Perhaps just being alive was the most important thing.

As a decision-maker without specific guidance from the dying person, you need as much information as possible on which to base your actions. You might ask the doctor:

- What might we expect to happen in the next few hours, days, or weeks if we continue our current course of treatment?

- Why is this new test being suggested?

- Will it change the current treatment plan?

- Will a new treatment help my relative get better?

- How would the new treatment change his or her quality of life?

- Will it give more quality time with family and friends?

- How long will this treatment take to make a difference?

- If we choose to try this treatment, can we stop it at any time? For any reason?

- What are the side effects of the approach you are suggesting?

- If we try this new treatment and it doesn't work, what then?

- If we don't try this treatment, what will happen?

- Is the improvement we saw today an overall positive sign or just something temporary?

It is a good idea to have someone with you when discussing these issues with medical staff. Having someone take notes or remember details can be very helpful. If you are unclear about something you are told, don't be afraid to ask the doctor or nurse to repeat it or to say it another way that does make sense to you. Keep asking questions until you have all the information you need to make decisions. Make sure you know how to contact a member of the medical team if you have a question or if the dying person needs something.

Sometimes, the whole family wants to be involved in every decision. Maybe that is the family's cultural tradition. Or, maybe the person dying did not pick one person to make healthcare choices before becoming unable to do so. That is not unusual, but it makes sense to choose one person to be the contact when dealing with medical staff. The doctors and nurses will appreciate having to phone only one person.

Even if one family member is named as the decision-maker, it is a good idea, as much as possible, to have family agreement about the care plan. If you can't agree on a care plan, a decision-maker, or even a spokesperson, the family might consider a mediator, someone trained to bring people with different opinions to a common decision.

In any case, as soon as it is clear that the patient is nearing the end of life, the family should try to discuss with the medical team which end-of-life care approach they want for their family member. That way, decision making for crucial situations can be planned and may feel less rushed.

Issues You May Face

Maybe you are now faced with making end-of-life choices for someone close to you. You've thought about that person's values and opinions, and you've asked the healthcare team to explain the treatment plan and what you can expect to happen.

But, there are other issues that are important to understand in case they arise. What if the dying person starts to have trouble breathing and a doctor says a ventilator might be needed? Maybe one family member wants the healthcare team to do everything possible to keep this relative alive. What does that involve? Or, what if family members can't agree on end-of-life care or they disagree with the doctor? What happens then?

Here are some other common end-of-life issues. They will give you a general understanding and may help your conversations with the doctors.

If we say do everything possible, what does that mean? This means that if someone is dying, all measures that might keep vital organs working will be tried—for example, using a ventilator to support breathing or starting dialysis for failing kidneys. Such life support can sometimes be a temporary measure that allows the body to heal itself and begin to work normally again. It is not intended to be used indefinitely in someone who is dying.

What can be done if someone's heart stops beating (cardiac arrest)? CPR (cardiopulmonary resuscitation) can sometimes restart a stopped heart. It is most effective in people who were generally healthy before their heart stopped. During CPR, the doctor repeatedly pushes on the chest with great force and periodically puts air into the lungs. Electric shocks (called defibrillation) may also be used to correct an abnormal heart rhythm, and some medicines might also be given. Although not usually shown on television, the force required for CPR can cause broken ribs or a collapsed lung. Often, CPR does not succeed in older adults who have multiple chronic illnesses or who are already frail.

What if someone needs help breathing or completely stops breathing (respiratory arrest)? If a patient has very severe breathing problems or has stopped breathing, a ventilator may be needed. A ventilator forces the lungs to work. Initially, this involves intubation, putting a tube attached to a ventilator down the throat into the trachea or windpipe. Because this tube can be quite uncomfortable, people are often sedated with very strong intravenous medicines. Restraints may be used to prevent them from pulling out the tube. If the person needs ventilator support for more than a few days, the doctor might suggest a tracheotomy, sometimes called a "trach" (rhymes with "make"). This tube is then attached to the ventilator. This is more comfortable than a tube down the throat and may not require sedation. Inserting the tube into the trachea is a bedside surgery. A tracheotomy can carry risks, including a collapsed lung, a plugged tracheotomy tube, or bleeding.

How can I be sure the medical staff knows that we don't want efforts to restore a heartbeat or breathing? Tell the doctor in charge as soon as the patient or person making healthcare decisions decides that CPR or other life-support procedures should not be performed. The doctor will then write this on the patient's chart using terms such as DNR (Do Not Resuscitate), DNAR (Do Not Attempt to Resuscitate), AND (Allow Natural Death), or DNI (Do Not Intubate). DNR forms vary by State and are usually available online.

If end-of-life care is given at home, a special nonhospital DNR, signed by a doctor, is needed. This ensures that if emergency medical technicians (EMTs) are called to the house, they will respect your wishes. Make sure it is kept in a prominent place so EMTs can see it. Without a nonhospital DNR, in many States EMTs are required to perform CPR and similar techniques. Hospice staff can help determine whether a medical condition is part of the normal dying process or something that needs the attention of EMTs.

DNR orders do not stop all treatment. They only mean that CPR and a ventilator will not be used. These orders are not permanent—they can be changed if the situation changes.

What about pacemakers (or similar devices)—should they be turned off? A pacemaker is a device implanted under the skin on the chest that keeps a heartbeat regular. It will not keep a dying person alive. Some people have an implantable cardioverter defibrillator (ICD) under the skin. An ICD shocks the heart back into regular rhythm when needed. The ICD should be turned off at the point when life support is no longer wanted. This can be done at the bedside without surgery.

What if the doctor suggests a feeding tube? If a patient can't or won't eat or drink, the doctor might suggest a feeding tube. While a patient recovers from an illness, getting nutrition temporarily through a feeding tube can be helpful. But, at the end of life, a feeding tube might cause more discomfort than not eating. For people with dementia, tube feeding does not prolong life or prevent aspiration.

As death approaches, loss of appetite is common. Body systems start shutting down, and fluids and food are not needed as before. Some experts believe that at this point few nutrients are absorbed from any type of nutrition, including those received through a feeding tube. Further, after a feeding tube is inserted, the family might need to make a difficult decision about when, or if, to remove it.

If tube feeding will be tried, there are two methods that could be used. In the first, a feeding tube, known as a nasogastric or NG tube, is threaded through the nose down to the stomach to give nutrition for a short time. Sometimes, the tube is uncomfortable. Someone with an NG tube might try to remove it. This usually means the person has to be restrained, which could mean binding his or her hands to the bed.

If tube feeding is required for an extended time, then a gastric or G tube is put directly into the stomach through an opening made in the side or abdomen. This second method is sometimes called a PEG (percutaneous endoscopic gastrostomy) tube. It carries risks of infection, pneumonia, and nausea.

Hand feeding (sometimes called assisted oral feeding) is an alternative to tube feeding. This approach may have fewer risks, especially for people with dementia.

Should someone who is dying be sedated? Sometimes, for patients very near the end of life, the doctor might suggest sedation to manage symptoms that are not responding to other treatments and are still making the patient uncomfortable. This means using medicines to put the patient in a sleep-like state. Many doctors suggest continuing to use comfort care measures like pain medicine even if the dying person is sedated. Sedatives can be stopped at any time. A person who is sedated may still be able to hear what you are saying—so try to keep speaking directly to, not about, him or her. Do not say things you would not want the patient to hear.

What about antibiotics? Antibiotics are medicines that fight infections caused by bacteria. Lower respiratory infections (such as pneumonia) and urinary tract infections are often caused by bacteria and are common in older people who are dying. Many antibiotics have side effects, so the value of trying to treat an infection in a dying person should be weighed against any unpleasant side effects. If someone is already dying when the infection began, giving antibiotics is probably not going to prevent death but might make the person feel more comfortable.

Is refusing treatment legal? Choosing to stop treatment that is not curing or controlling an illness, or deciding not to start a new treatment, is completely legal—whether the choice is made by the person who is dying or by the person making healthcare decisions. Some people think this is like allowing death to happen. The law does not consider refusing such treatment to be either suicide or euthanasia, sometimes called mercy killing.

What happens if the doctor and I have different opinions about care for someone who is dying? Sometimes medical staff, the patient, and family members disagree about a medical care decision. This can be especially problematic when the dying person can't tell the doctors what kind of end-of-life care he or she wants. For example, the family might want more active treatment, like chemotherapy, than the doctors think will be helpful. If there is an advance directive explaining the patient's preferences, those guidelines should determine care.

Without the guidance of an advance directive, if there is a disagreement about medical care, it may be necessary to get a second opinion from a different doctor or to consult the ethics committee or patient representative, also known as an ombudsman, of the hospital or facility. Palliative care consultation may also be helpful. An arbitrator (mediator) can sometimes assist people with different views to agree on a plan.

The doctor does not seem familiar with our family's views about dying. What should we do? America is a rich melting pot of religions, races, and cultures. Ingrained in each tradition are expectations about what should happen as a life nears its end. It is important for everyone involved in a patient's care to understand how each family background may influence expectations, needs, and choices.

Your background may be different from that of the doctor with whom you are working. Or, you might be used to a different approach to making healthcare decisions at the end of life than your medical team. For example, many healthcare providers look to a single person—the dying person or his or her chosen representative—for important healthcare decisions at the end of life. But, in some cultures, the entire immediate family takes on that role.

It is helpful to discuss your personal and family traditions with your doctors and nurses. If there are religious or cultural customs surrounding death that are important to you, make sure to tell your healthcare providers.

Knowing that these practices will be honored could comfort the dying person. Telling the medical staff ahead of time may also help avoid confusion and misunderstanding when death occurs. Make sure you understand how the available medical options presented by the healthcare team fit into your family's desires for end-of-life care.

Questions to Ask the Medical Staff about Healthcare Decisions

- What is the care plan? What are the benefits and risks?

- How often should we reassess the care plan?

- If we try using the ventilator to help with breathing and decide to stop, how will that be done?

- If my family member is dying, why does he or she have to be connected to all those tubes and machines? Why do we need more tests?

- What is the best way for our family to work with the care staff?

- How can I make sure I get a daily update on my family member's condition?

- Will you call me if there is a change in his or her condition?

Make sure the healthcare team knows what is important to your family surrounding the end of life. You might say:

- In my religion, we . . . (then describe your religious traditions regarding death).

- Where we come from . . . (tell what customs are important to you at the time of death).

- In our family when someone is dying, we prefer . . . (describe what you hope to have happen).

Section 44.4

What to Do after Someone Dies

This section includes text excerpted from "End-of-Life—What to Do after Someone Dies," National Institute on Aging (NIA), National Institutes of Health (NIH), August 16, 2017.

Nothing has to be done immediately after a person's death. Take the time you need. Some people want to stay in the room with the body; others prefer to leave. You might want to have someone make sure the body is lying flat before the joints become stiff and cannot be moved. This rigor mortis begins sometime during the first hours after death.

After the death, how long you can stay with the body may depend on where death happens. If it happens at home, there is no need to move the body right away. This is the time for any special religious, ethnic, or cultural customs that are performed soon after death.

If the death seems likely to happen in a facility, such as a hospital or nursing home, discuss any important customs or rituals with the staff early on, if possible. That will allow them to plan so you can have the appropriate time with the body.

Some families want time to sit quietly with the body, console each other, and maybe share memories. You could ask a member of your religious community or a spiritual counselor to come. If you have a list of people to notify, this is the time to call those who might want to come and see the body before it is moved.

As soon as possible, the death must be officially pronounced by someone in authority like a doctor in a hospital or nursing facility or a hospice nurse. This person also fills out the forms certifying the cause, time, and place of death. These steps will make it possible for an official death certificate to be prepared. This legal form is necessary for many reasons, including life insurance and financial and property issues.

If hospice is helping, a plan for what happens after death is already in place. If death happens at home without hospice, try to talk with the doctor, local medical examiner (coroner), your local health department, or a funeral home representative in advance about how to proceed.

Arrangements should be made to pick up the body as soon as the family is ready and according to local laws. Usually this is done by a funeral home. The hospital or nursing facility, if that is where the death took place, may call the funeral home for you. If at home, you will need to contact the funeral home directly or ask a friend or family member to do that for you.

The doctor may ask if you want an autopsy. This is a medical procedure conducted by a specially trained physician to learn more about what caused the death. For example, if the person who died was believed to have Alzheimer disease, a brain autopsy will allow for a definitive diagnosis. If your religion or culture objects to autopsies, talk to the doctor. Some people planning a funeral with a viewing worry about having an autopsy, but the physical signs of an autopsy are usually hidden by clothing.

Part Six

Legal and Economic Issues Related to Aging

Chapter 45

Advance Care Planning

Advance care planning is not just about old age. At any age, a medical crisis could leave someone too ill to make his or her own healthcare decisions. Even if you are not sick now, making healthcare plans for the future is an important step toward making sure you get the medical care you would want, even when doctors and family members are making the decisions for you.

Many older Americans face questions about medical treatment near the end of life but are not capable of making those decisions.

What Is Advance Care Planning?

Advance care planning involves learning about the types of decisions that might need to be made, considering those decisions ahead of time, and then letting others know about your preferences. These preferences are often put into an advance directive, a legal document that goes into effect only if you are incapacitated and unable to speak for yourself. This could be the result of disease or severe injury—no matter how old you are. It helps others know what type of medical care you want. It also allows you to express your values and desires related to end-of-life care. You might think of an advance directive as a living document—one that you can adjust as your situation changes because of new information or a change in your health.

This chapter includes text excerpted from "Advance Care Planning: Health-care Directives," National Institute on Aging (NIA), National Institutes of Health (NIH), August 16, 2017.

Medical Research and Advance Care Planning

Research shows that advance directives can make a difference and that people who document their preferences in this way are more likely to get the care they prefer at the end of life than people who do not.

Decisions That Could Come Up Near Death

Sometimes when doctors believe a cure is no longer possible and you are dying, decisions must be made about the use of emergency treatments to keep you alive. Doctors can use several artificial or mechanical ways to try to do this. Decisions that might come up at this time include:

- CPR (cardiopulmonary resuscitation)

- Ventilator use

- Artificial nutrition (tube feeding) or artificial hydration (intravenous fluids)

- Comfort care

CPR. CPR (cardiopulmonary resuscitation) might restore your heartbeat if your heart stops or is in a life-threatening abnormal rhythm. The heart of a young, otherwise healthy person might resume beating normally after CPR. An otherwise healthy older person, whose heart is beating erratically or not beating at all, might also be helped by CPR. CPR is less likely to work for an older person who is ill, can't be successfully treated, and is already close to death. It involves repeatedly pushing on the chest with force, while putting air into the lungs. This force has to be quite strong, and sometimes ribs are broken or a lung collapses. Electric shocks known as defibrillation and medicines might also be used as part of the process.

Ventilator use. Ventilators are machines that help you breathe. A tube connected to the ventilator is put through the throat into the trachea (windpipe) so the machine can force air into the lungs. Putting the tube down the throat is called intubation. Because the tube is uncomfortable, medicines are used to keep you sedated (unconscious) while on a ventilator. If you can't breathe on your own after a few days, a doctor may perform a tracheotomy or "trach" (rhymes with "make"). During this bedside surgery, the tube is inserted directly into the trachea through a hole in the neck. For long-term help with breathing, a trach is more comfortable, and sedation is not needed. People using such a breathing tube aren't able to speak without special help because exhaled air goes out of the trach rather than past their vocal cords.

Artificial nutrition or artificial hydration. A feeding tube and/ or intravenous (IV) liquids are sometimes used to provide nutrition when a person is not able to eat or drink. These measures can be helpful if you are recovering from an illness. However, if you are near death, these could actually make you more uncomfortable. For example, IV liquids, which are given through a plastic tube put into a vein, can increase the burden on failing kidneys. Or if the body is shutting down near death, it is not able to digest food properly, even when provided through a feeding tube. At first, the feeding tube is threaded through the nose down to the stomach. In time, if tube feeding is still needed, the tube is surgically inserted into the stomach.

Comfort care. Comfort care is anything that can be done to soothe you and relieve suffering while staying in line with your wishes. Comfort care includes managing shortness of breath; offering ice chips for dry mouth; limiting medical testing; providing spiritual and emotional counseling; and giving medication for pain, anxiety, nausea, or constipation. Often this is done through hospice, which may be offered in the home, in a hospice facility, in a skilled nursing facility, or in a hospital.

Getting Started

Start by thinking about what kind of treatment you do or do not want in a medical emergency. It might help to talk with your doctor about how your present health conditions might influence your health in the future. For example, what decisions would you or your family face if your high blood pressure leads to a stroke?

If you don't have any medical issues now, your family medical history might be a clue to thinking about the future. Talk with your doctor about decisions that might come up if you develop health problems similar to those of other family members.

In considering treatment decisions, your personal values are key. Is your main desire to have the most days of life, or to have the most life in your days? What if an illness leaves you paralyzed or in a permanent coma and you need to be on a ventilator? Would you want that?

What makes life meaningful to you? If your heart stops or you have trouble breathing, would you want to undergo life-saving measures if it meant that, in the future, you could be well enough to spend time with your family? Even if the emergency leaves you simply able to spend your days listening to books on tape or gazing out the window watching the birds and squirrels compete for seeds in the bird feeder, you might be content with that.

But, there are many other scenarios. Here are a few. What would you decide?

- If a stroke leaves you paralyzed and then your heart stops, would you want CPR? What if you were also mentally impaired by a stroke—does your decision change?

- What if you become unable to feed yourself near the end of life? Would you want a feeding tube used to give you nutrition?

- What if you are permanently unconscious and then develop pneumonia? Would you want antibiotics and a ventilator used?

For some people, staying alive as long as medically possible is the most important thing. An advance directive can help make sure that happens.

Your decisions about how to handle any of these situations could be different at age 40 than at age 85. Or they could be different if you have an incurable condition as opposed to being generally healthy. An advance directive allows you to provide instructions for these types of situations and then to change the instructions as you get older or if your viewpoint changes.

Do You or a Family Member Have Alzheimer Disease?

Many people are unprepared to deal with the legal and financial consequences of a serious illness such as Alzheimer disease. Advance planning can help people with Alzheimer and their families clarify their wishes and make well-informed decisions about healthcare and financial arrangements.

Making Your Wishes Known

There are two main elements in an advance directive—a living will and a durable power of attorney for healthcare. There are also other documents that can supplement your advance directive. You can choose which documents to create, depending on how you want decisions to be made. These documents include:

- Living will

- Durable power of attorney for healthcare

- Other documents discussing DNR (do not resuscitate) orders, organ and tissue donation, dialysis, and blood transfusions

- Physician Orders for Life-Sustaining Treatment (POLST)

Living will. A living will is a written document that helps you tell doctors how you want to be treated if you are dying or permanently unconscious and cannot make decisions about emergency treatment. In a living will, you can say which of the procedures you would want, which ones you wouldn't want, and under which conditions each of your choices applies.

Durable power of attorney for healthcare. A durable power of attorney for healthcare is a legal document naming a healthcare proxy, someone to make medical decisions for you when you are unable to do so. Your proxy, also known as a representative, surrogate, or agent, should be familiar with your values and wishes. This means that he or she will be able to decide as you would when treatment decisions need to be made. A proxy can be chosen in addition to or instead of a living will. Having a healthcare proxy helps you plan for situations that cannot be foreseen, like a serious auto accident.

Some people are reluctant to put specific health decisions in writing. For them, naming a healthcare agent might be a good approach, especially if there is someone they feel comfortable talking with about their values and preferences. In this case, the proxy can evaluate each situation or treatment option independently.

Other advance care planning documents. You might also want to prepare documents to express your wishes about a single medical issue or something not covered in your advance directive. A living will usually covers only the specific life-sustaining treatments discussed earlier. You might want to give your healthcare proxy specific instructions about other issues, such as blood transfusion or kidney dialysis. This is especially important if your doctor suggests that, given your health condition, such treatments might be needed in the future.

Two medical issues that might arise at the end of life are DNR orders and organ and tissue donation.

A ***DNR (do not resuscitate) order*** tells medical staff in a hospital or nursing facility that you do not want them to try to return your heart to a normal rhythm if it stops or is beating unevenly. Even though a living will might say CPR is not wanted, it is helpful to have a DNR order as part of your medical file if you go to a hospital. Posting a DNR next to your bed might avoid confusion in an emergency situation. Without a DNR order, medical staff will make every effort to restore the normal rhythm of your heart. A nonhospital DNR will alert emergency medical personnel to your wishes regarding CPR and other measures to restore your heartbeat if you are not in the hospital. A similar document that is less familiar is called a DNI (do not intubate) order. A DNI tells medical staff in a hospital or nursing facility that you do not want to be put on a breathing machine.

Organ and tissue donation allows organs or body parts from a generally healthy person who has died to be transplanted into people who need them. Commonly, the heart, lungs, pancreas, kidneys, corneas, liver, and skin are donated. There is no age limit for organ and tissue donation.

At the time of death, family members may be asked about organ donation. If those close to you, especially your proxy, know how you feel about organ donation, they will be ready to respond. There is no cost to the donor's family for this gift of life. If the person has requested a DNR order but wants to donate organs, he or she might have to indicate that the desire to donate supersedes the DNR. That is because it might be necessary to use machines to keep the heart beating until the medical staff is ready to remove the donated organs.

What Are POLST and MOLST?

A number of States use an advance care planning form known as POLST (Physician Orders for Life-Sustaining Treatment) or MOLST (Medical Orders for Life-Sustaining Treatment). This form provides more detailed guidance about your medical care preferences.

The form is filled out by your doctor, or sometimes a nurse practitioner or physician's assistant, after discussing your wishes with you and your family. Once signed by your doctor, this form has the same authority as any other medical order. Check with your State department of health to find out if this form is available where you live.

What about Pacemakers and ICDs?

Some people have pacemakers to help their hearts beat regularly. If you have one and are near death, it may not necessarily keep you alive. But, you might have an ICD (implantable cardioverter-defibrillator) placed under your skin to shock your heart back into regular beatings if the rhythm becomes irregular. If other life-sustaining measures are not used, the ICD may also be turned off. You need to state in your advance directive what you want done if the doctor suggests it is time to turn it off.

Selecting Your Healthcare Proxy

If you decide to choose a proxy, think about people you know who share your views and values about life and medical decisions. Your proxy might be a family member, a friend, your lawyer, or someone with whom you worship. It's a good idea to also name an alternate proxy. It is especially important to have a detailed living will if you choose not to name a proxy.

You can decide how much authority your proxy has over your medical care—whether he or she is entitled to make a wide range of decisions or only a few specific ones. Try not to include guidelines that make it impossible for the proxy to fulfill his or her duties. For example, it's probably not unusual for someone to say in conversation, "I don't want to go to a nursing home," but think carefully about whether you want a restriction like that in your advance directive. Sometimes, for financial or medical reasons, that may be the best choice for you.

Of course, check with those you choose as your healthcare proxy and alternate before you name them officially. Make sure they are comfortable with this responsibility.

Making It Official

Once you have talked with your doctor and have an idea of the types of decisions that could come up in the future and whom you would like as a proxy, if you want one at all, the next step is to fill out the legal forms detailing your wishes. A lawyer can help but is not required. If you decide to use a lawyer, don't depend on him or her to help you understand different medical treatments. That's why you should start the planning process by talking with your doctor.

Many states have their own advance directive forms. The American Bar Association has a list of advance care planning forms by state. Your local Area Agency on Aging can help you locate the right forms. You can find your area agency phone number by calling the Eldercare Locator toll-free at 800-677-1116 or by visiting www.eldercare.gov.

Some states want your advance directive to be witnessed; some want your signature notarized. A notary is a person licensed by the state to witness signatures. You might find a notary at your bank, post office, or local library, or call your insurance agent. Some notaries charge a fee.

Some people spend a lot of time in more than one state—for example, visiting children and grandchildren. If that's your situation also, you might consider preparing an advance directive using forms for each state—and keep a copy in each place, too.

After You Set Up Your Advance Directive

Give copies of your advance directive to your healthcare proxy and alternate proxy. Give your doctor a copy for your medical records. Tell key family members and friends where you keep a copy. If you have to go to the hospital, give staff there a copy to include in your records. Because you might change your advance directive in the future, it's a good idea to keep track of who receives a copy.

Review your advance care planning decisions from time to time—for example, every 10 years, if not more often. You might want to revise your preferences for care if your situation or your health changes. Or, you might want to make adjustments if you receive a serious diagnosis; if you get married, separated, or divorced; if your spouse dies; or if something happens to your proxy or alternate. If your preferences change, make sure your doctor, proxy, and family know about them.

What happens if you have no advance directive or have made no plans and you become unable to speak for yourself? In such cases, the state where you live will assign someone to make medical decisions on your behalf. This will probably be your spouse, your parents if they are available, or your children if they are adults. If you have no family members, the state will choose someone to represent your best interests.

Always remember, an advance directive is only used if you are in danger of dying and need certain emergency or special measures to keep you alive but are not able to make those decisions on your own. An advance directive allows you to continue to make your wishes about medical treatment known.

Nobody can predict the future. You may never face a medical situation where you are unable to speak for yourself and make your wishes known. But having an advance directive may give you and those close to you some peace of mind.

Advance Directive Wallet Card

You might want to make a card to carry in your wallet indicating that you have an advance directive and where it is kept. Here is a slightly revised example of the wallet card offered by the Office of the

Attorney General in Maryland. It uses the phrase “healthcare agent” instead of “healthcare proxy.”

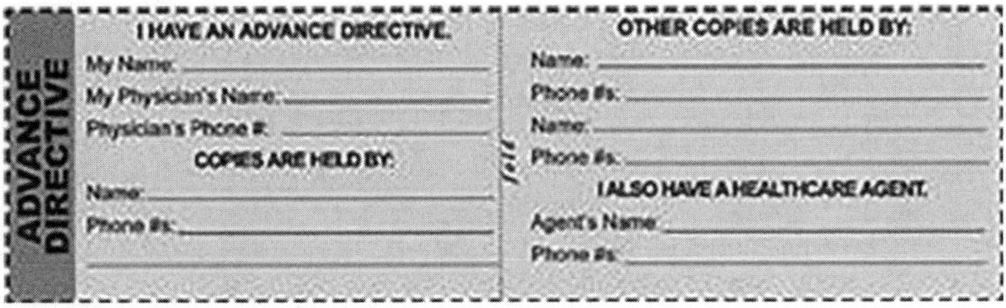
ADVANCE DIRECTIVE

I HAVE AN ADVANCE DIRECTIVE.

My Name:

My Physician's Name:

Physician's Phone #:

COPIES ARE HELD BY:

Name:

Phone #s:

fold

OTHER COPIES ARE HELD BY:

Name:

Phone #s:

Name:

Phone #s:

I ALSO HAVE A HEALTHCARE AGENT.

Agent's Name:

Phone #s:

Figure 45.1. *Advance Directive Wallet Card*

Chapter 46

Getting Your Affairs in Order

Plan for the Future

No one ever plans to be sick or disabled. Yet, it's this kind of planning that can make all the difference in an emergency.

What Exactly Is an "Important Paper"?

The answer to this question may be different for every family. Remember, this is a starting place. You may have other information to add. For example, if you have a pet, you will want to include the name and address of your veterinarian. Include complete information about:

Personal Records

- Full legal name
- Social Security number
- Legal residence
- Date and place of birth
- Names and addresses of spouse and children

This chapter includes text excerpted from "Getting Your Affairs in Order," National Institute on Aging (NIA), National Institutes of Health (NIH), August 16, 2017.

- Location of birth and death certificates and certificates of marriage, divorce, citizenship, and adoption

- Employers and dates of employment

- Education and military records

- Names and phone numbers of religious contacts

- Memberships in groups and awards received

- Names and phone numbers of close friends, relatives, doctors, lawyers, and financial advisors

- Medications taken regularly (be sure to update this regularly)

- Location of living will and other legal documents

Financial Records

- Sources of income and assets (pension from your employer, IRAs, 401(k)s, interest, etc.)

- Social Security and Medicare/Medicaid information

- Insurance information (life, health, long-term care, home, car) with policy numbers and agents' names and phone numbers

- Names of your banks and account numbers (checking, savings, credit union)

- Investment income (stocks, bonds, property) and stockbrokers' names and phone numbers

- Copy of most recent income tax return

- Location of most up-to-date will with an original signature

- Liabilities, including property tax—what is owed, to whom, and when payments are due

- Mortgages and debts—how and when they are paid

- Location of original deed of trust for home

- Car title and registration

- Credit and debit card names and numbers

- Location of safe deposit box and key

Steps for Getting Your Affairs in Order

Put your important papers and copies of legal documents in one place. You can set up a file, put everything in a desk or dresser drawer, or list the information and location of papers in a notebook. If your papers are in a bank safe deposit box, keep copies in a file at home. Check each year to see if there's anything new to add.

Tell a trusted family member or friend where you put all your important papers. You don't need to tell this friend or family member about your personal affairs, but someone should know where you keep your papers in case of an emergency. If you don't have a relative or friend you trust, ask a lawyer to help.

Give permission in advance for your doctor or lawyer to talk with your caregiver as needed. There may be questions about your care, a bill, or a health insurance claim. Without your consent, your caregiver may not be able to get needed information. You can give your okay in advance to Medicare, a credit card company, your bank, or your doctor. You may need to sign and return a form.

Legal Documents

There are many different types of legal documents that can help you plan how your affairs will be handled in the future. Many of these documents have names that sound alike, so make sure you are getting the documents you want. Also, State laws vary, so find out about the rules, requirements, and forms used in your State.

Wills and **trusts** let you name the person you want your money and property to go to after you die.

Advance directives let you make arrangements for your care if you become sick. There are two ways to do this:

- A **living will** gives you a say in your healthcare if you become too sick to make your wishes known. In a living will, you can state what kind of care you do or don't want. This can make it easier for family members to make tough healthcare decisions for you.

- A *durable power of attorney for healthcare* lets you name the person you want to make medical decisions for you if you can't make them yourself. Make sure the person you name is willing to make those decisions for you.

For legal matters, there are two ways to give someone you trust the power to act in your place:

- A **general power of attorney** lets you give someone else the authority to act on your behalf, but this power will end if you are unable to make your own decisions.

- A **durable power of attorney** allows you to name someone to act on your behalf for any legal task, but it stays in place if you become unable to make your own decisions.

Who Can Help Me Put My Legal and Financial Affairs in Order?

You may want to talk with a lawyer about setting up a general power of attorney, durable power of attorney, joint account, trust, or advance directive. Be sure to ask about the lawyer's fees before you make an appointment.

You should be able to find a directory of local lawyers at your library, or you can contact your local bar association for lawyers in your area. Your local bar association can also help you find what free legal aid options your State has to offer. An informed family member may be able to help you manage some of these issues.

Chapter 47

Beware of Health Scams

You'll never see these warnings on health products, but that's what you ought to be thinking when you see claims like "miracle cure," "revolutionary scientific breakthrough," or "alternative to drugs or surgery."

Health fraud scams have been around for hundreds of years. The snake oil salesmen of old have morphed into the deceptive, high-tech marketers of today. They prey on people's desires for easy solutions to difficult health problems—from losing weight to curing serious diseases like cancer.

According to the U.S. Food and Drug Administration (FDA), a health product is fraudulent if it is deceptively promoted as being effective against a disease or health condition but has not been scientifically proven safe and effective for that purpose.

Scammers promote their products through newspapers, magazines, TV infomercials, and cyberspace. You can find health fraud scams in retail stores and on countless websites, in popup ads and spam, and on social media sites like Facebook and Twitter.

Not Worth the Risk

Health fraud scams can do more than waste your money. They can cause serious injury or even death, says Gary Coody, R.Ph., FDA's national health fraud coordinator. "Using unproven treatments can

This chapter includes text excerpted from "6 Tip-offs to Rip-offs: Don't Fall for Health Fraud Scams," U.S. Food and Drug Administration (FDA), March 4, 2013. Reviewed September 2017.

delay getting a potentially life-saving diagnosis and medication that actually works. Also, fraudulent products sometimes contain hidden drug ingredients that can be harmful when unknowingly taken by consumers."

Coody says fraudulent products often make claims related to:

- weight loss

- sexual performance

- memory loss

- serious diseases such as cancer, diabetes, heart disease, arthritis, and Alzheimer disease.

A Pervasive Problem

Fraudulent products not only won't work—they could cause serious injury. In the past few years, FDA laboratories have found more than 100 weight-loss products, illegally marketed as dietary supplements, that contained sibutramine, the active ingredient in the prescription weight-loss drug Meridia. In 2010, Meridia was withdrawn from the U.S. market after studies showed that it was associated with an increased risk of heart attack and stroke.

Fraudulent products marketed as drugs or dietary supplements are not the only health scams on the market. FDA found a fraudulent and expensive light therapy device with cure-all claims to treat fungal meningitis, Alzheimer, skin cancer, concussions and many other unrelated diseases. Generally, making health claims about a medical device without FDA clearance or approval of the device is illegal.

"Health fraud is a pervasive problem," says Coody, "especially when scammers sell online. It's difficult to track down the responsible parties. When we do find them and tell them their products are illegal, some will shut down their website. Unfortunately, however, these same products may reappear later on a different website, and sometimes may reappear with a different name."

Tip-Offs

FDA offers some tip-offs to help you identify rip-offs.

- **One product does it all.** Be suspicious of products that claim to cure a wide range of diseases. A New York firm claimed its products marketed as dietary supplements could treat or cure senile dementia, brain atrophy, atherosclerosis, kidney dysfunction, gangrene, depression, osteoarthritis, dysuria, and lung, cervical and prostate cancer. In October 2012, at FDA's request, U.S. marshals seized these products.

- **Personal testimonials.** Success stories, such as, "It cured my diabetes" or "My tumors are gone," are easy to make up and are not a substitute for scientific evidence.

- **Quick fixes.** Few diseases or conditions can be treated quickly, even with legitimate products. Beware of language such as, "Lose 30 pounds in 30 days" or "eliminates skin cancer in days."

- **"All natural."** Some plants found in nature (such as poisonous mushrooms) can kill when consumed. Moreover, FDA has found numerous products promoted as "all natural" but that contain hidden and dangerously high doses of prescription drug ingredients or even untested active artificial ingredients.

- **"Miracle cure."** Alarms should go off when you see this claim or others like it such as, "new discovery," "scientific breakthrough" or "secret ingredient." If a real cure for a serious disease were discovered, it would be widely reported through the media and prescribed by health professionals—not buried in print ads, TV infomercials or on Internet sites.

- **Conspiracy theories.** Claims like "The pharmaceutical industry and the government are working together to hide information about a miracle cure" are always untrue and unfounded. These statements are used to distract consumers from the obvious, common-sense questions about the so-called miracle cure.

Even with these tips, fraudulent health products are not always easy to spot. If you're tempted to buy an unproven product or one with questionable claims, check with your doctor or other healthcare professional first.

Chapter 48

Paying for Care

Many older adults and caregivers worry about the cost of medical care. These expenses can use up a significant part of monthly income, even for families who thought they had saved enough.

How people pay for long-term care—whether delivered at home or in a hospital, assisted living facility, or nursing home—depends on their financial situation and the kinds of services they use. Often, they rely on a variety of payment sources, including personal funds, government programs, and private financing options.

Personal Funds

At first, many older adults pay for care in part with their own money. They may use personal savings, a pension or other retirement fund, income from stocks and bonds, or proceeds from the sale of a home.

Much home-based care is paid for using personal funds ("out of pocket"). Initially, family and friends often provide personal care and other services, such as transportation, for free. But as a person's needs increase, paid services may be needed.

Many older adults also pay out-of-pocket to participate in adult day service programs, meals, and other community-based services provided by local governments and nonprofit groups. These services help them remain in their homes.

This chapter includes text excerpted from "Paying for Care," National Institute on Aging (NIA), National Institutes of Health (NIH), August 17, 2017.

Professional care given in assisted living facilities and continuing care retirement communities is almost always paid for out of pocket, though, in some states, Medicaid may pay some costs for people who meet financial and health requirements.

Government Programs

Older adults may be eligible for some government healthcare benefits. Caregivers can help by learning more about possible sources of financial help and assisting older adults in applying for aid as appropriate. The Internet can be a helpful tool in this search.

Several federal and state programs provide help with healthcare-related costs.

Centers for Medicare and Medicaid Services

The Centers for Medicare and Medicaid Services (CMS) offers several programs. Over time, the benefits and eligibility requirements of these programs can change, and some benefits differ from State to State. Check with CMS or the individual programs directly for the most recent information.

Medicare

Medicare is a Federal Government health insurance program that pays some medical costs for people age 65 and older, and for all people with late-stage kidney failure. It also pays some medical costs for those who have gotten Social Security Disability Income for 24 months. It does not cover ongoing personal care at home. Here are brief descriptions of what Medicare will pay for:

Medicare Part A:

- Hospital costs after you pay a certain amount, called the "deductible"

- Short stays in a nursing home for certain kinds of illnesses

- Hospice care in the last 6 months of life

Medicare Part B:

- Part of the costs for doctor's services, outpatient care, and other medical services that Part A does not cover

- Some preventive services, such as flu shots and diabetes screening

Medicare Part D:

- Some medication costs

Medicaid

Some people may qualify for Medicaid, a combined Federal and State program for low-income people and families. This program covers the costs of medical care and some types of long-term care for people who have limited income and meet other eligibility requirements. Who is eligible and what services are covered vary from State to State.

Program of All-Inclusive Care for the Elderly (PACE)

Some States have PACE, Program of All-Inclusive Care for the Elderly, a Medicare program that provides care and services to people who otherwise would need care in a nursing home. PACE covers medical, social service, and long-term care costs for frail people. It may pay for some or all of the long-term care needs of a person with Alzheimer disease. PACE permits most people who qualify to continue living at home instead of moving to a long-term care facility. You will need to find out if the person who needs care qualifies for PACE. There may be a monthly charge. PACE is available only in certain States and locations within those States.

State Health Insurance Assistance Program

SHIP, the State Health Insurance Assistance Program is a national program offered in each State that provides counseling and assistance to people and their families on Medicare, Medicaid, and Medicare supplemental insurance (Medigap) matters.

Department of Veterans Affairs

The U.S. Department of Veterans Affairs (VA) may provide long-term care or at-home care for some veterans. If your family member or relative is eligible for veterans' benefits, check with the VA or get in touch with the VA medical center nearest you. There could be a waiting list for VA nursing homes.

Social Security Disability Income

This type of Social Security is for people younger than age 65 who are disabled according to the Social Security Administration's definition.

For a person to qualify for Social Security Disability Income, he or she must be able to show that:

- The person is unable to work

- The condition will last at least a year

- The condition is expected to result in death

Social Security has "compassionate allowances" to help people with Alzheimer disease, other dementias, and certain other serious medical conditions get disability benefits more quickly.

National Council on Aging

The National Council on Aging, a private group, has a free service called BenefitsCheckUp® (www.benefitscheckup.org). This service can help you find Federal and State benefit programs that may help your family. After providing some general information about the person who needs care, you can see a list of possible benefit programs to explore. These programs can help pay for prescription drugs, heating bills, housing, meal programs, and legal services. You don't have to give a name, address, or Social Security number to use this service.

Private Financing Options

In addition to personal and government funds, there are several private payment options, including long-term care insurance, reverse mortgages, certain life insurance policies, annuities, and trusts. Which option is best for a person depends on many factors, including the person's age, health status, personal finances, and risk of needing care.

Long-Term Care Insurance

Long-term care insurance covers many types of long-term care and benefits, including palliative and hospice care. The exact coverage depends on the type of policy you buy and what services are covered. You can purchase nursing home-only coverage or a comprehensive policy that includes both home care and facility care.

Many companies sell long-term care insurance. It is a good idea to shop around and compare policies. The cost of a policy is based on the type and amount of services, how old you are when you buy the policy, and any optional benefits you choose.

Buying long-term care insurance can be a good choice for younger, relatively healthy people at low risk of needing long-term care. Costs go up for people who are older, have health problems, or want more benefits. Someone who is in poor health or already receiving end-of-life care services may not qualify for long-term care insurance.

Reverse Mortgages

A reverse mortgage is a special type of home loan that lets a homeowner convert part of the ownership value in his or her home into cash. Unlike a traditional home loan, no repayment is required until the borrower sells the home, no longer uses it as a main residence, or dies.

There are no income or medical requirements to get a reverse mortgage, but you must be age 62 or older. The loan amount is tax-free and can be used for any expense, including long-term care. However, if you have an existing mortgage or other debt against your home, you must use the funds to pay off those debts first.

Life Insurance

Some life insurance policies can help pay for long-term care. Some policies offer a combination product of both life insurance and long-term care insurance.

Policies with an "accelerated death benefit" provide tax-free cash advances while you are still alive. The advance is subtracted from the amount your beneficiaries (the people who get the insurance proceeds) will receive when you die.

You can get an accelerated death benefit if you live permanently in a nursing home, need long-term care for an extended time, are terminally ill, or have a life-threatening diagnosis such as AIDS (acquired immune deficiency syndrome). Check your life insurance policy to see exactly what it covers.

You may be able to raise cash by selling your life insurance policy for its current value. This option, known as a "life settlement," is usually available only to people age 70 and older. The proceeds are taxable and can be used for any reason, including paying for long-term care.

A similar arrangement called a "viatical settlement," allows a terminally ill person to sell his or her life insurance policy to an insurance company for a percentage of the death benefit on the policy. This option is typically used by people who are expected to live 2 years or less. A viatical settlement provides immediate cash, but it can be hard to get.

Annuities

You may choose to enter into an annuity contract with an insurance company to help pay for long-term care services. In exchange for a single payment or a series of payments, the insurance company will send you an annuity, which is a series of regular payments over a specified period of time. There are two types of annuities: immediate annuities and deferred long-term care annuities.

Trusts

A trust is a legal entity that allows a person to transfer assets to another person, called the trustee. Once the trust is established, the trustee manages and controls the assets for the person or another beneficiary. You may choose to use a trust to provide flexible control of assets for an older adult or a person with a disability, which could include yourself or your spouse. Two types of trusts can help pay for long-term care services: charitable remainder trusts and Medicaid disability trusts.

Chapter 49

Health Coverage for Retirees

The Health Insurance Marketplace

Health Insurance Marketplace—also known as the Health Insurance Exchange—is the place where people without healthcare insurance can find information about health insurance options and also purchase healthcare insurance. Information can also be found regarding eligibility for help with paying premiums and reducing out-of-pocket costs. Each year the Marketplace has an open enrollment period.

In addition to the federally-facilitated Marketplace, HealthCare.gov, there are also state-based Marketplaces. Whether you use the federally-facilitated Marketplace or a state-based Marketplace depends on the state in which you live. If you visit HealthCare.gov, you will be asked to provide your ZIP code. If you live in an area served by a state-based Marketplace, you'll then be redirected to the website of your state-based Marketplace.

This chapter contains text excerpted from the following sources: Text under the heading "The Health Insurance Marketplace" is excerpted from "The Health Insurance Marketplace," Internal Revenue Service (IRS), August 27, 2017; Text under the heading "If You Retire Before Age 65 without Health Coverage" is excerpted from "Health Coverage for Retirees," Centers for Medicare and Medicaid Services (CMS), April 11, 2015.

If You Retire Before Age 65 without Health Coverage

If you retire before you're 65 and lose your job-based health plan when you do, you can use the Health Insurance Marketplace to buy a plan.

Losing health coverage qualifies you for a Special Enrollment Period. This means you can enroll in a health plan even if it's outside the annual Open Enrollment Period.

When you fill out a Marketplace application, you'll find out if you qualify for a private plan with premium tax credits and lower out-of-pocket costs. This will depend on your income and household size.

You'll also find out if you qualify for free or low-cost coverage through the Medicaid program in your state.

If You Have Retiree Health Benefits

If you have retiree health benefits, you're considered covered under the healthcare law. You don't have to pay the penalty that people without insurance must pay.

If you have retiree coverage and want to buy a Marketplace plan instead, you can. But:

- You can't get premium tax credits and other savings based on your income. This is true only if you're actually enrolled in retiree coverage. If you're **eligible for but not enrolled** in retiree coverage, you may qualify for premium tax credits and lower out-of-pocket costs based on your household size and income.

- If you voluntarily drop your retiree coverage, you won't qualify for a Special Enrollment Period to enroll in a new Marketplace plan. You won't be able to enroll in health coverage through the Marketplace until the next Open Enrollment period.

More Answers: Coverage for Retirees without Medicare

What if I turn 65 in the middle of the year? Can I get Marketplace coverage to carry me over until I'm eligible for Medicare?

Yes. You can get a Marketplace plan to cover you before your Medicare begins. You can then cancel the Marketplace plan once your Medicare coverage starts.

What if I'm 65 or older but not eligible for Medicare?

You may be able to buy insurance in the Marketplace and get lower costs on monthly premiums and out-of-pocket costs based in your household size and income. If you don't have health coverage, you may have to pay the penalty that most people without coverage must pay.

What if I retire from my job and am self-employed?

If you have retiree insurance, see "If you have retiree health benefits."

If you don't have retiree insurance or Medicare, you have the same insurance choices and responsibilities as anyone else who's self-employed.

What if I had job-based insurance but lost it when I retired? Do I qualify for a Special Enrollment Period?

Yes. Losing job-based coverage qualifies you for a Special Enrollment Period. This means you can enroll in a health plan outside of Open Enrollment. You can apply to the Marketplace with a Special Enrollment Period any time from 60 days before and 60 days after your separation date.

Do my IRA or 401k withdrawals count as income?

Generally, yes. Learn more about reporting income from retirement savings funds from the IRS.

Can I drop COBRA and get Marketplace coverage instead and qualify for lower costs based on my income?

It depends.

- **If your COBRA coverage runs out outside Open Enrollment,** you qualify for a Special Enrollment Period. This means you can enroll in a Marketplace plan outside the annual Open Enrollment Period.

- **But you can't choose to drop your COBRA coverage** outside **Open Enrollment and enroll in a Marketplace plan instead.** The Special Enrollment Period applies only if your COBRA coverage runs out.

- **During the annual Open Enrollment Period, you can drop your COBRA coverage even if it's not running out and replace it with a Marketplace plan.**

Chapter 50

Pension Counseling

A predictable and secure pension provides peace of mind and improves your life in many ways. Pension income increases your financial freedom and expands choices related to your health, lifestyle, and independence well beyond retirement age. Pension counseling and information projects provide free legal assistance and can help you understand your rights, make informed decisions, and claim earned benefits.

Run by local nonprofits, pension counseling and information projects are funded in 30 states under the Older Americans Act through a grant from the U.S. Administration on Aging (AOA). Legal training and support are provided by the National Pension Assistance Resource Center, an initiative of the Pension Rights Center.

Counseling Benefits

Pension plans and laws are complex and difficult to navigate without assistance from a knowledgeable source. Corporate mergers, bankruptcies, and changes in personal circumstances can complicate things further. Pension counseling projects fill a unique and unmet need — direct, specialized assistance provided at no charge and regardless of

This chapter contains text excerpted from the following sources: Text in this chapter begins with excerpts from "Pension Counseling and Information Projects," Eldercare Locator, U.S. Administration on Aging (AOA), October 30, 2015; Text under the heading "Protecting Your Private Pension Benefits" is excerpted from "Retirement," USA.gov, May 18, 2017.

your age or income. Trustworthy counselors are professional and well trained.

Plan Diversity

Pension counseling projects can help you regardless of the type of work you performed and the type of pension plan you have. Counselors can assist with retirement income plans offered by private and government employers, including the common plans below.

- Traditional "defined benefit" pension plan

- Cash balance or other "hybrid" pension plan

- 401(k), 403(b), or 457 "defined contribution" plan

- Money purchase or other profit-sharing plan

Personalized Assistance

Pension counselors provide assistance based on your unique needs. In addition to tracking down benefits from past employers, they can correct pension miscalculations and help you appeal denied claims. Counselors can also obtain and explain complex retirement plan publications and forms. They can address questions about pension laws and provide referrals to lawyers, actuaries, and other professionals as needed.

Common Questions

Pension counseling projects can address a vast range of questions, including:

- Am I entitled to a pension?

- What happens to my pension when I change employers?

- Can I claim my pension from a company that has merged with another or gone bankrupt?

- What happens to my pension when I die? What happens to my spouse's pension?

- Can I receive pension benefits from my ex-spouse?

- What if my pension is miscalculated or denied?

Protecting Your Private Pension Benefits

Avoiding Errors and Getting Help

If your job is covered by a traditional pension plan, make sure you get the pension amount you're owed.

- Find ways to protect yourself by reading these 10 common causes of errors in pension calculation.

- Get free legal help if you're experiencing a problem with your pension plan.

- Find out whether your pension or annuity income is taxable.

- If you have questions or complaints about your employer-sponsored pension plan, contact your human resources office or locate the Employee Benefits Security Administration (EBSA) regional office near you.

Federal Insurance for Private Pensions

If you've earned a traditional pension, you're likely to receive it even if your company runs into financial problems.

The Pension Benefit Guaranty Corporation (PBGC):

- Insures most private-sector defined-benefit pensions that typically pay a certain amount each month after you retire.

- Covers most cash-balance plans, a type of defined-benefit pension that allows you to take a lump-sum distribution.

- Does not cover government and military pensions, 401k plans, IRAs, and certain other plans.

Part Seven

Additional Help and Information

Chapter 51

Glossary of Aging Terms

abdomen: The part of the body between the ribs and pelvis that holds the stomach, intestines, liver, and other organs.

abstinence: Not having sexual intercourse.

activities of daily living (ADLs): Activities of daily living are basic activities that support survival, including eating, bathing, and toileting.

acupuncture: A form of complementary and alternative medicine that involves inserting thin needles through the skin at specific points on the body to control pain and other symptoms.

acute: Brief, not ongoing. Usually also implies relatively high intensity. For example, acute asthma symptoms may be ones that last a short time but are worse than a person's usual symptoms.

addiction: A chronic, relapsing disease, characterized by compulsive drug seeking and use accompanied by neurochemical and molecular changes in the brain.

aerobic exercise: A type of physical activity that burns fat, gets your heart rate going (you will be able to feel it beating faster), and makes your heart muscle stronger.

alcoholism: A disease characterized by a dependency on alcohol. Excessive alcohol use can have a negative impact on bone health.

This glossary contains terms excerpted from documents produced by several sources deemed reliable.

allergy: A type of excessive immune system reaction to a substance in a person's environment. (Can also be called "hypersensitivity reaction.") Allergies can be triggered by eating, touching, or breathing in an allergen. Allergies are often associated with asthma, especially in children.

Alzheimer disease: Progressive, degenerative form of dementia that causes severe intellectual deterioration. First symptoms are impaired memory, followed by impaired thought and speech, and finally complete helplessness.

anemia: A condition in which the number of red blood cells is less than normal, resulting in less oxygen carried to the body's cells.

anesthesia: A drug that makes you sleepy or can numb a part of your body before surgery so that you don't feel pain.

aneurysm: A weak or thin spot on an artery wall that has stretched or ballooned out from the wall and filled with blood, or damage to an artery leading to pooling of blood between the layers of the blood vessel walls.

angioplasty: A medical procedure used to open a blocked artery.

antibiotic: A drug that can destroy or prevent the growth of bacteria.

antibodies: Proteins made by the immune system that bind to structures (antigens) they recognize as foreign to the body.

anticoagulants: A drug therapy used to prevent the formation of blood clots that can become lodged in cerebral arteries and cause strokes.

antidepressant: Drugs given by your doctor to treat depression.

anxiety disorder: Any of a group of illnesses that fill people's lives with overwhelming anxieties and fears that are chronic and unremitting. Anxiety disorders include panic disorder, obsessive-compulsive disorder, posttraumatic stress disorder, phobias, and generalized anxiety disorder.

arrhythmia: A problem with the rate or rhythm of the heartbeat. During an arrhythmia, the heart can beat too fast, too slow, or with an irregular rhythm.

artery: Any of the thick-walled blood vessels that carry blood away from the heart to other parts of the body.

arthritis: Literally means joint inflammation. Arthritis causes joint swelling, pain, and stiffness.

assisted living facility: Residential living arrangement that provides individualized personal care, assistance with Activities of Daily Living, help with medications, and services such as laundry and housekeeping. Facilities may also provide health and medical care, but care is not as intensive as care offered at a nursing home. Types and sizes of facilities vary, ranging from small homes to large apartment-style complexes. Levels of care and services also vary. Assisted living facilities allow people to remain relatively independent.

atherosclerosis: A blood vessel disease characterized by deposits of lipid material on the inside of the walls of large to medium-sized arteries which make the artery walls thick, hard, brittle, and prone to breaking.

autoimmune disease: A disease in which the body's defense system malfunctions and attacks a part of the body itself rather than foreign matter.

basal cell: A small, round cell found in the lower part (or base) of the epidermis, the outer layer of the skin.

biopsy: To remove cells or tissues from the body for testing and examination under a microscope.

bipolar disorder: A depressive disorder in which a person alternates between episodes of major depression and mania (periods of abnormally and persistently elevated mood). Also referred to as manic depression.

bladder: The organ in the human body that stores urine. It is found in the lower part of the abdomen.

blood cholesterol: Cholesterol that travels in the serum of the blood as distinct particles containing both lipids and proteins (lipoproteins). Also referred to as serum cholesterol.

blood glucose level: Also called blood sugar level, it is the amount of glucose, or sugar, in the blood. Too much glucose in the blood for a long time can cause diabetes and damage many parts of the body, such as the heart, blood vessels, eyes, and kidneys.

blood pressure: The force of blood against the walls of arteries.

blood vessel: A tube-shaped part of the circulatory system which helps blood move through the body.

body mass index (BMI): This is a measure of body weight adjusted for height that correlates with body fat. A tool for indicating weight status in adults, BMI is generally computed using metric units and is defined as weight divided by height or kilograms/meters.

brain stem: The portion of the brain that connects to the spinal cord and controls automatic body functions, such as breathing, heart rate, and blood pressure.

breast cancer: A disease in which abnormal tumor cells develop in the breast. Women who have had breast cancer may be at increased risk for osteoporosis and fracture because of possible reduced levels of estrogen, chemotherapy or surgery, or early menopause.

calcium: A mineral that is an essential nutrient for bone health. It is also needed for the heart, muscles and nerves to function properly and for blood to clot.

calorie: When talking about food, a calorie is a measure of the amount of energy you get from eating a certain amount of food. When talking about physical activity, a calorie is a measure of the energy that your body uses in performing the activity.

carbohydrate: A "carb" is a major source of energy for your body. Your digestive system changes carbohydrates into blood glucose (sugar).

carcinoma: Cancer that begins in the skin or in tissues that line or cover internal organs.

cardiac rehabilitation: A medically supervised program that helps improve the health and well-being of people who have heart problems.

cardiopulmonary resuscitation (CPR): Combination of rescue breathing (mouth-to-mouth resuscitation) and chest compressions used if someone isn't breathing or circulating blood adequately. CPR can restore circulation of oxygen-rich blood to the brain.

cardiovascular disease: Disease of the heart and blood vessels.

carotid artery disease: Carotid artery disease is a disease in which a waxy substance called plaque builds up inside the carotid arteries.

chickenpox: A disease caused by the varicella-zoster virus, which results in a blister-like rash, itching, tiredness, and fever.

chlamydia: A common sexually transmitted disease caused by the bacterium *Chlamydia trachomatis*.

cholesterol: A waxy substance, produced naturally by the liver and also found in foods, that circulates in the blood and helps maintain tissues and cell membranes.

cognitive behavioral therapy (CBT): CBT helps people focus on how to solve their current problems. The therapist helps the patient learn how to identify distorted or unhelpful thinking patterns, recognize and change inaccurate beliefs, relate to others in more positive ways, and change behaviors accordingly.

cognitive impairment: Deficiency in short or long-term memory, orientation to person, place and time, deductive or abstract reasoning, or judgment as it relates to safety awareness. Alzheimer's Disease is an example of a cognitive impairment.

coma: A state of profound unconsciousness caused by disease, injury, or poison.

computed tomography (CT): A type of diagnostic imaging that uses X-rays and computer technology to produce two-dimensional images of organs, bones, and tissues.

coronary heart disease: Coronary heart disease is a disease in which a waxy substance called plaque builds up inside the coronary arteries.

cortex: Part of the brain responsible for thought, perception, and memory. HD affects the basal ganglia and cortex; see basal ganglia.

counselor: A person who usually has a master's degree in counseling and has completed a supervised internship.

dehydration: Excessive loss of body water that the body needs to carry on normal functions at an optimal level. Signs include increasing thirst, dry mouth, weakness or lightheadedness (particularly if worse on standing), and a darkening of the urine or a decrease in urination.

delusion: When a person believes something that is not true and that person keeps the belief even though there is strong evidence against it. Delusions can be the result of brain injury or mental illness.

dementia: Deterioration of mental faculties due to a disorder of the brain.

deoxyribonucleic acid (DNA): The substance of heredity containing the genetic information necessary for cells to divide and produce proteins. DNA carries the code for every inherited characteristic of an organism; see gene.

depression: A disorder marked by sadness, inactivity, difficulty with thinking and concentration, significant increase or decrease in appetite and time spent sleeping, feelings of dejection and hopelessness, and, sometimes, suicidal thoughts or an attempt to commit suicide.

diabetes: A condition characterized by high blood glucose, resulting from the body's inability to use blood glucose for energy.

dialysis: The process of filtering wastes from the blood artificially.

dopamine: A neurotransmitter present in regions of the brain that regulate movement, emotion, motivation, and the feeling of pleasure.

epilepsy: A physical disorder that involves recurrent seizures. It is caused by sudden changes in how the brain works.

exercise: A type of physical activity that is planned and structured.

fat: A source of energy used by the body to make substances it needs.

fatigue: A condition that results when the body cannot provide enough energy for the muscles to perform a task.

gene: The basic unit of heredity. Genes play a role in how high a person's risk is for certain diseases.

genital warts: A sexually transmitted disease caused by the human papillomavirus.

heart attack: It happens when the flow of oxygen-rich blood to a section of heart muscle suddenly becomes blocked and the heart can't get oxygen.

heart failure: A serious condition that occurs when the heart can't pump enough blood to meet the body's needs. It does not mean that the heart has stopped but that muscle is too weak to pump enough blood.

hemorrhoids: Veins around the anus or lower rectum that are swollen and inflamed.

high blood pressure: Blood pressure is the force of blood pushing against your blood vessel walls. High blood pressure is when that force, as measured by a blood pressure cuff, is elevated above normal limits.

hormone: A substance that stimulates the function of a gland.

human immunodeficiency virus (HIV): The virus that causes AIDS, which is the most advanced stage of HIV infection.

human papilloma virus (HPV): The virus that causes human papillomavirus infection, the most common sexually transmitted infection.

hypertension: Characterized by persistently high arterial blood pressure defined as a measurement greater than or equal to 140 mm/Hg systolic pressure over 90 mm/Hg diastolic pressure.

hypnosis: A focused state of concentration used to reduce pain. With self-hypnosis, you repeat a positive statement over and over. With guided imagery, you create relaxing images in your mind.

immune system: The complex group of organs and cells that defends the body against infections and other diseases.

immunosuppressant: A drug given to stop the natural responses of the body's immune system.

incontinence: The inability to control urination.

influenza: A highly contagious viral infection characterized by sudden onset of fever, severe aches and pains, and inflammation of the mucous membrane.

insomnia: Not being able to sleep

invasive cancer: Cancer that has spread beyond the layer of tissue in which it developed and is growing into surrounding, healthy tissues.

ischemia: A loss of blood flow to tissue, caused by an obstruction of the blood vessel, usually in the form of plaque stenosis or a blood clot.

jaundice: A condition in which the skin and the whites of the eyes become yellow, urine darkens, and the color of stool becomes lighter than normal.

kidney stone: Hard mass developed from crystals that separate from the urine and build up on the inner surfaces of the kidney.

lobe: A portion of an organ, such as the liver, lung, breast, thyroid, or brain.

lupus: A chronic inflammatory disease that occurs when the body's immune system attacks its own tissues and organs.

lymph nodes: Small glands that help the body fight infection and disease. They filter a fluid called lymph and contain white blood cells.

magnetic resonance imaging (MRI): A type of imaging involving the use of magnetic fields to detect subtle changes in the water content of tissues.

massage therapy: It encompasses many different techniques. In general, therapists press, rub, and otherwise manipulate the muscles and other soft tissues of the body. They most often use their hands and fingers, but may use their forearms, elbows, or feet.

melanoma: A form of cancer that begins in melanocytes (cells that make the pigment melanin).

mental illness: A health condition that changes a person's thinking, feelings, or behavior (or all three) and that causes the person distress and difficulty in functioning.

metabolism: It refers to all of the processes in the body that make and use energy, such as digesting food and nutrients and removing waste through urine and feces.

musculoskeletal disorders: A group of conditions that involve the nerves, tendons, muscles, and supporting structures such as intervertebral discs.

mutation: Any change in the DNA of a cell. Mutations may be caused by mistakes during cell division, or they may be caused by exposure to DNA-damaging agents in the environment.

nervous system: The system that coordinates an organism's response to the environment.

obesity: Having too much body fat. Obesity is more extreme than being overweight, which means weighing too much.

osteoarthritis: A painful, degenerative joint disease that often involves the hips, knees, neck, lower back, or small joints of the hands.

osteoporosis: Literally means "porous bone." This disease is characterized by too little bone formation, excessive bone loss, or a combination of both, leading to bone fragility and an increased risk of fractures of the hip, spine, and wrist.

pancreas: A large gland that helps digest food and also makes some important hormones.

panic disorder: An anxiety disorder in which a person suffers from sudden attacks of fear and panic. The attacks may occur without a known reason, but many times they are triggered by events or thoughts that produce fear in the person, such as taking an elevator or driving.

plaque: Fatty cholesterol deposits found along the inside of artery walls that lead to atherosclerosis and stenosis of the arteries.

plasma: The liquid portion of the blood that is involved in controlling infection.

psychosis: A mental disorder characterized by delusional or disordered thinking detached from reality; symptoms often include hallucinations.

radiation: The emission of energy in waves or particles. Often used to treat cancer cells.

resection: Surgery to remove tissue, an organ, or part of an organ.

rheumatoid arthritis (RA): An inflammatory disease that causes pain, swelling, stiffness, and loss of function in the joints.

scabies: An infestation of the skin by the human itch mite (Sarcoptes scabiei var. hominis). The most common symptoms of scabies are intense itching and a pimple-like skin rash.

sexually transmitted disease: An infectious disease that spreads from person to person during sexual contact.

sleep disorder: Clinical conditions that are a consequence of a disturbance in the ability to initiate or maintain the quantity and quality of sleep needed for optimal health, performance and well being.

soft tissues: Tissues that connect, support, or surround other structures and organs of the body.

stroke: It occurs when blood flow to your brain stops.

suicide: Death caused by self-directed injurious behavior with any intent to die as a result of the behavior.

tendons: Fibrous cords that connect muscle to bone.

tumor: An abnormal growth of body tissue. Tumors can be cancerous (malignant) or noncancerous (benign). Cancerous tumors can have uncontrolled growth and may spread to other parts of the body. Noncancerous tumors do not grow or spread.

ulcer: An open lesion on the surface of the skin or a mucosal surface, caused by superficial loss of tissue, usually with inflammation.

ultrasound: A type of test in which sound waves too high to hear are aimed at a structure to produce an image of it.

urinalysis: A test of a urine sample that can reveal many problems of the urinary tract and other body systems.

urinary tract: The path that urine takes as it leaves the body. It includes the kidneys, ureters, bladder, and urethra.

vaccine: A substance meant to help the immune system respond to and resist disease.

vasculitis: A condition that involves inflammation in the blood vessels.

ventilator: In medicine, a machine used to help a patient breathe. Also called a respirator.

virus: A microscopic infectious agent that requires a living host cell in order to replicate.

X-ray: A type of high-energy radiation. In low doses, X-rays are used to diagnose musculoskeletal problems by making pictures of the inside of the body. In high doses, X-rays are used to treat cancer.

yoga: A combination of breathing exercises, physical postures, and meditation used to calm the nervous system and balance the body, mind, and spirit.

Chapter 52

Directory of Resources That Provide Information about Aging

General Aging-Related Resources

Agency for Healthcare Research and Quality (AHRQ)
Office of Communications and Knowledge Transfer
5600 Fishers Ln.
Seventh Fl.
Rockville, MD 20857
Phone: 301-427-1364
Website: www.ahrq.gov

American Academy of Family Physicians (AAFP)
11400 Tomahawk Creek Pkwy
Leawood, KS 66211-2680
Toll-Free: 800-274-2237
Phone: 913-906-6000
Fax: 913-906-6075
Website: www.aafp.org

American Academy of Hospice and Palliative Medicine (AAHPM)
8735 W. Higgins Rd., Ste. 300
Chicago, IL 60631
Phone: 847-375-4712
Fax: 847-375-6475
Website: www.aahpm.org
E-mail: info@aahpm.org

Resources in this chapter were compiled from several sources deemed reliable; all contact information was verified and updated in September 2017.

American Autoimmune-Related Diseases Association, Inc. (AARDA)
22100 Gratiot Ave.
Eastpointe, MI 48021
Toll-Free: 800-598-4668
Phone: 586-776-3900
Fax: 586-776-3903
Website: www.aarda.org

American Society on Aging (ASA)
575 Market St.
Ste. 2100
San Francisco, CA 94105-2869
Toll-Free: 800-537-9728
Phone: 415-974-9600
Fax: 415-974-0300
Website: www.asaging.org
E-mail: info@asaging.org

Centers for Disease Control and Prevention (CDC)
1600 Clifton Rd.
Atlanta, GA 30329-4027
Toll-Free: 800-CDC-INFO
(800-232-4636)
Phone: 404-639-3311
Toll-Free TTY: 888-232-6348
Website: www.cdc.gov

Centers for Medicare and Medicaid Services (CMS)
7500 Security Blvd.
Baltimore, MD 21244
Toll-Free: 800-MEDICARE
(800-633-4227)
Phone: 410-786-3000
Toll-Free TTY: 877-486-2048
Website: www.cms.gov

Eldercare.gov
Toll-Free: 800-677-1116
TTY: 800-677-1116
Website: www.eldercare.gov/
Eldercare.NET/Public/About/
Contact_Info/Index.aspx
E-mail: eldercarelocator@n4a.
org

Healthcare.gov
Website: www.healthcare.gov/
contact-us

Healthfinder®
National Health Information
Center (NHIC)
1101 Wootton Pkwy
Rockville, MD 20852
Website: www.healthfinder.gov
E-mail: healthfinder@hhs.gov

Immune Deficiency Foundation (IDF)
110 W. Rd.
Ste. 300
Towson, MD 21204
Toll-Free: 800-296-4433
Fax: 410-321-9165
Website: www.primaryimmune.
org
E-mail: info@primaryimmune.
org

National Center for Complementary and Integrative Health (NCCIH)
9000 Rockville Pike
Bethesda, MD 20892
Toll-Free: 888-644-6226
TTY: 866-464-3615
Website: www.nccih.nih.gov/
tools/contact.htm

National Hospice and Palliative Care Organization (NHPCO)
1731 King St.
Alexandria, VA 22314
Toll-Free: 800-658-8898
Phone: 703-837-1500
Fax: 703-837-1233
Website: www.nhpco.org
E-mail: nhpco_info@nhpco.org

National Immunization Program (NIP)
NIP Public Inquiries
1600 Clifton Rd.
Mailstop E-05
Atlanta, GA 30333
Toll-Free: 800-232-2522
Website: www.cdc.gov/nip
E-mail: nipinfo@cdc.gov

National Institute of Dental and Craniofacial Research (NIDCR)
Bethesda, MD 20892-2190
Toll-Free: 866-232-4528
Phone: 301-496-4261
Website: www.nidcr.nih.gov
E-mail: nidcrinfo@mail.nih.gov

National Institute on Aging (NIA)
31 Center Dr. MSC 2292
Bldg. 31 Rm. 5C27
Bethesda, MD 20892
Toll-Free: 800-222-2225
Phone: 301-496-1752
Toll-Free TTY: 800-222-4225
Website: www.nia.nih.gov
E-mail: niaic@nia.nih.gov

National Institute on Deafness and Other Communication Disorders (NIDCD)
31 Center Dr. MSC 2320
Bethesda, MD 20892-2320
Toll-Free: 800-241-1044
Phone: 301-827-8183
TTY: 800-241-1055
Fax: 301-402-0018
Website: www.nidcd.nih.gov
E-mail: nidcdinfo@nidcd.nih.gov

National Institutes of Health (NIH)
9000 Rockville Pike
Bethesda, MD 20892
Phone: 301-496-4000
Website: www.nih.gov
E-mail: NIHinfo@od.nih.gov

Office on Women's Health (OWH)
Office on Women's Health (OWH)
200 Independence Ave. S.W.
Rm. 712E
Washington, DC 20201
Toll-Free: 800-994-9662
Phone: 202-690-7650
Toll-Free TDD: 888-220-5446
Fax: 202-205-2631
Website: www.womenshealth.gov

U.S. Department of Health and Human Services (HHS)
200 Independence Ave. S.W.
Washington, DC 20201
Toll-Free: 877-696-6775
Website: www.hhs.gov

U.S. Department of Veterans Affairs (VA)
810 Vermont Ave. N.W.
Washington, DC 20420
Toll-Free: 800-827-1000
Website: www.va.gov

U.S. National Library of Medicine (NLM)
8600 Rockville Pike
Bethesda, MD 20894
Toll-Free: 888-FIND-NLM
(888-346-3656)
Phone: 301-594-5983
Website: www.nlm.nih.gov
E-mail: custserv@nlm.nih.gov

Allergies and Asthma

Allergy & Asthma Network
8229 Boone Blvd.
Ste. 260
Vienna, VA 22182
Toll-Free: 800-878-4403
Fax: 703-288-5271
Website: www.
allergyasthmanetwork.org/main

American Academy of Allergy, Asthma & Immunology (AAAAI)
555 E. Wells St.
Ste. 1100
Milwaukee, WI 53202-3823
Toll-Free: 800-822-2762
Phone: 414-272-6071
Website: www.aaaai.org

American College of Allergy, Asthma & Immunology (ACAAI)
85 W. Algonquin Rd.
Ste. 550
Arlington Heights, IL 60005
Toll-Free: 800-842-7777
Phone: 847-427-1200
Fax: 847-427-1294
Website: www.acaai.org

Association of Asthma Educators (AAE)
70 Buckwalter Rd.
Ste. 900
Royersford, PA 19468
Toll-Free: 888-988-7747
Website: www.asthmaeducators.
org
E-mail: admin@
asthmaeducators.org

Asthma and Allergy Foundation of America (AAFA)
8201 Corporate Dr.
Ste. 1000
Landover, MD 20785
Toll-Free: 800-7-ASTHMA
(800-727-8462)
Website: www.aafa.org
E-mail: info@aafa.org

Asthma Center Education and Research Fund
205 N. Broad St.
Ste. 300
Philadelphia, PA 19107
Phone: 215-569-1111
Website: www.theasthmacenter.
org

Food Allergy Research & Education
7925 Jones Branch Dr.
Ste. 1100
McLean, VA 22102
Toll-Free: 800-929-4040
Phone: 703-691-3179
Fax: 703-691-2713
Website: www.foodallergy.org

National Institute of Allergy and Infectious Diseases (NIAID)
5601 Fishers Ln.
MSC 9806
Bethesda, MD 20892-9806
Toll-Free: 866-284-4107
Phone: 301-496-5717
TDD: 800-877-8339
Fax: 301-402-3573
Website: www.niaid.nih.gov
E-mail: ocpostoffice@niaid.nih.gov

Alzheimer Disease

Alzheimer's Drug Discovery Foundation (ADDF)
57 W. 57th St.
Ste. 904
New York, NY 10019
Phone: 212-901-8000
Website: www.alzdiscovery.org
E-mail: info@alzdiscovery.org

Alzheimer's Foundation of America (AFA)
322 Eighth Ave.
Seventh Fl.
New York, NY 10001
Toll-Free: 866-232-8484
Phone: 646-638-1542
Fax: 646-638-1546
Website: www.alzfdn.org
E-mail: info@alzfdn.org

Arthritis and Musculoskeletal Disorders

American Academy of Orthopaedic Surgeons (AAOS)
9400 W. Higgins Rd.
Rosemont, IL 60018
Phone: 847-823-7186
Fax: 847-823-8125
Website: www.aaos.org
E-mail: custserv@aaos.org

American Academy of Physical Medicine and Rehabilitation (AAPM&R)
9700 W. Bryn Mawr Ave.
Ste. 200
Rosemont, IL 60018
Phone: 847-737-6000
Website: www.aapmr.org
E-mail: info@aapmr.org

American College of Rheumatology (ACR)
2200 Lake Blvd. N.E.
Atlanta, GA 30319
Phone: 404-633-3777
Fax: 404-633-1870
Website: www.rheumatology.org/Contact
E-mail: website@rheumatology.org

American Council on Exercise (ACE)
4851 Paramount Dr.
San Diego, CA 92123
Toll-Free: 888-825-3636
Phone: 858-576-6500
Fax: 858-576-6564
Website: www.acefitness.org
E-mail: support@acefitness.org

American Physical Therapy Association (APTA)
1111 N. Fairfax St.
Alexandria, VA 22314-1488
Toll-Free: 800-999-2782
Phone: 703-684-APTA
(703-684-2782)
TDD: 703-683-6748
Fax: 703-684-7343
Website: www.apta.org
E-mail: Research-dept@apta.org

American Running Association (ARA)
4405 E.W. Hwy
Ste. 405
Bethesda, MD 20814
Toll-Free: 800-776-2732
Fax: 301-913-9520
Website: www.americanrunning.org

Arthritis Foundation
1355 Peachtree St. N.E.
Ste. 600
Atlanta, GA 30309
Toll-Free: 800-283-7800
Phone: 404-872-7100
Website: www.arthritis.org/about-us/contact-us.php

National Institute of Arthritis and Musculoskeletal and Skin Diseases (NIAMS)
1 AMS Cir.
Bethesda, MD 20892-3675
Toll-Free: 877-22-NIAMS
(877-226-4267)
Phone: 301-495-4484
TTY: 301-565-2966
Fax: 301-718-6366
Website: www.niams.nih.gov
E-mail: NIAMSinfo@mail.nih.gov

National Osteoporosis Foundation (NOF)
1150 17th St. N.W.
Ste. 850
Washington, DC 20036
Toll-Free: 800-231-4222
Phone: 202-223-2226
Fax: 202-223-2237
Website: www.nof.org/privacy-policy
E-mail: info@nof.org

Brain and Mental Health Disorders

American Academy of Neurology (AAN)
201 Chicago Ave.
Minneapolis, MN 55415
Toll-Free: 800-879-1960
Phone: 612-928-6000
Fax: 612-454-2746
Website: www.aan.com
E-mail: memberservices@aan.com

American Psychiatric Association (APA)
1000 Wilson Blvd.
Ste. 1825
Arlington, VA 22209
Toll-Free: 888-357-7924
Phone: 703-907-7300
Website: www.psych.org
E-mail: apa@psych.org

American Psychological Association (APA)
750 First St. N.E.
Washington, DC 20002-4242
Toll-Free: 800-374-2721
Phone: 202-336-5500
TDD/TTY: 202-336-6123
Website: www.apa.org

Brain Injury Association of America (BIAA)
1608 Spring Hill Rd.
Ste. 110
Vienna, VA 22182
Toll-Free: 800-444-6443
Phone: 703-761-0750
Fax: 703-761-0755
Website: www.biausa.org
E-mail: braininjuryinfo@biausa.org

Brain Trauma Foundation
1 Bdwy.
Sixth Fl.
New York, NY 10004
Phone: 212-772-0608
Fax: 212-772-0357
Website: www.braintrauma.org

Depression and Bipolar Support Alliance (DBSA)
55 E. Jackson Blvd.
Ste. 490
Chicago, IL 60604
Toll-Free: 800-826-3632
Fax: 312-642-7243
Website: www.dbsalliance.org

National Brain Tumor Society (NBTS)
55 Chapel St.
Ste. 200
Newton, MA 02458
Phone: 617-924-9997
Fax: 617-924-9998
Website: www.braintumor.org

National Institute of Mental Health (NIMH)
6001 Executive Blvd.
Rm. 6200 MSC 9663
Bethesda, MD 20892-9663
Toll-Free: 866-615-6464
Phone: 301-443-4513
TTY: 301-443-8431
Toll-Free TTY: 866-415-8051
Fax: 301-443-4279
Website: www.nimh.nih.gov
E-mail: nimhinfo@nih.gov

National Institute of Neurological Disorders and Stroke (NINDS)
P.O. Box 5801
Bethesda, MD 20824
Toll-Free: 800-352-9424
Phone: 301-496-5751
Website: www.ninds.nih.gov

National Stroke Association
9707 E. Easter Ln.
Ste. B
Centennial, CO 80112
Toll-Free: 800-STROKES
(800-787-6537)
Fax: 303-649-1328
Website: www.stroke.org
E-mail: info@stroke.org

Stroke Awareness
Foundation
51 E. Campbell Ave.
Ste. 106-M
Campbell, CA 95008
Phone: 408-370-5282
Website: www.strokeinfo.org
E-mail: noemi@strokeinfo.org

Cancers

American Cancer Society
(ACS)
250 Williams St. N.W.
Atlanta, GA, 30303
Toll-Free: 800-227-2345
Website: www.cancer.org

CancerCare
275 Seventh Ave.
22nd Fl.
New York, NY 10001
Toll-Free: 800-813-4673
Website: www.cancercare.org
E-mail: info@cancercare.org

Colorectal Cancer Control
Program (CRCCP)
4770 Buford Hwy N.E.
Atlanta, GA 30341
Toll-Free: 800-232-4636
Fax: 888-232-6348
Website: www.cdc.gov/cancer/
crccp
E-mail: cdcinfo@cdc.gov

Foundation for Women's
Cancer (FWC)
230 W. Monroe St.
Ste. 710
Chicago, IL 60606-4902
Toll-Free: 800-444-4441 (hotline)
Phone: 312-578-1439
Fax: 312-235-4059
Website: www.
foundationforwomenscancer.org/
contact-us
E-mail: FWCinfo@sgo.org

National Cancer Institute
(NCI)
Public Inquiries Office
9609 Medical Center Dr.
Bethesda, MD 20892-9760
Toll-Free: 800-4-CANCER
(800-422-6237)
Website: www.cancer.gov
E-mail: cancergovstaff@mail.nih.
gov

The Skin Cancer Foundation
(SCF)
149 Madison Ave.
Ste. 901
New York, NY 10016
Phone: 212-725-5176
Website: www.skincancer.org/
contact-us

Cardiovascular Disorders

American Association of Cardiovascular and Pulmonary Rehabilitation (AACVPR)
330 N. Wabash Ave., Ste. 2000
Chicago, IL 60611
Phone: 312-321-5146
Fax: 312-673-6924
Website: www.aacvpr.org
E-mail: aacvpr@aacvpr.org

American College of Cardiology (ACC)
Heart House
2400 N. St. N.W.
Washington, DC 20037
Toll-Free: 800-253-4636
Phone: 202-375-6000
Fax: 202-375-7000
Website: www.acc.org
E-mail: resource@aac.org

American College of Chest Physicians (ACCP)
3300 Dundee Rd.
Northbrook, IL 60062-2348
Toll-Free: 800-343-2227
Phone: 847-498-1400
Fax: 847-498-5460
Website: www.chestnet.org

American Heart Association (AHA)
7272 Greenville Ave.
Dallas, TX 75231
Toll-Free: 800-AHA-USA-1
(800-242-8721)
Phone: 214-570-5978
Fax: 214-706-1551
Website: www.heart.org

Cardiovascular Research Foundation (CRF)
1700 Bdwy.
Ninth Fl.
New York, NY 10019
Phone: 646-434-4500
Website: www.crf.org
E-mail: info@crf.org

Heart Rhythm Society (HRS)
1325 G St. N.W.
Ste. 400
Washington, DC 20005
Phone: 202-464-3400
Fax: 202-464-3401
Website: www.hrsonline.org
E-mail: info@HRSonline.org

National Heart, Lung, and Blood Institute (NHLBI)
P.O. Box 30105
Bethesda, MD 20824-0105
Phone: 301-592-8573
Website: www.nhlbi.nih.gov
E-mail: nhlbiinfo@nhlbi.nih.gov

Diabetes

American Diabetes Association (ADA)
Center for Information
2451 Crystal Dr.
Ste. 900
Arlington, VA 22202
Toll-Free: 800-DIABETES
(800-342-2383)
Website: www.diabetes.org/
about-us/contact-us/center-for-
information.html
E-mail: askada@diabetes.org

National Diabetes Education Program (NDEP)
1 Diabetes Way
Bethesda, MD 20814-9692
Toll-Free: 888-693-NDEP
(888-693-6337)
TTY: 866-569-1162
Fax: 703-738-4929
Website: www.ndep.nih.gov
E-mail: ndep@mail.nih.gov

National Diabetes Information Clearinghouse (NDIC)
1 Information Way
Bethesda, MD 20892-3560
Toll-Free: 800-860-8747
TTY: 866-569-1162
Fax: 703-738-4929
Website: www.diabetes.niddk.
nih.gov
E-mail: ndic@info.niddk.nih.gov

National Institute of Diabetes and Digestive and Kidney Diseases (NIDDK)
31 Center Dr. MSC 2560
Bldg. 31 Rm. 9A06
Bethesda, MD 20892-2560
Phone: 301-496-3583
Website: www.niddk.nih.gov

Diet and Nutrition

Center for Nutrition Policy and Promotion (CNPP)
3101 Park Center Dr.
10th Fl.
Alexandria, VA 22302-1594
Toll-Free: 866-632-9992
Phone: 703-305-3300
Fax: 703-305-3300
Website: www.cnpp.usda.gov
E-mail: john.webster@cnpp.
usda.gov

Food and Nutrition Information Center (FNIC)
USDA Agriculture Research Service
10301 Baltimore Ave.
Beltsville, MD 20705-2351
Toll-Free: 888-624-8373
Phone: 301-504-5414
TTY: 301-504-6856
Fax: 301-504-6409
Website: www.fnic.nal.usda.gov
E-mail: FNIC@ars.usda.gov

International Food Information Council Foundation (IFIC)
1100 Connecticut Ave. N.W.
Ste. 430
Washington, DC 20036
Phone: 202-296-6540
Website: www.foodinsight.org
E-mail: foodinfo@ific.org

Office of Dietary
Supplements (ODS)
National Institutes of Health
(NIH)
6100 Executive Blvd.
Rm. 3B01 MSC 7517
Bethesda, MD 20892-7517
Toll-Free: 888-723-3366
Phone: 301-435-2920
Fax: 301-480-1845
Website: www.ods.od.nih.gov
E-mail: ods@nih.gov

U.S. Food and Drug
Administration (FDA)
10903 New Hampshire Ave.
Silver Spring, MD 20993
Toll-Free: 888-INFO-FDA
(888-463-6332)
Website: www.fda.gov

Weight-Control Information
Network (WIN)
31 Center Dr.
Rm. 9A06 MSC 2560
Bethesda, MD 20892-2560
Toll-Free: 800–860–8747
Phone: 301-496-3583
Website: www.niddk.nih.gov
E-mail: healthinfo@niddk.nih.
gov

Drug Abuse

National Council on
Alcoholism and Drug
Dependence, Inc. (NCADD)
217 Bdwy.
Ste. 712
New York, NY 10007
Toll-Free: 800-NCACALL
(800-622-2255)
Phone: 212-269-7797
Fax: 212-269-7510
Website: www.ncadd.org
E-mail: national@ncadd.org

National Institute on Drug
Abuse (NIDA)
6001 Executive Blvd.
Rm. 5213 MSC 9561
Bethesda, MD 20892-9561
Website: www.drugabuse.gov
E-mail: media@nida.nih.gov

Substance Abuse and
Mental Health Services
Administration (SAMHSA)
5600 Fishers Ln.
Rockville, MD 20857
Toll-Free: 877-SAMHSA-7
(877-726-4727)
Toll-Free TDD: 800-487-4889
Website: www.samhsa.gov

Eye Injuries

American Academy of
Ophthalmology (AAO)
655 Beach St.
San Francisco, CA 94109
Phone: 415-561-8500
Fax: 415-561-8533
Website: www.aao.org

National Eye Institute (NEI)
Information Office
31 Center Dr.
MSC 2510
Bethesda, MD 20892-2510
Phone: 301-496-5248
Website: www.nei.nih.gov
E-mail: 2020@nei.nih.gov

Prevent Blindness
211 W. Wacker Dr.
Ste. 1700
Chicago, IL 60606
Toll-Free: 800-331-2020
Website: www.preventblindness.
org
E-mail: info@preventblindness.
org

Gastrointestinal and Digestive Disorders

Academy of Nutrition and Dietetics
120 S. Riverside Plaza
Ste. 2190
Chicago, IL 60606-6995
Toll-Free: 800-877-1600
Phone: 312-899-0040
Website: www.eatrightpro.org/
resource/about-us/academy-
vision-and-mission/who-we-are/
contact-us
E-mail: knowledge@eatright.org

American Celiac Disease Alliance (ACDA)
2504 Duxbury Pl.
Alexandria, VA 22308
Phone: 703-622-3331
Website: www.americanceliac.org
E-mail: info@americanceliac.org

American College of Gastroenterology (ACG)
6400 Goldsboro Rd.
Ste. 200
Bethesda, MD 20817
Phone: 301-263-9000
Website: www.gi.org
E-mail: info@gi.org

American Gastroenterological Association (AGA)
4930 Del Ray Ave.
Bethesda, MD 20814
Phone: 301-654-2055
Fax: 301-654-5920
Website: www.gastro.org/
contact/contact-aga
E-mail: member@gastro.org

Celiac Disease Foundation (CDF)
20350 Ventura Blvd.
Ste. 240
Woodland Hills, CA 91364
Phone: 818-716-1513
Toll-Free Fax: 818-267-5577
Website: www.celiac.org
E-mail: cdf@celiac.org

National Digestive Diseases Information Clearinghouse (NDDIC)
2 Information Way
Bethesda, MD 20892-3570
Toll-Free: 800-891-5389
TTY: 866-569-1162
Fax: 703-738-4929
Website: www.digestive.niddk.
nih.gov
E-mail: nddic@info.niddk.nih.gov

Kidney, Liver, and Urologic Diseases

American Liver Foundation (ALF)
39 Bdwy.
Ste. 2700
New York, NY 10006
Toll-Free: 800-GO-LIVER
(800-465-4837)
Phone: 212-668-1000
Fax: 212-483-8179
Website: www.liverfoundation.org

American Urological Association (AUA)
1000 Corporate Blvd.
Linthicum, MD 21090
Toll-Free: 866-RING AUA
(866-746-4282)
Phone: 410-689-3700
Fax: 410-689-3800
Website: www.auanet.org/about-us/contact-us
E-mail: aua@AUAnet.org

National Kidney and Urologic Diseases Information Clearinghouse (NKUDIC)
3 Information Way
Bethesda, MD 20892
Toll-Free: 800-891-5390
Toll-Free TTY: 866-569-1162
Fax: 301–634–0176
Website: www.kidney.niddk.nih.gov
E-mail: nkdep@info.niddk.nih.gov

National Kidney Foundation (NKF)
30 E. 33rd St.
New York, NY 10016
Toll-Free: 800-622-9010
Phone: 212-889-2210
Website: www.kidney.org
E-mail: info@kidney.org

Prostatitis Foundation (PF)
1063 30th St.
Smithshire, IL 61478
Phone: 309-325-7184
Fax: 309-325-7189
Website: www.prostatitis.org
E-mail: info@prostatitis.org

Urology Care Foundation
1000 Corporate Blvd.
Linthicum, MD 21090
Toll-Free: 800-828-7866
Phone: 410-689-3700
Fax: 410-689-3998
Website: www.urologyhealth.org
E-mail: info@UrologyCareFoundation.org

Parkinson Disease

American Parkinson Disease Association (APDA)
135 Parkinson Ave.
Staten Island, NY 10305-1425
Toll-Free: 800-223-2732
Phone: 718-981-8001
Fax: 718-981-4399
Website: www.apdaparkinson.org
E-mail: apda@apdaparkinson.org

Parkinson's Disease Foundation (PDF)
1359 Bdwy., Ste. 1509
New York, NY 10018
Toll-Free: 800-457-6676
Phone: 212-923-4700
Fax: 212-923-4778
Website: www.pdf.org
E-mail: info@pdf.org

Parkinson's Institute and Clinical Center
675 Almanor Ave.
Sunnyvale, CA 94085
Toll-Free: 800-655-2273
Phone: 408-734-2800
Fax: 408-734-8522
Website: www.thepi.org
E-mail: info@thepi.org

Suicide

American Association of Suicidology (AAS)
5221 Wisconsin Ave. N.W.
Washington, DC 20015
Toll-Free: 800-273-TALK
(800-273-8255)
Phone: 202-237-2280
Fax: 202-237-2282
Website: www.suicidology.org

Suicide Prevention Resource Center (SPRC)
43 Foundry Ave.
Waltham, MA 02453-8313
Toll-Free: 877-GET-SPRC
(877-438-7772)
TTY: 617-964-5448
Fax: 617-969-9186
Website: www.sprc.org
E-mail: info@sprc.org

Support Groups

Administration for Community Living (ACL)
330 C St. S.W.
Washington, DC 20201
Toll-Free: 800-677-1116
Phone: 202-401-4634
Website: www.acl.gov/contact
E-mail: aclinfo@acl.hhs.gov

Family Caregiver Alliance (FCA)
785 Market St.
Ste. 750
San Francisco, CA 94103
Toll-Free: 800-445-8106
Phone: 415-434-3388
Website: www.caregiver.org
E-mail: eldercarelocator@
spherix.com

GriefShare
P.O. Box 1739
Wake Forest, NC 27588-1739
Toll-Free: 800-395-5755
Phone: 919-562-2112
Website: www.griefshare.org
E-mail: info@griefshare.org

National Association for Home Care (NAHC)
228 Seventh St. S.E.
Washington, DC 20003
Phone: 202-547-7424
Fax: 202-547-3540
Website: www.nahc.org
E-mail: hospice@nahc.org

Index

Index

605